The Patient with End Stage Renal Disease

The Patient with End Stage Renal Disease

Edited by

LARRY E. LANCASTER R.N., M.S.N.

Clinical Specialist, Nephrology
Vanderbilt University Medical Center
Assistant Professor of Medical-Surgical Nursing
Vanderbilt University School of Nursing
Nashville, Tennessee

A WILEY MEDICAL PUBLICATION
JOHN WILEY & SONS
New York • Chichester • Brisbane • Toronto

Copyright © 1979 by John Wiley & Sons, Inc.

All rights reserved. Published simultaneously in Canada.

Reproduction or translation of any part of this
work beyond that permitted by Sections 107 or 108
of the 1976 United States Copyright Act without the
permission of the copyright owner is unlawful. Requests
for permission or further information should be addressed
to the Permissions Department, John Wiley & Sons, Inc.

Library of Congress Cataloging in Publication Data:

Main entry under title:

The Patient with end stage renal disease.

(A Wiley medical publication)
1. Renal insufficiency—Nursing. 2. Renal insufficiency—Social aspects. 3. Hemodialysis. 4. Kidneys—
Transplantation. I. Lancaster, Larry E. II. Title.
[DNLM: 1. Kidney diseases—Nursing. 2. Terminal
care. WY164 L244p]

RC918.R4P34   616.6′1   78–23659
ISBN 0-471-03564-5

Printed in the United States of America

10 9 8 7 6 5 4 3

To
ESRD patients and the nurses who care for them,
To
Our families and friends,
And of course,
To
Brompton

L.E.L.

Contributors

CAROLYN J. BESS, R.N., M.S.N., Clinical Specialist, Medical-Surgical Nursing, Vanderbilt University Medical Center; and Associate Professor of Medical-Surgical Nursing, Vanderbilt University School of Nursing, Nashville, Tennessee

LOWANNA S. BINKLEY, R.N., M.A., Coordinator, Dialysis Unit, Veterans Administration Hospital; and Assistant Professor of Medical-Surgical Nursing, Vanderbilt University School of Nursing, Nashville, Tennessee

MARY ECCARD, R.N., M.S.N., Clinical Specialist, Psychiatric-Mental Health Nursing, Associate Director for Medical Nursing, Vanderbilt University Medical Center; and Assistant Professor of Psychiatric-Mental Health Nursing, Vanderbilt University School of Nursing, Nashville, Tennessee

H. EARL GINN, M.D., Professor of Medicine and Chief, Division of Nephrology, Vanderbilt University Medical Center, Nashville, Tennessee

SUSAN A. HOPPER, R.N., M.S.N., Organ Donor Coordinator, Transplant Service, University of California, San Francisco, California

VICTORIA R. LIDDLE, R.D., Dietitian, Dialysis Clinic, Inc., Nashville, Tennessee

EDITH T. OBERLEY, M.A., Health Writing Consultant, Health Planning Council, Inc., Madison, Wisconsin

TERRY D. OBERLEY, M.D., Ph.D., Assistant Professor of Pathology, University of Wisconsin, Madison, Wisconsin. The Oberleys have been home dialysis partners since 1973. They are co-authors of *Understanding Your New Life on Dialysis.*

SHARON R. PARKER, R.N., Medical Specialist, Artificial Organs Division, Travenol Laboratories, Deerfield, Illinois

PENNY PIERCE, R.N., M.S.N., Assistant Professor of Medical-Surgical Nursing, Yale University School of Nursing, New Haven, Connecticut

JUDITH HEFFRON TAYLOR, R.N., M.S.N., Clinical Specialist, Renal Transplantation, Vanderbilt University Medical Center; and Assistant Professor of Medical-Surgical Nursing, Vanderbilt University School of Nursing, Nashville, Tennessee

Foreword

The care of the patient with end stage renal disease is complex and calls upon a variety of disciplines. As techniques have been developed in recent decades to prolong the lives of this patient population, nurses have been significant participants in the care system. The earlier focus was on mastering the procedural aspects of dialysis and transplantation, and the treatment modalities were new enough that long-term experiences were simply not available. It is, therefore, no wonder that for a long time the nursing literature has provided only sparse information about total patterns and plans of care for the patient with renal disease.

As this patient population has expanded, probably as a result of additional funding in the early 1970s as well as the experiences gained, and as many of these people have lived longer and fuller lives, much information has been obtained that can be of assistance to health care professionals entering, interested in, or presently working in nephrology.

It is interesting to note not only the depth this field has achieved but also the breadth. A chronic illness that can affect all age groups offers several sophisticated treatment options, has many acute phases as part of the continuum, and seeks rehabilitation as its goal is bound to touch many areas of both health and illness, patient and family, institution and community. Within the area of treatment of renal disease many issues are continually confronted: quality of life, funding for catastrophic illness, self and/or home care, criteria for death, organ donor selection, and patient choice in treatment options, to name but a few. In essence, the amount of baseline data we need in order to understand the complexities of care for this patient population is quite extensive.

The nurse has over the years assumed many new roles with regard to the patient with renal failure. Many nurses have pursued educational endeavors to become not only outstanding nephrology nurses but specialists within the field of nephrology as well. It is, therefore, significant that persons with individual expertise are collectively drawn together here to share their ideas, knowledge, and experiences so as to stimulate the reader and provide more comprehensive background for delivery of patient care. Through this text one is introduced to subjects the members of various disciplines address as well as their participating roles, is exposed to concepts regarding the patient's and family's involvement in care, and is also privileged to gain insight into the patient's and spouse's perception of the treatment process.

Nurses and other health care providers should find this text a valuable resource both for information and for an appreciation of the multidisciplinary approach to the care of the patient with end stage renal disease.

MARCIA CLARK, R.N., M.S.N.
Past President, American Association of
    Nephrology Nurses and Technicians
Renal Coordinator, Northwest Kidney Center
Seattle, Washington

Preface

During the past twenty years, dramatic medical and technical advances have occurred in the care of the patient with end stage renal disease. Knowledge about the effects of uremia on the body has greatly increased. Dialysis and transplantation have become widely accepted methods of treatment for patients with renal failure. Because patients are living longer, the psychosocial effects of chronic illness may be more closely studied. As a result of federal funding for dialysis and transplantation, patient selection for maintenance dialysis is no longer a salient issue. In the United States about 38,000 patients are now receiving dialysis or transplantation therapy. It is anticipated that this number will reach a peak of 50,000 to 60,000 in 1980.

The increasing renal disease–dialysis–transplant population needs an increasing number of knowledgeable nursing personnel to administer care throughout the renal disease/treatment continuum. Hence this book is written primarily for nurses who have chosen nephrology nursing as a specialty. However, the content will also prove useful to other members of the renal health care team. For our present purposes, the nephrology nurse specialist is defined as any nurse who has knowledge and clinical skill in one or more aspects of renal disease and its treatment—early diagnosis and treatment, acute and chronic dialysis therapy, and/or transplantation.

The person who has chosen nephrology nursing as a specialty has a challenging role to develop. The nurse must not wait for that role to be delegated by other health team members. Instead, the nephrology nurse specialist must actively define the parameters of that role for herself and for the health care team. This book offers a basis for the development of a knowledgeable nurse specialist who can delineate such a role and who, in cooperation with other members of the renal health care team, can deliver quality care to patients and families.

This book is written by several authors representing various health care disciplines. This multiple authorship gives the nurse detailed coverage of end stage renal disease, dialysis, and transplantation from different perspectives. Also, it will help the nurse understand the unique contributions of each discipline to total patient care. All contributors emphasize biopsychosocial principles rather than techniques and procedures. Specific procedures are rapidly outdated with medical and technological advances, but principles will continue to guide medical and nursing care. Procedures are, however, outlined as necessary to illustrate certain points.

The book does not include separate chapters on anatomy, physiology, diagnostic examinations, or causes of renal failure, because that information is adequately covered in other medical and nursing texts.

I am fortunate in having so many capable contributors to this book. I express my deepest appreciation to them for their cooperation and hard work. I am also indebted to Fred Hall for the illustrations and to Ellen Longworth for the typing of the manuscript. I would like to thank the staff of John Wiley & Sons, Inc., Publishers, for their patience and assistance in preparing the manuscript.

LARRY E. LANCASTER

Contents

The Patient
with End Stage
Renal Disease

1

Total Body Manifestations of End Stage Renal Disease and Related Medical and Nursing Management

Larry E. Lancaster, R.N., M.S.N.

Penny Pierce, R.N., M.S.N.

A patient in the end stage of renal failure presents a myriad of challenges to the nephrology nurse. As the kidneys fail, all body systems eventually become involved. Normal body functions are drastically altered in ways that redefine a person's quality of life. Hardly an aspect of physical, social, or psychological performance is left untouched by this disease process.

Because the process of renal degeneration is often slow and stormy, the patient reaches the end stage with a variety of illness experiences. The very nature of the disease requires close medical management, numerous interventions, and relationships with a variety of medical personnel. As with other chronic illnesses, periodic crises and frequent hospital admissions document a worsening of symptoms. These cumulative stressors diminish the patient's resources to such an extent that the nurse-patient relationship becomes very important.

Until the kidneys fail and dialysis or transplantation is imminent, nursing is highly involved in the conservative management of the patient.

Brundage states, "[T]he goals of conservative management of chronic renal failure are to: *1*) preserve renal function, *2*) postpone or eliminate the need for definitive treatment (dialysis and transplatation), *3*) improve body chemistries, *4*) reverse organ system alterations where possible, and *5*) provide comfort and an improved quality of life" (1).

The patient's response to conservative management depends to a great extent on nursing intervention. This includes such considerations as management of the patient's diet and medications; symptomatic relief of uremic symptoms; treatment of infection; alterations in body chemistry and alterations in organ systems; and teaching the patient to live within the limitations imposed by his disease (2).

Because the nature of the illness is chronic with intermittent acute episodes, the nurse may see the patient in the outpatient setting as well as in the hospital. Understandably the patient's needs will vary, depending upon the progression of the illness with its uremic manifestations and the presence or absence of life-threatening complications.

Nursing of the uremic patient focuses upon the assessment and management of fluid and electrolyte alterations, disordered regulatory functions, and the effects of an accumulation of uremic toxins upon every system of the body. Concurrently, one also attends to the needs of the person who is struggling with the illness, seeking to find some understanding of how he can learn to live within the boundaries of chronic illness (3).* The nurse-patient-family relationship develops in a meaningful way as the nurse sustains the patient when in crisis, promotes a maximum level of functioning when stable, and allows time for anticipatory guidance to prepare for the predictable outcomes of the patient's disease.

The task of prescribing comprehensive care is often difficult, owing to the complexity and fluidity of the physical well-being of the uremic patient. The purposes of this chapter are to discuss selected methods of assessment of renal function, to describe the effects of renal failure on various organ systems and physiological processes, to discuss the related medical management, and to present a nursing problem-oriented approach to the management of clinical problems presented by the uremic patient.

NURSING PROCESS

The patient's need for comprehensive management depends upon the nurse's ability to deliver care in a deliberative way. Patients' needs and concerns can best be addressed through developing a clear conceptualization of the nursing process. The steps of the process include: 1) assessment, 2) intervention, and 3) evaluation. For purposes of this discussion, a basic working knowledge of nursing process is assumed. How-

*Though educational needs and psychological support are not addressed in the chapter, it is understood that the plan of care would include these considerations.

ever, many resources are available to the nurse who wishes to study the process further (4,5,6).

Assessment

Assessment of a patient's status is an ongoing process, which begins with an initial collection of pertinent data. Many suitable data collection tools are available. Whether it is a nursing history (3) or one of a number of assessment tools, the purpose is to collect relevant information in a systematic way concerning the patient and his response to and understanding of the illness. Data are also solicited from the medical record and laboratory data, from other health workers involved in the care of the patient, and from family members. Assessment* also includes skill in physical examination, namely, inspection, palpation, percussion, and auscultation. Besides helping the nurse assess the initial status of the patient, these skills are most valuable in evaluating the patient's progress toward stated goals.

Identification of nursing problems or nursing diagnosis (7,8) flows from the initial data base. These problems include actual as well as potential or anticipated health problems. It is particularly important to identify these potential problems in a chronically ill population in order to educate, support, and prepare patients for inevitable occurrences with end stage renal disease.

Synthesis of the data and identification of a problem list focuses the nurse's attention on prescribing a plan of care. The plan must define and articulate its objectives so that the care is consistent and achieves the expected outcomes in a measurable way. Evaluation of the nursing intervention depends upon a clear statement of the treatment goals and the process in terms of nursing actions that lead to the desired outcome.

Lewis (9) adds, "This step includes the making of clinical judgments, establishing priorities of care, predicting potentialities for wholeness, and estimating progress toward wholeness." Consideration of wholeness is pertinent to planning long-term care in this chronically ill population.

In summary, assessment includes the collection of data, the recording of a nursing history, the identification of nursing problems in diagnosis, and the formulation of nursing objectives.

Intervention

Nursing objectives formulated at the assessment level define the nursing actions that have the greatest probability of relieving the patient's prob-

*A basic knowledge of physical assessment skill is understood.

lem. A nursing care plan is a written record of the nurse's actual and proposed actions. Each objective must be directed by clear nursing orders so that consistency is maintained from nurse to nurse, inpatient setting to outpatient, institution to institution. It is particularly important for chronically ill persons to have as much consistency as possible, as this reduces stress and helps reinforce trust in their care givers. Direction for writing nursing objectives, nursing orders, and care plans may be found in a variety of sources on the nursing process.

Evaluation

As the final step of the nursing process, evaluation is the true test of the adequacy of the intervention. At this point the nurse discovers whether or not her plan of action actually met the patient's needs. In order for evaluation to take place, the nursing objectives must have stated criteria. Lewis (9) states, "These criteria should be observable indications that the nursing care given either proved or disproved the hypotheses set up in the intervention phase, thereby achieving or failing to achieve the nursing objectives formulated in the assessment step."

Summary

Use of the nursing process is an effective approach to the delivery of nursing care. Carlson (5) writes, "The nursing process is basically set up for one purpose: to encourage the nurse to use a problem-solving approach in assisting the patient to understand his life process or style so that he can better control and cope with his illness." Meaningful long-term management of the uremic patient requires a systematic approach to solving his multiple physical and psychosocial problems throughout the course of treatment.

CONCEPTS BASIC TO AN UNDERSTANDING OF RENAL FAILURE

Papper defines renal failure as "that stage of renal function in which the kidney is no longer able to maintain the integrity of the internal environment of the organism" (10). For purposes of this book, _end stage renal disease_ is defined as irreversible kidney disease causing chronic abnormalities in the internal environment and necessitating treatment with dialysis or kidney transplantation for survival.

The constellation of signs and symptoms and physiochemical changes that occurs with renal failure is referred to as *uremia* or the uremic syndrome. These changes are related to fluid and electrolyte abnormalities; disordered regulatory functions (anemia, hypertension, renal osteodystrophy, and metastatic calcification); and accumulation of uremic toxins, which causes physiological changes and alters the function of various organ systems (10).

Urea nitrogen is a major end product of protein metabolism and is a major component of the urine. *Blood urea nitrogen* (BUN) refers to the level of urea in the serum. Blood urea nitrogen is normally excreted by the kidneys to maintain a serum level of 20 to 25 mg/100 ml. A rough determination of glomerular filtration rate may be obtained by measuring the BUN; however, there are limitations to its use for this purpose. First, urea is filtered and absorbed in relation to urine flow. The BUN level is also affected by several variables: *1*) high-protein diets result in an increased BUN; *2*) blood in the gastrointestinal tract increases the BUN; *3*) when there is a catabolic state (injury, infection, temperature elevation, poor nutrition), the BUN rises (10).

Serum creatinine is superior to BUN in determining glomerular filtration rate. Serum creatinine is liberated from muscle tissue at a constant rate and excreted at the same rate. The diet and metabolic state have little influence on serum creatinine. A normal range is 1 to 2 mg/100 ml. Since women have less muscle mass than men, their serum creatinine is usually slightly lower (10).

There is an advantage to using BUN and serum creatinine determinations together. For example, a normal serum creatinine and an elevated BUN might suggest blood in the gastrointestinal tract, high intake of protein, or a catabolic state, rather than decreased renal function (10).

Clearance is the rate at which a substance is excreted in terms of its plasma concentration. Because creatinine is an endogenous product and its production is not influenced by the metabolic state, *endogenous creatinine clearance* is an excellent clinical guide to glomerular filtration rate (GFR).

For an accurate determination of creatinine clearance both nurse and patient must understand and rigidly adhere to the following procedure (1):

1. The patient empties his bladder, and the exact time is marked on his record.
2. *All* urine is saved for 24 hours.
3. Exactly 24 hours after the start of the procedure the patient voids again and the specimen is saved.
4. The total volume of urine and the urine creatinine is measured.

5. A serum creatinine is collected at the end of the 24-hour period.

Creatinine clearance is computed using the formula:

$$\text{Creatinine clearance (ml/min)} = \frac{\text{Urine creatinine (mg/100 ml)} \times \text{Urine flow (ml/min)}}{\text{Serum creatinine (mg/100 ml)}}$$

This formula may be abbreviated to:

$$C_{Cr} = \frac{UV}{P}$$

Table 1.1 shows the range for serum creatinine and creatinine clearance for men and women. After age 40, GFR slowly declines; and by age 80 it may be 50% that in the normal young adult. Table 1.2 shows an approximate correlation among creatinine clearance, serum creatinine, and degree of renal failure.

Relationship Between GFR and Uremia

When considering renal failure it is helpful to keep in mind the relationship between glomerular filtration rate (as measured by creatinine clearance) and blood urea nitrogen. This relationship is shown by the graph

Table 1.1. Range for Serum Creatinine and Creatinine Clearance

Serum creatinine	Men	0.85–1.5 mg/100 ml
	Women	0.70–1.25 mg/100 ml
Creatinine clearance	Men	100–150 ml/min
	Women	85–125 ml/min

Table 1.2. Correlation Among Creatinine Clearance, Serum Creatinine, and Renal Failure

Creatinine Clearance (ml/min)	Serum Creatinine (mg/100 ml) (approximate)	Degree of Renal Failure
85–150	1.0–1.4	Normal
50–84	1.5–2.0	Mild
10–49	2.1–6.5	Moderate
< 10	> 6.5	Severe
0	> 12	Anuric (end stage)

in Figure 1.1. BUN is represented on the vertical axis, and GFR with corresponding percent of normal is shown on the horizontal axis. The curve representing change in BUN as GFR decreases is an average of many patients rather than an absolute for all patients. The graph shows that as much as 75% of renal function must be lost before there is a significant rise in BUN. When more than 75% of function is lost, further small decrements in renal function cause large increases in BUN. The length of time for the GFR to decrease to 25% of normal varies with disease processes and with individual patients; it may be a matter of weeks or months, depending on the severity of the pathology and the individual patient's response to the disease (10).

Two theories help explain overall renal pathophysiology and partially explain the kidney's ability to maintain homeostasis despite 75–80% loss of function. These theories are referred to as the "all nephron disease" hypothesis and the "intact nephron" or Bricker hypothesis.

The "all nephron disease" hypothesis explains renal failure in terms of all nephrons being involved in whole or in part by the pathological process (10). The remaining renal function is a result of any part or parts of the nephron that remain functional. For example, the tubule of all nephrons may become nonfunctional, but the glomerulus may remain intact and maintain some degree of renal function (10).

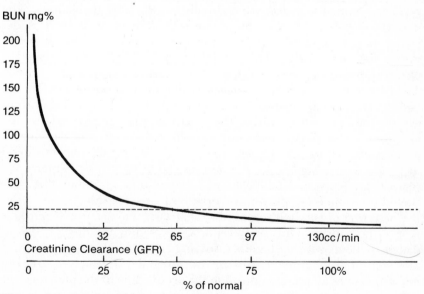

Figure 1.1. Relationship between glomerular filtration rate (as measured by creatinine clearance) and blood urea nitrogen. See text for explanation.

More current and more readily accepted is Bricker's "intact nephron" hypothesis. Bricker's observations led to the belief that in the event of disease there are two types of nephrons: *1*) those that are affected by the pathological process and are nonfunctional, and *2*) those that remain disease free and function normally. Homeostasis is maintained until late renal failure by hypertrophy of the normal nephrons (10).

The reader should keep in mind that the pathophysiological changes discussed in this chapter arise when overall renal function is less than 20–25% of normal (75–80% of renal function is lost), at which point the kidneys have lost their ability to regulate the internal environment. These changes may often be managed conservatively (diet and fluid control and medications) until GFR decreases to 10–15% of normal. Maintenance dialysis must then be implemented or renal transplantation performed to sustain life.

CHANGES IN THE INTEGUMENT
Skin

The skin of uremic persons has a characteristic pallid, grayish-bronze color and is unusually dry and scaly. The cause of the discoloration is retained pigments, which are normally excreted by the kidney. The underlying pallor is caused by the anemia common to uremia. A decrease in activity of oil glands and a decrease in size of sweat glands causes diminished perspiration and dryness of the skin. A combination of dry skin and deposition of phosphate crystals causes severe itching. The patient is compelled to scratch, and the skin may become excoriated and infected. An antipruritic such as trimeprazine tartrate (Temaril) or cyproheptadine hydrochloride (Periactin) is often prescribed for the itching. The use of bath oil and/or a lanolin-base lotion may alleviate the dryness and itching. During periods of intense itching the patient should be taught to rub lanolin into the skin instead of scratching. Superfatted soaps (e.g., Basis) and oatmeal baths may also be of value. The nails should be trimmed to prevent excoriation from scratching.

Correction of elevated serum phosphate and dialysis usually partially relieve the pruritis. One study reports successfully treating pruritis in dialysis patients with parenteral lidocaine (11). The therapy consists of 200 mg of lidocaine in 100 ml of normal saline given during hemodialysis as an infusion through the arterial line of the dialyzer over a 20-minute period. The treatment may be repeated only once after one hour if the pruritis is not relieved by the first dose. Slow infusion and a limited total dose are necessary for safe therapy. The relief of pruritis may last into the day following dialysis but often recurs by the second day.

Because of abnormal blood clotting activity and increased capillary fragility in uremia, minor blows to the skin may cause ecchymoses and purpura. The patient must be very careful to avoid falls or any minor trauma to the skin. If the patient is confined to bed, the side rails should be padded. Because the skin integrity of the uremic patient is poor, frequent turning and proper positioning are necessary to prevent prolonged pressure on bony prominences and subsequent decubiti formation. An eggshell mattress or flotation pad is a valuable aid to prevent pressure sores. Uremic frost formation on the skin (a white powdery substance, composed chiefly of urates) is a rare occurrence with modern management of uremia; however, if it does appear, it should be removed with soap and water.

Nails

Protein wasting in uremia often causes the nails to become thin and brittle. Red bands (Terry's nails) often develop at the end of the nail, or multiple red bands (Muercke's lines) develop along the nail. These signs cause no problems and may clear with proper management of uremia.

Hair

The hair of uremic patients frequently becomes dry, brittle, and may change color. It may fall out easily, leading to sparseness though not to total baldness. Shampoos and/or hair conditioners may alleviate the dryness, and the hair usually returns to normal after initiation of dialysis.

Uremic manifestations in the skin present some of the most distressing symptoms the patient will experience. Relentless itching and scratching predispose the patient to infection while making him irritable, restless, and frustrated. Since the causes are not well understood, treatment is symptomatic and left to the nurse's ingenuity. Frequently, one approach is tried after another until the nurse and patient find a satisfactory solution. Persistence in these cases serves to support the patient when his resources are most taxed, while communicating the nurse's willingness to make him comfortable. Her consistent response to complaints of this nature serves to establish trust in what may become a long-term relationship. As patients begin to perceive themselves differently in light of their changing bodies, it is important for them to have a nurse upon whom they can depend. Further discussion of the nurse-patient relationship and the psychological care of the uremic patient can be found in Chapter 2.

Nursing Approach

Problem No. 1:   Alterations in color, turgor, vascularity, and integrity of the integument.

SUBJECTIVE
Skin
Rough skin
Dry, itchy skin
Rash
Pain
Bleeding or bruising
Swelling
Infection
Nails
Thin, brittle nails
Hair
Dry hair
Color change
Hair loss

OBJECTIVE
Note changes in the following (12):
Color
Vascularity and evidence of bleeding or bruising
Lesions
Edema
Moisture
Temperature
Texture
Thickness
Mobility and turgor

ASSESSMENT
Inspection
Skin
Alteration in skin color.
Increase in pigmentation.
Yellow to gray color caused by the retention of urinary chromogens. Most evident in exposed areas, may be generalized; does not involve sclerae or mucous membranes (12).

Pallor secondary to underlying anemia.

Alteration in texture, due possibly to hypothyroidism, dehydration, or a decrease in oil gland activity.

Pruritus, occurring possibly because of hyperparathyroidism and the presence of calcium in the skin (13,14).

Superficial *Candida albicans* infection, often due to no known cause and treated symptomatically.

Dermatitis, most frequently a maculopapular eruption on the limbs and anterior chest (14).

Subcutaneous calcifications secondary to hyperparathyroidism.

Purpura secondary to abnormal clotting activity and increased capillary fragility.

Increased susceptibility to infection secondary to poor circulation and exacerbated by scratching.

Nails

Changes in the nails occur with inadequate nutrition or following a serious illness. Changes specific to the uremic patient include Terry's nails and Muercke's lines.

PLAN

Objective 1A: Patient's skin will remain intact, clean, and free from infection.

Nursing orders

1. Assess skin periodically for changes in color, texture, turgor, and vascularity.
2. Inspect for bruises, purpura, and signs of infection.
3. Inspect conjunctiva, mouth, nails for pallor of anemia.
4. Inspect dependent areas and periorbital spaces for edema.
5. Keep skin clean while relieving itching and dryness using one of the following methods: Basis soap, sodium bicarbonate in bath water, oatmeal baths, starch, bath oil.
6. Apply ointments or creams for comfort (Lanolin, Aquaphor).
7. Keep nails trimmed to avoid splitting as well as scratching.
8. Bathe patient every other day to reduce drying.
9. Administer drugs for relief of itching as ordered and/or indicated (Temaril, Periactin, antihistamines, phosphate binders).
10. Monitor serum phosphate levels (2–4.5 mg/100 ml).
11. Monitor serum calcium levels (8.5–10.5 mg/100 ml).
12. Monitor intake and output, avoiding overhydration and dehydration.

Objective 1B: Given an explanation of the manifestations of uremia, the patient will understand the symptoms expressed in the skin, hair, and nails.

Nursing orders

1. Describe (at the patient's level of understanding*) that toxic materials in the serum get into the skin and irritate nerve fibers.
2. Explain that itching may occur because of hyper-parathyroidism and that the presence of calcium phosphate deposits in the skin also causes irritation.
3. Begin to prepare the patient for the eventuality of dialysis (where feasible).
4. Answer patient's questions frankly, being supportive to the expression of negative affects.

GASTROINTESTINAL PROBLEMS

From mouth to anus, the gastrointestinal system is affected by uremia. It is not uncommon for uremic patients to suffer from stomatitis, *fetor uremicus,* esophagitis, gastritis, duodenal ulcers, nausea, vomiting, diarrhea, anorexia, lesions of the small and large bowel, and proctitis. The cause of these problems is elevated serum uremic toxins that cause inflammation and ulceration of the gastrointestinal mucosa. The management of selected problems is discussed in the following sections.

Oral Cavity

The concentration of urea in the saliva is approximately three-fourths that of the serum. In renal failure, the excessive salivary urea is coverted by the enzyme urease (from teeth bacteria) to ammonia. The ammonia is thought to be responsible for the *fetor uremicus* (smell of urine and ammonia to the breath), gum ulceration, bleeding, metallic taste, and generalized stomatitis common to advanced uremia (1). These symptoms usually clear after the initiation of dialysis. Until the symptoms clear, good oral hygiene may alleviate many of the problems. If the patient is unable to do his own mouth care, assistance must be provided. Measures that may be helpful include: *1*) Brushing the teeth several times a day to remove bacteria that cause urease production. A soft brush should be used and rigorous brushing should be avoided to prevent gum injury and bleeding. *2*) Frequent use of mouthwash, sour balls, lemon juice, or

*Determined by the nurse's knowledge and assessment of the patient. Consider physical status of the patient (uremic) in terms of ability to learn as well as patient's readiness to accept physical changes.

gum to improve taste and alleviate thirst. A vinegar mouthwash helps neutralize the ammonia formed by bacterial action. *3*) Dry, cracked mucous membranes and lips may be kept moistened with Vaseline or mineral oil. Glycerin is not advised since it causes a long-term drying effect on mucous membranes. *4*) Bland, soft foods are better tolerated than foods that are spicy and difficult to chew. *5*) A dental referral is indicated if cavities or calculus formation is present.

Anorexia, Nausea, Vomiting

The nausea and vomiting of uremia usually occur in the early morning and resemble the morning sickness of pregnancy. If the uremic person does not allow for part of his fluid to be taken during the night, a nocturnal dehydration may cause an increase in serum uremic toxins. This elevation in serum uremic toxins is thought to be one cause of early morning nausea and vomiting (10). The prescribed 24-hour fluid intake must be scheduled such that not all of the allowed fluid is consumed before bedtime. If the patient finds food repulsive on first arising, he should be encouraged to avoid food for 2–3 hours and then attempt to eat small servings. If the patient requests special foods, they should be included in his 24-hour dietary prescription. If these measures fail, an antiemetic such as prochlorperazine (Compazine) or promethazine hydrochloride (Phenergan) may be ordered. Remission of the early morning nausea and vomiting often occurs after initiation of dialysis.

Gastritis, Ulcers, Bowel Lesions

Patients with signs and symptoms of gastrointestinal inflammation and ulceration must be observed for bleeding. Since anemia is a problem of all uremic patients, blood loss in any amount, small or large, must not be overlooked. All vomitus and stools must be examined for gross or occult blood. The serum urea nitrogen will become more elevated if blood remains in the gastrointestinal tract; therefore, cleansing enemas are indicated to remove blood from the bowel.

If the patient has diarrhea, an antidiarrheic such as diphenoxylate hydrochloride (Lomotil) may be given. The anal area must be cleaned meticulously to prevent excoriation.

If the patient has constipation, a bulk-forming laxative (Metamucil) or a stool softener (Colace, Doxidan) should be ordered. Magnesium-containing laxatives (Milk of Magnesia) must be avoided because of the possibility of hypermagnesemia. Aluminum hydroxide gels (Amphojel, Basajel) given as phosphate binders to treat renal osteodystrophy may also cause constipation and require concomitant administration of a stool softener (15).

The problem of viral hepatitis in relation to hemodialysis will be discussed in a subsequent chapter.

SELECTED METABOLIC PROBLEMS

The metabolic consequences of chronic renal failure and uremia are numerous. Carbohydrate intolerance, hyperlipidemia, and protein metabolism are discussed.

Carbohydrate Intolerance

Causes of glucose intolerance in chronic renal failure are insensitivity of peripheral tissues to insulin, delayed production of insulin by the pancreas, and an increased half-life of insulin. Some researchers believe that the peripheral resistance to insulin is caused by an enzyme abnormality associated with uremia, but this has not been clearly demonstrted by research (16). There is probably an *adequate* production of insulin by the pancreas in response to glucose, but there seems to be a *delayed* production in uremia. The serum level of insulin is often elevated in uremia because of an increased half-life due to slowed insulin degradation by the kidney. Even though the level is elevated, the insulin cannot be effective because of the peripheral resistance. Extreme hyperglycemia and ketoacidosis are not associated with the glucose intolerance of chronic renal failure. Insulin and glucose metabolism are improved, but do not completely normalize, after implementation of regular hemodialysis.

Hyperlipidemia

Except in the nephrotic syndrome serum cholesterol remains normal in renal failure. Because of increased production and decreased removal, serum triglycerides are elevated in uremia. The increased production of triglycerides is related to the peripheral resistance to insulin and elevated serum insulin, which cause an increased hepatic output of glycerides (16). Reduction in activity of the enzyme, lipoprotein lipase, also due to insulin resistance, contributes to the abnormality.

The serum level of triglycerides does not decrease after hemodialysis is started. In fact, the condition often worsens, and patients who did not have elevated triglycerides before hemodialysis will often develop elevated levels within weeks after the treatment is implemented.

The relationship between hyperlipoproteinemia (especially Type IV) and arteriosclerotic cardiovascular disease is well documented. Many uremic patients, especially those receiving chronic hemodialysis, develop this related heart and vascular disease and die from myocardial infarction.

Protein Metabolism

Because of decrease in renal function the end products of protein metabolism accumulate, as reflected by an increase in blood urea nitrogen. The elevated BUN and other uremic toxins are responsible, in part, for the development of the uremic syndrome with its various manifestations.

It is not surprising that patients are often placed on low-protein diets to decrease the nitrogenous load and to control uremia to some extent. When the overall protein intake is decreased, as much as possible should be high-biological-value (contains more essential amino acids) and as little as possible should be low-biological-value protein (contains few essential amino acids). The essential amino acids are vital for protein synthesis in the body and must be included in the daily dietary intake. Low-biological-value proteins provide few essential amino acids and furnish more urea nitrogen than high-biological-value proteins during metabolism, thus increasing the BUN. Further discussion of protein in the diet will be found in Chapter 5.

FLUID-ELECTROLYTE AND ACID-BASE DISORDERS

Problems related to body water and metabolic acidosis are discussed in this section. Problems pertaining to sodium are discussed in relation to hypertension; potassium in relation to the cardiovascular system; and calcium and phosphorus in relation to the skeletal system and parathyroid gland.

Body Water

The patient with chronic renal failure may be either dehydrated or fluid overloaded depending on the basic pathological process and the degree of renal failure. Large urinary losses of water and dehydration may be found in early renal failure and in late renal failure caused by a disease such as polycystic kidneys. When the creatinine clearance is less than 4–5 ml/min, volume overload is usually the major problem. Volume overload is managed by limiting intake of fluid and by ultrafiltration during hemodialysis. The 24-hour fluid intake is individualized based on weight change, serum sodium concentration, urine volume, and maintenance of maximum GFR (10). The fluid intake should be distributed over 24 hours to prevent nocturnal dehydration. (Control and calculation of fluid intake will be discussed in more detail in Chapter 5.)

Metabolic Acidosis

Acidosis in renal failure develops because of several factors (10,17):

1. The kidney's inability to excrete excessive hydrogen ions.
2. Reduction in ammonia production by the kidney.
3. Retention of acid end products of protein metabolism, which use available buffers.
4. Loss of bicarbonate in the urine.

The respiratory system partially compensates by increasing the rate and depth to excrete carbon dioxide via the lungs. Demineralization of bone also helps buffer hydrogen ions. For this reason acidosis contributes to the development of renal osteodystrophy, which will be discussed in a later section.

The only clinical finding characteristic of metabolic acidosis is hyperventilation. Lethargy and coma may be seen in severe acidosis, but it is difficult to decide whether these result from the acidosis per se or from the underlying disease (such as uremia or diabetic acidosis). Laboratory findings include a low plasma bicarbonate and low pH of arterial blood.

Patients with symptoms of acidosis or a plasma bicarbonate level less than 15 mEq/L (normal 25 to 28 mEq/L) are treated (10). An oral alkalizing agent such as Shohl's solution is often beneficial in controlling acidosis. If the acidosis is severe and Kussmaul respirations are present, intravenous sodium bicarbonate is often administered. If acidosis is severe, rapid correction by intravenous sodium bicarbonate may precipitate hypocalcemic tetany. The degree of ionization of calcium is determined by the pH; the more acid the plasma, the more ionized calcium present. If acidosis is rapidly corrected, the plasma ionized calcium level decreases as it binds to plasma proteins. Ten to 30 grams of calcium gluconate given intravenously slowly at the time of sodium bicarbonate administration may prevent hypocalcemic tetany.

Hemodialysis corrects acidosis by removal of hydrogen ions and by the addition of acetate, a bicarbonate precursor, to buffer acids.

Nursing Approach

Problem No. 2:   Inadequate nutrition.

SUBJECTIVE

Pleasure of food diminished, owing to dry mucous membranes, sour or metallic taste in mouth, painful chewing and swallowing, nausea, and loss of appetite.

OBJECTIVE

Inflammation and ulcerations in the mouth contribute to unpleasant taste; uremic patients often have dental problems related to altered calcium and phosphorus metabolism and bleeding of soft tissues in mouth.

ASSESSMENT

Adequate nutrition is essential to sustain life; additional considerations are directed toward particular needs of the uremic patient to avoid negative nitrogen imbalance, long periods of fasting to avoid endogenous protein breakdown, and dehydration.

Problem related to high levels of ammonia due to breakdown of salivary urea by bacterial urease (1,14); *Candida albicans* infection occurs in this susceptible host.

Important to establish ideal weight for each patient considering actual weight (versus fluid) and nutritional requirements of activity, stressor of chronic illness.

PLAN

Objective 2A: Adequate nutrition will be maintained as evidenced by *1*) the intake of the prescribed diet (see Chapter 5), *2*) maintaining the patient's ideal weight, *3*) maintaining the BUN, creatinine, and potassium levels within acceptable limits.*

Nursing orders
1. Inspect mucous membranes for ulcerations (see Objective No. 2B if ulcerations are present).
2. Offer small, frequent, attractive meals.
3. Consult dietitian to assist patient with particular nutritional problems and begin diet instruction.

*Acceptable limits are defined for each patient.

4. Monitor patient's weight accurately by a) measuring weight at the same time of the day, b) wearing the same amount of clothing, c) using the same scales.
5. Monitor BUN, creatinine, and serum potassium levels as an indirect indicator of dietary compliance.
6. Question patient regarding factors that may contribute to inadequate nutrition, such as anorexia, vomiting, nausea, noncompliance, others.
7. Keep other team members informed of nutritional status of patient.

Objective 2B: Given prescribed mouth care, patient's mucous membranes will be clean, moist, and free from ulcerations or infection.

Nursing orders
1. Inspect mucous membranes.
2. Give thorough and gentle mouth care using a soft toothbrush, Q-tips, or padded tongue blade.
3. Avoid trauma to delicate tissues when administering treatments.
4. Refer patient for correction of any dental problems identified on oral examination.
5. Advise patient to inform dentist of illness in terms of bleeding difficulties, medications, etc.
6. Treat infections immediately:
   a. Inform physician of finding.
   b. Treat *Candida albicans* in one of a variety of ways:
      1) Nystatin suspension
      2) Amphotericin lozenges
      3) 1% gentian violet three times a day
   c. Evaluate effectiveness of treatment daily.
7. Keep mucous membranes moist using Vaseline or mineral oil.
8. Give one of the following to improve altered taste:
   a. 25% acetic acid in cool water used as a mouthwash (neutralizes ammonia),
   b. Sour balls or cool liquids (caution for patients on a fluid restriction).
9. Discuss symptoms with patient and provide support as needed. (For predialysis patients, it may be helpful to know that most of these symptoms are relieved with dialysis.)

Problem No. 3:   Gastrointestinal inflammation or bleeding secondary to ulcerations resulting in blood loss.

SUBJECTIVE

Patients may be unaware of bleeding, yet experience pain, alterations in bowel patterns, weight loss, or excessive fatigue.

OBJECTIVE

Pain located in epigastrium, midsternal area (with or without radiation), midabdominal, or lower abdominal area. Since pain is a subjective complaint, it is important to question the patient further in terms of location, character, onset, cause, duration, frequency, severity, precipitating factors, and attenuating factors (18). Alterations in bowel habits include constipation, diarrhea, presence of blood, or painful elimination.

Weight loss may be identified while evaluating objective no. 1 (nutrition) before the patient becomes aware of the problem. Excessive fatigue is difficult to evaluate in a chronically ill person but should be pursued when presented by the patient. Monitoring hematocrit and hemoglobin often assists in identifying blood loss.

ASSESSMENT

Abdominal exam

Inspect for symmetry of abdomen; gaseous distention or obstruction of the bowel would be reflected by asymmetry.

Auscultation of bowel sounds: Inflammation is represented by decreased or absent bowel sounds of peristalsis. Sounds increased in intensity and frequency may be caused by increased intestinal motility due to diarrhea, laxatives, gastroenteritis, and possibly bleeding peptic ulcer. With mucosal irritation, the increased sounds are not heard in rushes and are of lesser intensity (18).

Percussion: normal sounds may vary if free air is present.

Palpation detects areas of tenderness and abnormal areas of fluid.

Laboratory data

Hematocrit indicates anemia associated with blood loss.

WBC may indicate infection.

PLAN

Objective 3:   Patient's usual pattern of elimination will be maintained (or restored) without complications of pain, weight loss, or blood loss.

Nursing orders

1. Determine patient's usual pattern of elimination from the nursing history.
2. Identify those aids patient uses to help maintain usual pattern.

3. Consult dietitian if dietary modifications are required.
4. Consult physician if drugs are required:
    a. Stool softeners.
    b. Bulk-forming laxatives.
    c. Avoid drugs containing magnesium.
5. Evaluate side effects of prescribed drugs as possible causative factor:
    a. Constipation may be caused by phosphate binders taken by patients for renal osteodystrophy.
6. Observe for gross blood in stool or vomitus.
7. Test for occult blood in stool and vomitus.
8. Monitor serum urea nitrogen levels (elevates when blood remains in the gastrointestinal tract).
9. Give cleansing enemas to remove blood from the gastrointestinal tract to prevent bacterial action that raises urea levels.
10. Monitor serum calcium levels.
11. Keep rectal area clean to promote comfort and prevent irritation and infection.
12. Monitor weight.
13. Monitor fluid and electrolyte losses associated with diarrhea:
    a. Monitor serum potassium levels (normal 3.5–5.5 mEq/100 ml).
    b. Keep patient hydrated and avoid dehydration.

Problem No. 4:   Nausea and vomiting.

SUBJECTIVE
Nausea frequently occurs in the morning and at the sight of food. Vomiting may or may not be preceded by nausea.

OBJECTIVE
Vomitus may contain gross or occult blood.

ASSESSMENT
Nausea is thought to be a result of an elevation in serum uremic toxins. Evaluate as a possible side effect of digitalis for patients who are taking the drug.
Vomiting contributes to loss of fluids and electrolytes and contributes to metabolic alkalosis. Consider the possibility of cerebral edema if vomiting is projectile.

PLAN
Objective 4:   When nausea and vomiting cannot be avoided, owing to uremia, the patient will receive symptomatic relief

of symptoms as evidenced by verbal report and ability to eat and drink. (Maintain nutrition.)

Nursing orders

1. Offer small, frequent meals.
2. Avoid serving foods early in the morning.
3. Encourage patient to ease waves of nausea by finding suitable distractions or taking deep breaths.
4. Prepare a fluid schedule that provides for a balanced intake throughout the day and allows for fluid during the night to avoid nocturnal dehydration.
5. Consult physician for possible use of antiemetics.
6. Avoid fluid and electrolyte imbalances:
    a. Monitor serum potassium levels.
    b. Measure intake and output.
    c. Consider insensible fluid loss.
7. Replace fluids as necessary.
8. Treat metabolic alkalosis when present.
9. Assess relief of nausea and resultant ability to eat and drink by asking patient.
10. Determine those factors patient has found helpful in alleviating nausea.

PULMONARY PROBLEMS

Pulmonary problems in chronic renal failure include pulmonary edema, pleuritic pain, pleural rub, pleural effusions, uremic pleuritis, and a condition referred to as "uremic lung" or uremic pneumonitis. The sputum is tenacious, the cough reflex is depressed, and there is an increased susceptibility to infections because the pulmonary macrophage activity is reduced in uremia. The respiratory system attempts to compensate for the metabolic acidosis of renal failure by increasing the rate to eliminate carbon dioxide, thus decreasing the body's carbonic acid (hydrogen ion) concentration.

Uremic pneumonitis, which is one manifestation of fluid overload, usually disappears following fluid removal during two or three dialyses. Frequent chest x-rays are necessary to detect changes in pneumonitis. Antibiotics may be administered to prevent a superimposed bacterial infection in the "wet," uremic lung.

The objective of therapy is to reduce the amount of excess fluid, thereby reducing the risk of cardiopulmonary complications while promoting the patient's comfort.

Nursing Approach

Problem No. 5:   Dyspnea secondary to pulmonary edema.

SUBJECTIVE
> Patient is uncomfortable, restless, and dyspneic. Difficulty with respirations causes a fright response, which increases dyspnea.

OBJECTIVE
> Respirations are difficult and labored. When hyperventilation results in hypocapnia, patient may experience psychomotor impairment, numbness and tingling of hands and feet, and dizziness.

ASSESSMENT
> Fluid overload may be caused by heart failure, sodium and fluid retention. When renal function is less than 15% of normal and serum creatinine is less than 5 mg/100 ml, the control of sodium input controls body water (1). Serum sodium levels are monitored closely, while usually restricted along with fluid. Overhydration may lead to hyponatremia and water intoxication manifested by headache, delirium progressing to lethargy, coma, and convulsions.

PLAN
> *Objective 5:*   Given supportive treatment, the patient's comfort and well-being will be maintained until his respiratory status returns to normal.

> *Nursing orders*
> 1. Observe for changes in respiratory rate, depth, and character.
> 2. Auscultate chest for rales and/or rhonchi.
> 3. Observe amount and character of sputum.
> 4. Prevent pulmonary congestion by encouraging deep breathing and coughing in a way that avoids fatigue.
> 5. Maintain good oral hygiene.
> 6. Provide patient with rest periods and an atmosphere conducive to rest.
> 7. Consult with dietitian and provide a diet with adequate calories to compensate for additional catabolism.
> 8. Carefully monitor additional fluids that may be prescribed to avoid further overload.
> 9. Monitor fluid and sodium restriction when indicated.
> 10. Administer medications as indicated (diuretics, digitalis).
>   *a.* Observe for possible side effects of diuretics: nausea, vomiting, anorexia, diarrhea, constipation, orthostatic

hypotension, electrolyte imbalance (potassium depletion). Thiazide diuretics may cause serious side effects of hyperglycemia, hyperuricemia, hypokalemia.

  b. Monitor serum potassium levels of patients receiving digitalis (patients with excess serum potassium require more drug for the same effect than a patient with normal potassium).

  c. Observe for possible toxic effects of digitalis:
    1) Nausea, vomiting, disturbances of color vision.
    2) EKG changes including: prolongation of P–R interval, VPCs, bigeminy, various other arrhythmias.

  d. Take apical pulse before administering drug; withhold if pulse is below 60 beats per minute.

  e. Notify physician at notation of any side effect.

 11. Observe for orthopnea, distention of neck veins, pallor, cool skin, or diaphoresis.

 12. Administer antibiotics as ordered to prevent a superimposed bacterial infection.

Problem No. 6:   Increased suceptibility to infection.

SUBJECTIVE

Patient may report a frequency of colds and flu as well as skin infections that require a long time to heal.

OBJECTIVE

Thick, tenacious sputum with upper respiratory infections. Vital signs are often misleading, as patients with uremia may have a low body temperature even with an infection. Also, the patient may have an elevated WBC without having an infection. One must be alert for other less specific symptoms of infection; a disparity between pulse and temperature or in leukocyte count may be a guide to infection (2,14).

ASSESSMENT

Response to infection in the uremic patient is altered. White blood cell counts (granulocytes and lymphocytes) are usually normal. The increase in WBC count in response to infection is less than normal. Immune responsiveness of the lymphoreticular system is depressed, but immunoglobulin levels are normal. Cell-mediated responses are altered, but the formation of antibodies to red and white cell antigens is not inhibited (1).

PLAN

  Objective 6:   Given that the uremic patient is a compromised host, he will be protected from infection.

Nursing orders
1. Teach patient to avoid exposure to those who are ill and avoid crowds during flu and cold epidemics.
2. Maintain adequate nutritional status.
3. Provide for rest.
4. Avoid unnecessary procedures and instrumentation that would break barriers of defense.
5. Use sterile technique for all procedures.
6. Advise patient to discuss necessity for flu vaccine during winter months.
7. Observe for changes in sputum amount or character or presence of blood.
8. Advise patient to stop smoking.
9. Observe for other signs of infection: malaise, listlessness, rapid heart, and rapid respiration.
10. Review medications patient may have been given for previous infections and caution against using any drugs without consulting physician.
    a. Nitrofurantoin and methenamine mandelate are not effective if azotemia is present.
    b. Tetracycline causes a rise in BUN concentration and should not be used.
    c. Aminoglycoside antibiotics (gentamycin, kanamycin, neomycin, and streptomycin) are nephrotoxic (3).

NEUROLOGICAL PROBLEMS

Nervous system changes occur in virtually all uremic patients. The signs and symptoms are numerous and vary according to the degree of uremia and the part of the nervous system affected—central, peripheral, or autonomic. Changes may occur in mental function, muscle function, behavior, and sensory and motor nerves.

Changes in mentation include shortened memory and attention span, lack of interest in the environment, confusion, stupor, coma, and convulsions. Electroencephalographic changes are indicative of a metabolic encephalopathy. These changes are characterized by disturbances of cortical background rhythm, and normal alpha waves are replaced by a slow irregular rhythm.

Depending on the patient's premorbid personality, behavior changes may range from slight irritability to complete withdrawal. Other changes include psychosis, delusions, decreased or absent libido, agitation, and depression. As these symptoms are expressed, the patient becomes more and more difficult to manage for both his family and care takers. Exacerbated by other manifestations of uremia, the patient's quality of life suffers. The patient uses his limited strength and resources to deal only with living on a day-to-day basis. Soon the patient realizes his world has become narrow and restricted to managing only his chronic illness.

A slowing of peripheral nerve conduction leads to peripheral neuropathy manifested by symmetrical numbness and burning, beginning in the toes and spreading up the legs; the "restless legs" syndrome; foot drop; and the "burning feet" syndrome.

The "restless legs" syndrome is one of the earliest signs of peripheral neuropathy. This syndrome consists of painful cramps and crawling, pricking, and itching sensations localized to the lower extremities and usually developing during the night. The symptoms are often relieved by movement, thus the name "restless legs" syndrome (19,20).

Symptoms of the "burning feet" syndrome include a bilateral painful, burning, prickling, tingling sensation of the feet. Insomnia and curtailment of ambulation may result from the pain and burning (16).

If dialysis is instituted before motor nerve dysfunction develops, these changes may be slowly reversed. Bilateral footdrop is the most common motor nerve abnormality of uremic neuropathy.

Autonomic nervous system changes in uremia include a decreased baroreceptor response. When the blood pressure increases, the usual bradycardia does not occur, nor does tachycardia occur when the blood pressure falls (16).

Nursing Approach

Caring for a chronically ill person demands tremendous strength, patience, and understanding for both family and care takers. It is a situation in which extraordinary amounts of time and energy are expended. An important function for nursing is to intervene early in the progression of the disease, assisting families to create an atmosphere wherein important communication can take place in regard to the individual's reactions to the ill member of the family. Recognizing the need for diversion, recreation, and the pursuit of one's own interests is an important step toward keeping the patient from feeling like a burden upon his family. Development of a meaningful nurse-patient-family relationship offers a ready counselor during difficult times. An important function of the nurse involves helping the patient and his family understand the symptoms as they occur and make necessary modifications in a way that is least disturbing to their daily life.

Following is a plan for caring for patients with the problems of altered mentation, personality changes, and peripheral neuropathy.

Problem No. 7:   Alterations in mentation.

SUBJECTIVE

Confusion.

Somnolence.

Lack of interest in the environment.

Shortened attention span.

Memory loss.

Disorientation.

Sensory disturbances including altered sense of smell, vision, and
hearing.

OBJECTIVE

Difficulty in carrying on a conversation.

Depressed motor activity.

Lack of orientation to person, place, or time.

ASSESSMENT

Alterations in central nervous system function are represented by
EEG changes characteristic of metabolic encephalopathy and
usually parallel the clinical disorders of uremia (13,16,27).

Direct toxicity to the central nervous system by toxic metabolites is
probably the main cause of impaired cerebral function. EEG
changes are present and are similar to those seen in hepatic
coma (14).

Careful assessment of the neurological status of the patient allows
the nurse to intervene early in the progression of neurological
involvement. Protecting the patient from seizures, excitation,
somnolence, or coma is of prime importance. One of the earliest signs of impaired function is an inability to concentrate.
Changes in mental functioning, behavior, and level of consciousness progress as uremia becomes more profound. It is
extremely important on these occasions for the nurse to have an
assessment of the patient's pre-illness personality structure.

PLAN

Objective 7:   Given an explanation of the relationship of uremia to
presenting symptoms, the patient and his family will
understand the need to modify the environment to
provide for the patient's comfort, safety, and acceptance.

Nursing orders

1. Explain the concept of metabolic encephalopathy: that impaired cerebral function is due to direct toxicity of the central
nervous system.

2. Help patient's family understand that his behavior is beyond his control.
3. Alter method of communication with patient:
   a. Allow additional time for patient to respond to questions.
   b. Assess ability to think and reason before asking patient to make decisions.
   c. Evaluate ability to learn before attempting to instruct the patient.
   d. Respond to patient in a calm, reassuring manner, avoiding confrontation.
4. Keep environmental stimuli to a minimum.
5. Avoid fatigue as much as possible and provide for adequate rest.
6. Encourage patient to maintain hobbies and interests that are not fatiguing yet keep him interested in his environment.
7. Discuss safety considerations with patient's family (such as leaving the patient alone with a lighted cigarette, providing a night light in the patient's room)
8. Orient patient to new surroundings.
9. Assist with meals, ambulation, or other activities as necessary.
10. When the patient is hospitalized, place bed in low position and use side rails.
11. Place handrail in bathroom of home.

Problem No. 8:   Peripheral neuropathy.

SUBJECTIVE

Decreased sensation in extremities (sensory neuropathy is one of the earliest signs).

Numbness and burning of the extremities beginning in the toes (restless leg syndrome).

Muscle cramps.

Loss in muscle strength.

OBJECTIVE

Footdrop (most common nerve abnormality of uremic neuropathy).

ASSESSMENT

Nervous system depression and neuromuscular irritability are closely associated. Peripheral neuropathy is an early sign of the metabolic disruption of uremia. Neurons are damaged by severe demyelination, particularly the distal portion. Progressive decrease in nerve conduction velocity appears to parallel the worsening of peripheral neuropathy (1). Decreased nerve conduction affects both motor and sensory function. Assessment of motor function usually reveals a decrease in deep tendon and vibratory reflexes. Sensory neuropathy can be assessed by the patient's ability to respond to a two-point discrimination test.

PLAN

Objective 8:   Given supportive therapy, the patient will be able to ambulate safely and comfortably.

Nursing orders

1. Consult physical therapy for initial assessment of muscle strength, gait, and degree of impairment.
2. Request physical therapy to develop an exercise regimen to maintain patient's level of activity.
3. Protect patient from leg and foot trauma:
   a. Check shoes for proper fit.
   b. Inspect feet for ingrown toenails, blisters, calluses, and the like, which may predispose patient to injury and infection.
4. Use footboard to avoid footdrop while hospitalized or bedridden.
5. Administer analgesics when indicated.
6. Administer Valium 5–10 mg, 3–4 times a day, for restless leg syndrome as indicated.
7. Encourage patient to maintain a moderate amount of activity.

With worsening of uremia the patient may experience extremes of neurological involvement including stupor, convulsions, or coma. When hospitalized, patients are observed closely for signs of these complications and are protected from predisposing factors: hypertension, cerebral edema, fluid and electrolyte disturbances. It is important to recognize that most uremic patients do not convulse in the absence of another underlying disorder. Most commonly, other precipitating disorders are epilepsy, malignant hypertension, or sepsis.

Problem No. 9:   Stupor, convulsions or coma secondary to neurological response to uremia.

PLAN

Objective 9:   When identified as a high risk, the patient will be protected from neurological complications as evidenced by the absence of stupor, convulsions, or coma.

Nursing orders

1. Observe frequently for alterations in behavior: agitation, excitation, depression, or somnolence.
2. Observe for cerebral edema.

3. Administer drugs as indicated to reduce blood pressure.
4. Administer drugs as indicated for agitation (paraldehyde or chloral hydrate).
5. Administer drugs cautiously, as most actions are potentiated by uremia.
6. Keep padded tongue blade, suction, O_2 equipment available.
7. Provide a quiet environment with minimal stimulation.
8. Avoid administration of opiates, phenobarbital, or long-acting barbiturates.
9. Monitor blood pressure closely.

CARDIOVASCULAR SYSTEM PROBLEMS

Problems of the cardiovascular system related to chronic renal failure include hypertensive heart disease, hyperkalemia, hypermagnesemia, hypocalcemia, myocardial calcification, cardiomyopathy, pericarditis, pericardial effusion, pericardial tamponade, arterial calcification, and hypertension. Hypertension, arterial calcification, hyperkalemia, pericarditis, and pericardial tamponade are discussed in the following sections.

Hypertension

The most common cardiovascular problem in chronic renal failure is hypertension, which has two basic causes: *1*) that caused by fluid and sodium overload, and *2*) that caused by the renin-angiotensin system (10,16,21).

The first cause is a result of the kidney's inability to excrete sodium and water. The retention of sodium and water causes a circulatory overload and elevated blood pressure. With a decrease in sodium and fluid intake and/or fluid removal during dialysis the blood pressure usually returns to normal.

The second cause of hypertension is a result of a malfunctioning renin-angiotensin system in renal failure. Figure 1.2 shows that in normal persons renin is released by the juxtaglomerular apparatus of the kidneys in response to renal ischemia. Renin is converted to angiotensin II, which causes an increase in blood pressure and a decrease in renal ischemia. Once renal ischemia decreases, renin production decreases. In renal failure, the kidneys apparently do not recognize the decrease in ischemia and may continue producing large quantities of renin. This type of hypertension does not respond well to fluid and sodium restrictions or to dialysis. In fact, significant ultrafiltration for fluid removal

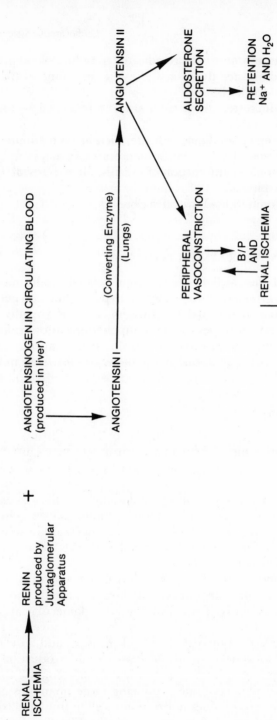

Figure 1.2. Schema of the renin-angiotensin mechanism.

30

during hemodialysis may increase renal ischemia, increase renin production, and aggravate hypertension. A β-adrenergic inhibitor such as propranolol (Inderal) may be helpful in decreasing renin release. A bilateral nephrectomy is often required to remove the source of renin production.

Many patients will require antihypertensive medications for blood pressure control. Table 1.3 is a summary of some oral antihypertensive drugs commonly used for patients with chronic renal failure (21). If drugs are required, effects must be carefully monitored. The blood pressure should be measured at intervals throughout the day (early morning, before arising; noon; and evening) in supine, sitting, and standing positions. The patient should be warned about the possibility of orthostatic hypotension and should be taught to move slowly from lying to standing positions. If ultrafiltration is to be used for fluid removal during hemodialysis, all antihypertensive medications must be withheld for 8–10 hours before the initiation of dialysis. The presence of antihypertensives in the serum during hemodialysis does not allow the vascular system to react normally to the decrease in circulating blood volume caused by extracorporeal blood volume and ultrafiltration; therefore, shock may develop. Furthermore, adequate amounts of fluid cannot be removed during dialysis, and excess body fluid will continue.

Arterial Calcification

A common vascular complication of chronic renal failure is arterial calcification from improper calcium and phosphorus metabolism and excretion. Coronary artery disease often ensues, and infarction of the myocardium is a cause of death in many patients. Arterial calcification does not respond to treatment but may be ameliorated by proper dosages of phosphate binding medications beginning early in the course of renal failure (16).

Hyperkalemia

Normal serum potassium levels (3.5–5.0 mEq/L) are maintained until the 24-hour urine output falls below 500 ml with a decreased GFR. There are few warning signs of hyperkalemia until the serum level reaches 7–8 mEq/L, and then severe electrocardiographic changes may rapidly progress to cardiac arrest and death.

Causes of hyperkalemia in renal failure include acidosis, ingestion of potassium in medication, failure to follow dietary regimen, blood transfusions, and bleeding.

Table 1.3. Examples of Antihypertensive Drugs Used in Chronic Renal Failure

Drug	Daily Dosage	Mode of Action	Side Effects
Methyldopa (Aldomet)	250–2000 mg orally	Decreases peripheral resistance by diminishing sympathetic outflow lowering renin release	Postural hypotension, drowsiness, constipation, fever, skin rash, decreased libido, hepatocellular dysfunction
Hydralazine (Apresoline)	40–200 mg orally	Relaxes smooth muscles of arterioles to decrease peripheral resistance	Angina pectoris, headache, palpitations, tachycardia, diarrhea, myalgia, urticaria
Guanethidine (Ismelin)	12.5–100 mg orally	Decreases peripheral resistance by inhibiting neurotransmission at adrenergic nerve endings and by decreasing cardiac output	Postural hypotension, muscular weakness, diarrhea
Propranolol (Inderal)	40–320 mg orally	Decreases cardiac output and renin release by inhibition of β-adrenergic activity	Bradycardia, muscle cramps, sleeplessness, diarrhea, bronchospasms in patients with COLD

EKG changes (which are the single most important indication of potassium intoxication) include elevated T wave, S-T segment depression, prolonged P-R interval (first degree heart block), and broadening of the QRS complex with eventual ventricular fibrillation and cardiac standstill. These changes are illustrated in Figure 1.3.

Acidosis increases serum potassium because the kidneys (if there is any kidney function) excrete hydrogen ions instead of potassium ions to maintain acid-base balance. The increased extracellular hydrogen ions diffuse into the cells and the abundant intracellular potassium ions diffuse out of the cell, thus increasing serum potassium.

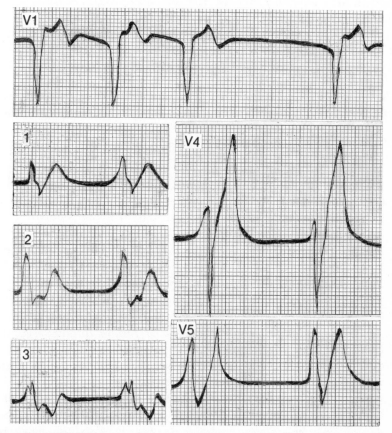

Figure 1.3. EKG indicative of hyperkalemia (serum potassium 8.5 mEq/L). Note tall peaked T waves, absent P waves, widened QRS complex, and irregular rhythm.

Management of hyperkalemia centers on prevention and treatment of emergencies.

Hyperkalemia may be prevented by closely monitoring intake of potassium in medications and food. The dietary intake of potassium is based on GFR and serum potassium levels. (Refer to Chapter 5 for further information.) Catabolic states must be minimized, since breakdown of tissue releases potassium as well as nitrogenous wastes. Medications that contain significant amounts of potassium must be avoided or substitutions may be made (such as sodium penicillin instead of potassium penicillin). Since patients are usually on a sodium-restricted as well as potassium-restricted diet, they should be warned *not* to use salt substitute that contains potassium or ammonium as the cation. Because whole blood transfusions may increase the serum potassium, washed packed cells should be used, and, if possible, they should be administered during dialysis so that any excess potassium may be removed by the dialysis treatment. Serial serum potassium levels and serial electrocardiograms should be available and used as a guide in observing for and treating potassium intoxication.

Since there are few warning signs, the patient with hyperkalemia often presents as a medical emergency. Emergency therapy includes:

1. *Administration of Sodium Bicarbonate Intravenously.* Two to three ampules (44–132 mEq) of sodium bicarbonate helps correct acidosis and causes potassium to shift back into cells. Serum potassium decreases within minutes after administration of adequate quantities of sodium bicarbonate. Administration of large amounts of sodium may precipitate congestive heart failure and/or a state of hyperosmolarity.

2. *Administration of Calcium Intravenously.* Ten to 30 milliliters of 10% calcium gluconate, given intravenously over a 1- to 5-minute period, antagonizes the effect of elevated potassium on the heart. Calcium may induce cardiac arrhythmias and should be administered with electrocardiographic monitoring. Calcium does not decrease serum potassium concentration (17).

3. *Administration of Hypertonic Glucose and Insulin Intravenously.* Two hundred to 500 milliliters of 10% glucose or smaller quantities of 20–50% glucose may be infused rapidly. Ten units of regular insulin may be added to the infusion or given subcutaneously. As glucose is transported across the cell membrane, potassium also moves into the cell.

4. *Administration of a Cation Exchange Resin* such as sodium polystyrene sulfonate (Kayexalate) either orally or as a retention enema helps remove potassium from the body. Kayexalate is usually administered

with Sorbitol to prevent constipation. Beneficial effects occur in 30 to 60 minutes when given rectally and in one to two hours when administered orally. This drug has an exchange capacity of approximately 1 mEq of potassium per gram. The sodium content is approximately 100 mg per gram of the drug. As the resin passes along the intestine or is retained in the colon after administration by enema, the sodium ions are partially released and replaced by potassium ions. For the most part, this action occurs in the large intestine, which excretes potassium ions to a greater degree than does the small intestine. Serious potassium deficiency can occur from Kayexalate therapy. It is imperative to determine potassium levels frequently. Intracellular potassium deficiency is not always reflected by serum potassium levels; therefore, the level at which treatment with Kayexalate should be discontinued must be determined individually for each patient. The patient's clinical condition and the electrocardiogram are important aids in making this determination. Marked hypokalemia may be manifested by severe muscle weakness. Severe hypokalemia is associated with a lengthened Q-T interval, change in the deflection of the T wave, and the appearance of U waves on the EKG. The toxic effects of digitalis are exaggerated in hypokalemia.

During the resin's action in the intestine sodium is released mole for mole with potassium uptake. A single dose (15 gm) of Kayexalate contains 60 mEq of sodium. The cation exchange process is approximately 33% efficient; therefore, about 20 mEq of sodium is actually exchanged. Caution is advised when Kayexalate is administered to patients who cannot tolerate small increases in sodium loads (congestive heart failure, hypertension, or marked edema).

Kayexalate is not totally selective in its actions, and small amounts of other cations such as magnesium and calcium may also be lost; therefore, patients must be monitored for all electrolyte imbalances.

Pericarditis, Pericardial Effusion, and Tamponade

Pericarditis occurs in approximately 30–50% of patients with chronic renal failure (16), and, if not treated, may lead to hemorrhagic effusion and cardiac tamponade.

Normally, a few milliliters of fluid are present between the visceral and parietal layers of the pericardium. This lubrication allows the layers to glide over each other during cardiac contraction. In renal failure the pericardial sac may become inflamed and irritated by uremic toxins; therefore, the layers do not glide, but rub together harshly during contraction. The pericardial friction rub may be heard as a harsh, loud "leathery" sound while auscultating the precordium and is often louder during systole. Other signs and symptoms of pericarditis include low-grade fever, hypotension, and chest pain of varying quality.

Often the inflammatory process of pericarditis will precipitate effusion of fluid and bleeding into the pericardial space (pericardial effusion). One of the early signs of an effusion is the disappearance of a preexisting pericardial friction rub. The rub disappears because the pericardial layers are separated by an accumulation of fluid and/or blood so that they cannot rub together and produce the harsh sound. A paradoxical pulse is often cited as specific for pericardial effusion. Normally, there is a decrease in arterial blood pressure of less than 10 mm Hg during inspiration. In the presence of pericardial effusion, the blood pressure drop may reach 15 to 20 mm Hg because inspiration increases venous return to the right heart and, since this increase in volume occurs inside the distended pericardium, it results in compression of the left heart and reduction in filling. Chest x-rays and echocardiographic studies are important to the diagnosis of pericardial effusion.

The treatment for pericarditis and/or pericardial effusion associated with chronic renal failure is intense dialysis, often on a daily basis until the condition improves. The patient must be monitored before, during, and after dialysis for any change in cardiac status. The chest must be carefully auscultated for the presence or disappearance of a pericardial friction rub. Special care must be taken during each blood pressure measurement to observe for auscultatory gaps of over 10 mm Hg, which indicate a paradoxical pulse. The patient must be dialyzed using regional heparinization to prevent an increased clotting time and possible bleeding into the pericardial space. When a regional heparinization is used, the possibility of heparin rebound must be considered for six to nine hours after the termination of dialysis. (Refer to Chapter 6 for an explanation of regional heparinization and heparin rebound.) Chest x-rays and echocardiograms are done on a regular basis to detect changes in effusion. If the patient is fluid overloaded, ultrafiltration is used during dialysis.

Some patients develop cardiac tamponade regardless of measures used to treat the effusion. Rapid bleeding into the pericardial space places pressure against the myocardium, and there is inadequate venous return during diastole, a weak systole, and a low cardiac output. If the condition is not treated rapidly, death will ensue.

Signs and symptoms of cardiac tamponade are increased venous pressure, bulging neck veins, hypotension, narrowing pulse pressure, weak peripheral pulses, muffled heart sounds, and a paradoxical pulse greater than 10 mm Hg.

A pericardiocentesis is the emergency treatment for rapidly progressing cardiac tamponade. A 14 to 16 gauge needle is inserted into the pericardial space through the fourth left intercostal space and the accumulated fluid is drained. Often 1 ml of air will be injected into the pericardial space for each 2 ml of fluid removed. The air prevents the inflamed membranes from rubbing together and may prevent recurrence of effusion (16,22).

One of the hazards of pericardiocentesis is a vago-vagal reaction in which extreme bradycardia and possible asystole accompany puncture of the pericardium. Atropine may be given before the procedure to prevent this complication. Another complication is laceration of the myocardium or coronary artery with the needle. These problems may be minimized or prevented by attaching the precordial lead of an EKG machine to the pericardial needle and observing for S-T segment elevation in the EKG when the needle tip touches the myocardium.

Often a subtotal pericardiectomy or pericardial "window" will be performed to prevent a recurrence of effusion and tamponade.

Nursing Approach

Problem No. 10:   Hypertension.

SUBJECTIVE
 Patients may be symptomatic and not present subjective complaints.
  Possible symptoms may include:
  Headache—morning, occipital.
  Dizziness or lightheadedness.
  Shortness of breath.
  Paroxysmal nocturnal dyspnea.
  Cough.
  Edema.
  Chest pain.

OBJECTIVE
 Blood pressure: *mild:* diastolic pressure 100 mmHg or less
       moderate: diastolic pressure 100 to 120 mmHg
       severe: diastolic pressure above 120 mmHg
       malignant: diastolic pressure above 140 mmHg

ASSESSMENT
 Inspection
  PMI—shift to the left indicates left ventricular enlargement.
  Pedal edema—indicates cardiac failure and salt overload.

Palpation

The apical impulse is normally located in or about the fifth intercostal space at the midclavicular line less than 10 cm from the left sternal border, encompassing an area no greater than 2–3 cm in diameter. Location is best determined with the patient in the sitting position.

Auscultation

Rales or rhonchi indicate congestive heart failure.

Laboratory data

Electrolytes—monitor carefully, particularly potassium, when patients are on diuretics.

Urinalysis—proteinuria, casts, or microscopic hematuria.

EKG—document and monitor cardiac status, particularly left-sided enlargement.

Chest x-ray—monitor cardiac size.

PLAN

Objective 10:   Following a therapeutic regimen, the patient's blood pressure will be maintained within an acceptable range,* avoiding complications involving other body systems and further renal damage.

Nursing orders

1. Monitor blood pressure accurately.
    a. Use correct size cuff.
    b. Place cuff so that lower border is about 2.5 cm above the antecubital crease.
    c. Place patient in a consistent position for long-term follow-up.
    d. Take blood pressure in supine, sitting, and standing positions (waiting at least five minutes between measurements).
    e. Help the patient relax.
    f. Record blood pressure readings, using a flow sheet, to monitor influence of medications, weight, diet, and possible stressors upon the blood pressure.
2. Monitor use of drugs.
    a. Question patient regarding possible side effects he may experience: depression, orthostatic hypotension, lethargy, nasal stuffiness, nightmares.
    b. Teach the patient about the particular drugs that have been prescribed.

*Range is defined for each patient.

    1) Caution patient about possible orthostatic hypotension:
       a) Change position slowly.
       b) Avoid standing too quickly.
    2) Monitor serum potassium levels when patient is pre-
       scribed drugs that deplete this cation.
  3. Request patient to report any change in status which may indi-
    cate fluid overload, hypertensive encephalopathy, vision
    changes, or hypokalemia.
    a. Observe for signs of fluid overload, particularly periorbital,
      sacral, and peripheral edema.
    b. Observe for signs of encephalopathy: increase in intracra-
      nial pressure, seizures, headaches, coma, or cerebrovascular
      accident.
    c. Observe for funduscopic changes (an early indicator of
      end-organ disease). Observe for A-V nicking, exudates or
      hemorrhages, diminution in the caliber of small vessels most
      distal from the disc. Papilledema is a serious sign and de-
      mands hospitalization and treatment (18).
    d. Observe for signs of hypokalemia (signs rarely develop be-
      fore serum potassium falls below 3.0 mEq/L unless the rate
      of fall has been rapid):
      1) *Neuromuscular disturbances*—weakness, hyporeflexia,
        paresthesias.
      2) *Cardiac abnormalities*—arrhythmias, increased sensitivity
        to digitalis, and EKG changes (flat or inverted T waves,
        prominent U waves, and depressed S-T segments,
        hypotension).
      3) *CNS symptoms*—nausea, paralytic ileus.

Problem No. 11:   Hyperkalemia secondary to metabolic acidosis, exces-
                  sive oral intake of fluids or medications, blood trans-
                  fusions and/or bleeding.

SUBJECTIVE
Weakness.
Muscle paralysis, usually first noted in the legs, trunk, and arms.
Paresthesia of face, tongue, feet, and hands.
OBJECTIVE
Serum potassium level greater than 5 mEq/L.
Cardiac manifestations are frequent when the serum potassium
    level exceeds 8.0 mEq/L and include bradycardia, hypotension,
    ventricular fibrillation, and cardiac arrest. EKG changes in-

clude tall, peaked T waves, depressed S-T segments, prolonged P-R interval, diminished to absent P waves, and widening of the QRS complexes with prolongation of the Q-T interval (23). (See Figure 1.3.) These changes usually occur when serum potassium concentration is 6.5–8 mEq/L. Cardiac arrhythmias and standstill are more likely as the serum level approaches 9 to 10 mEq/L. Serum sodium concentration usually is decreased; vibratory and position sense may be decreased or absent.

ASSESSMENT

Symptoms of muscle weakness or paralysis have no direct relationship to the serum potassium concentration. However, when the concentration reaches 10 to 12 mEq/L, ventricular fibrillations, cardiac arrest, and death usually occur (24).

PLAN

Objective 11:   Patient's serum potassium concentration will be maintained within a range of 3.5–5 mEq/L.

Nursing orders

1. Instruct patient about presence of potassium in food and medication.
2. Discuss importance of following prescribed diet, avoiding foods high in potassium.
3. Discuss relationship of potassium to diminished kidney function and importance of avoiding consequences of hyperkalemia.
4. Monitor blood transfusions to assure that washed red cells are used.
5. Avoid hypercatabolic states as potassium is released as tissues break down.
6. Monitor metabolic acidotic states as serum potassium increases as kidneys excrete hydrogen ions in an attempt to maintain acid-base balance.
7. Monitor serum potassium levels and notify physician as levels exceed 5.5 mEq/L.

Problem No. 12:   Lethal hyperkalemia (emergency treatment required).

SUBJECTIVE

Dull headache, abdominal pain, rapid respirations, weakness, nausea, general malaise, vomiting, muscle twitching.

OBJECTIVE

Serum potassium greater than 7.0 mEq/L.

Serum sodium may be normal or low.

Decreased temperature.

EKG changes, including the disappearance of P waves or QRS interval.

Urine: acid, pH 4.6 to 6.2 (may be normal); high ammonia content.

Blood pH: below 7.2

WBC: leukocytosis may be present.

Skin: warm, flushed.

Fruity odor to breath.

Hyperventilation usually does not occur until serum bicarbonate concentration falls below 10 mEq/L (24).

ASSESSMENT

Symptoms usually appear when CO_2 content falls to 18.2 mEq/L (40 vol.%) or lower (24).

Wide pulse pressure with bounding pulse and/or active apical pulses.

Dehydration usually accompanies metabolic acidosis.

PLAN

Objective 12:   Given emergency treatment, the complications of hyperkalemia will be prevented.

Nursing orders

1. Treat metabolic acidosis.

    a. Administer 2–3 ampules (44–132 mEq) sodium bicarbonate intravenously (forces potassium into cells) over five-minute period.

    1) Observe for cardiovascular overload.

    2) Monitor closely those patients who cannot tolerate increases in sodium loads (CHF, edema, hypertension).

    3) Observe for signs of decreased serum calcium: twitching and muscle spasm. Correction of acidosis may cause tetany if hypocalcemia is present.

    4) Monitor serum calcium levels of patients taking digitalis, as calcium acts synergistically with the drug.

    b. Administer 10–30 ml of 10% calcium gluconate intravenously over a two-minute period (antagonizes cardiac toxicity of hyperkalemia).

    1) Monitor EKG during administration.

    2) Do not give to patient receiving digitalis.

    c. Administer glucose-insulin infusion, one unit of insulin for each 2 gm glucose, over a 30- to 60-minute period (forces potassium to shift into cells).

       1) Observe for signs of hypoglycemia: nervousness, weakness, shaking, diaphoresis, or loss of consciousness.

       2) Check urine for glycosuria.

   d. Administer cation-exchange resins (Kayexalate) (exchanges 1.7 to 2.5 mEq sodium for each mEq potassium removed).

       1) Observe for side effects: anorexia, nausea, vomiting, severe constipation, hypocalcemia, and hypokalemia.

       2) Use cautiously in patients who are receiving digitalis preparations to avoid digitalis toxicity precipitated by hypokalemia.

   e. Avoid potassium deficiency by observing for EKG changes: lengthened Q-T interval, changes in the deflection of the T wave.

   f. Observe for signs of dehydration: thirst, dizziness, malaise, abdominal pain, weakness, restlessness, vomiting, level of consciousness. If dehydration is present:

       1) Monitor patient's weight.

       2) Monitor creatinine clearance, serum, creatinine, and urine sodium excretion.

Problem No. 13:   Pericarditis, pericardial effusion, and pericardial tamponade secondary to uremia.

SUBJECTIVE

Chest pain (left-sided or central) that increases on deep respiration. Character of pain altered with position change.

Nonproductive cough.

Chills.

Weakness.

Anxiety.

OBJECTIVE

Low-grade fever.

Hypotension.

Chest x-ray.

Echocardiogram.

EKG changes include S-T segment elevation; T waves become flattened, then inverted.

ASSESSMENT

Inspection:

Bulging neck veins

Palpation:

Paradoxical pulse (specific for pericardial effusion).

Auscultation

Friction rub heard throughout the cardiac cycle; location may be variable but best heard in the third interspace to the left of the sternum. Intensity may increase when the patient leans forward and exhales. High-pitched sound of a rasping, scratching nature.

PLAN

Objective 13:   Monitor patient closely to prevent complications of pericarditis: pericardial effusion and tamponade.

Nursing orders

1. Observe for auscultatory gap, changes in peripheral pulse rate and quality.
2. Auscultate chest to listen for heart sounds that become softer or diminished in volume.
3. Monitor patient for signs of cardiac tamponade: increased venous pressure, bulging neck veins, hypotension, narrowing pulse pressure, cold and poorly perfused extremities, weak peripheral pulse, muffled heart sounds, and a paradoxical pulse greater than 10 mmHg.

HEMATOLOGICAL SYSTEM PROBLEMS

Effects of chronic renal failure on the hematological system include anemia, a defect in the quality of platelets, an increased bleeding tendency, and a change in the physiology of red and white cells.

Four causes may be listed for anemia in chronic renal failure. (1) Decreased red blood cell production caused by the diseased kidney. In a normal state, erythropoietin, or its precursor, is produced by the kidney in response to hypoxia. This substance stimulates the bone marrow, and the rate of maturation of red blood cells is increased. (See Figure 1.4.) (2) Decreased survival time of RBC's due to elevated uremic toxins. (3) Loss of blood through gastrointestinal bleeding. (4) Blood loss during hemodialysis from membrane rupture, hemolysis, and residual dialyzer blood loss (16).

The hematocrit usually falls slowly over several months and stabilizes around 20%. One compensatory mechanism for the low hematocrit is an increase in the enzyme, 2,3-diphosphoglycerate (2,3-DPG), which causes the oxygen dissociation curve to shift to the right and hemoglobin to liberate oxygen to tissues more readily (16). Also, hypoxia may act as a direct stimulus for bone marrow to produce red blood cells.

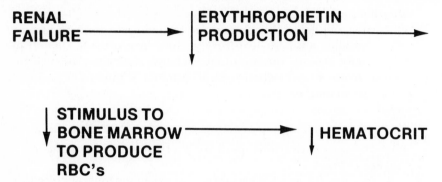

Figure 1.4. Schema of cause of anemia in chronic renal failure. See text for explanation.

Because of the problems related to blood transfusions, they are not given until the patient becomes symptomatic, showing dyspnea, fatigue, tachycardia, and palpitations. The disadvantages of blood transfusions are that bone marrow production of red blood cells is suppressed and the patient becomes transfusion-dependent to maintain his hematocrit; the dangers of transfusions reactions; transmission of diseases including hepatitis; and the development of cytotoxic antibodies.

Cytotoxic antibodies are those formed in response to an antigen contained in virtually all tissues of the body except red blood cells. If a patient receives a whole blood transfusion that contains red blood cells, white blood cells, and platelets, antibodies are formed against the white blood cells and platelets. When the patient eventually receives a kidney transplant, a hyperacute rejection may occur because of the presence of preformed antibodies (from previous blood transfusions) against the transplanted tissue. Leukocyte-poor blood and frozen blood are used to mitigate this problem. Leukocyte-poor blood is what remains after whole blood is allowed to sediment and the layer above the red blood cells is removed. The purpose is to remove the layer that contains the platelets and white blood cells and the source of the antigen that causes cytotoxic antibodies to form. This method is not extremely effective, and recently frozen blood has been used effectively for patients with chronic renal failure. Frozen blood is blood that is placed in a glycerol solution, which penetrates the RBC's and freezes them rapidly to −7°C. Before use, the red blood cells are washed in various solutions to remove the glycerol; in this process many platelets and white blood cells are also removed. The recipient receives blood with greatly decreased antigenic properties, and fewer cytotoxic antibodies are formed.

When dialysis is implemented and uremic toxins are decreased, the life span of red blood cells increases toward normal and the hematocrit usually stabilizes at about 20–25%.

If the patient is found to have an iron or folate deficiency, he is started on iron or folate supplements. Iron is customarily given with meals to prevent gastrointestinal irritation; however, iron cannot be given at mealtime to chronic renal patients who are also receiving phosphate binding medication as a major part of the iron will be bound with the phosphate binding medication and absorption greatly decreased. Iron may be given orally as ferrous fumerate, ferrous sulfate, or ferrocholinate, or it may be given parenterally as iron-dextran (Imferon). Folic acid will be removed by hemodialysis if it is administered before or during the treatment; therefore, the medication should be given post-dialysis for complete benefit (24).

The use of erythropoietin to treat anemia is not currently practicable because of the cost and the small quantities available (24).

Androgen therapy is used with some success to increase the hematocrit of patients with chronic renal failure. Androgens commonly administered at weekly intervals are testosterone or nandrolone decanoate (Deca-Durabolin). The side effects of these drugs are acne, hirsutism in women, and priapism in men (25).

Chronic renal patients usually have a mild thrombocytopenia and a defect in quality of platelets. The results are a prolonged bleeding time, decreased platelet adhesiveness, and abnormal prothrombin consumption. Purpura may result from a minor blow and bleeding may occur from body orifices.

White blood cell counts in chronic renal failure are usually normal, but the increase in response to infection is usually somewhat less than would be expected. Within minutes following the start of a hemodialysis treatment there is a profound decrease in the white blood cell count (neutropenia). The cause is unknown but may be stagnation of blood in the dialyzer (16) or migration of leukocytes to the lungs. The patient usually remains asymptomatic and the count returns to normal within one to two hours.

Nursing Approach

Problem No. 14:   Anemia.

SUBJECTIVE
    Dyspnea, fatigue, tachycardia, palpitations.
OBJECTIVE
    Pallor of nail beds and mucous membranes.

Hemoglobin: 8 gm/100 ml (severe anemia).
Reticulocyte count normal.
Presence of "burr cells."
WBC usually normal.
Platelets reduced.

ASSESSMENT

Anemia is usually normochronic, normocytic, and characterized by a shortened RBC survival and subnormal marrow response. Anemia does not usually cause symptoms until the hemoglobin falls below 7 gm/100 ml. The degree of anemia is roughly associated with the degree of renal insufficiency, though there is no good correlation between the degree of anemia and the severity of the renal disease as measured by the blood urea nitrogen (26). Hemoglobin decreases by about 1 gm per 100 ml for each 10 mg per 100 ml rise in blood urea nitrogen up to a level of 100 mg per 100 ml (14).

PLAN

Objective 14A: Given supportive therapy, the patient will experience symptomatic relief of the effects of anemia.

Nursing Orders
1. Administer iron or folate supplements as indicated.
   a. Avoid giving iron at the same time with phosphate binding medications.
   b. Give 30 to 60 minutes before meals for best results.
2. Administer androgens as indicated.
   a. Inform patient of possible side effects: fluid retention, masculinization, hirsutism, and skin infections.
3. Discuss the need for the patient to avoid fatigue.
4. Provide for rest periods when hospitalized.
5. Avoid unnecessary collection of blood specimens.

Objective 14B: Understanding the consequences of platelet deficiency, the patient will learn how to protect himself from trauma and excessive bleeding.

Nursing orders
1. Discuss the function of platelets and the alterations that occur in uremia.
2. Instruct patient to use a soft toothbrush, avoid vigorous noseblowing, constipation, and contact sports.
3. Demonstrate pressure method to control bleeding should it occur.
4. Advise patient to obtain a medical alert tag.

SELECTED ENDOCRINE PROBLEMS

Much controversial information has been published about abnormal endocrine function in chronic renal failure. Pituitary function in relation to growth hormone and gonadal function are considered in this section. Parathyroid function will be discussed in another section of this chapter.

Pituitary Function and Growth Hormone

There are conflicting studies regarding serum levels of growth hormone in chronic renal failure; most report an elevation of serum growth hormone. It is well known that children with chronic renal failure cease growth. Even though the serum level is elevated, there is a failure to respond to the growth hormone (22,27).

Gonadal Function

In advanced renal failure infertility often occurs in both men and women. Amenorrhea and cessation of ovulation take place in women. There is decreased libido in both sexes, and men are usually impotent. Decreased libido and impotence probably have a psychological as well as pathophysiological basis. Following implementation of dialysis, libido often improves in both sexes. Ovulation and menstruation may resume in women, and excessive bleeding may be a problem while heparinized during hemodialysis. Successful pregnancy for a female with chronic renal failure before or after regular hemodialysis is very rare.

Impaired Sexual Functioning

The impact of chronic illness upon the patient's life is extensive. This chapter has discussed the proliferative influence of uremia upon each body system. As the disease progresses, the patient experiences a narrowing of existence; mobility decreases, pain and discomfort become common, and there arise more and more treatment prescriptions with which to deal. A person's very identity is defined by an illness over which there is very little control. Nowhere is the personal loss so profound as it is in the patient's inability to live as a complete sexual being. Unfortunately, sexual functioning is an area of the patient's life that the nurse feels most uncomfortable with or incapable of helping the patient express (28,29).

One useful approach is to explore the meaning of sexuality with the patient and his or her "significant other." It is known that one of the first signs of neuropathy in males is an inability to have an erection. Females commonly report a decreased libido. An important issue to pursue is how the couple personally describe their needs, desires, and feelings. A focus for assessing sexual functioning may be directed by the following questions: How is the loss, depression, and loneliness of illness comforted by others? How does the patient express his needs for dependency, independency; intimacy or isolation? How is the loss of sexual potency related to other areas of functioning such as job, sports, or hobbies? How does one define himself or herself in light of a changing body image? Does one's view of masculine or feminine roles undergo changes? And, finally, is there enough trust, sharing, and communication between the partners and staff to deal with these personal issues?

Frequently, through the process of sharing the problem with a careful listener, the couple find they can work out many of their own difficulties. It is very helpful when discussing sexuality to change the focus of "performing" to "being." In so doing the nurse helps the couple recognize the human needs of touch, tenderness, and respect above, but not independent of, the masculine or feminine role. Setting personal values aside, the nurse also can legitimize the couple's personal style of giving and sharing affection. The strength, companionship, and comfort inherent in a healthy love or marital relationship serves the patient well in coping with the demands of life and chronic illness.

CALCIUM, PHOSPHORUS, VITAMIN D, PARATHYROID GLAND, AND SKELETAL PROBLEMS

There are very intricate interrelationships among calcium, phosphorus, vitamin D, parathyroid gland, bone, and kidneys. Before discussing the problems that occur in chronic renal failure, let us review the normal complex interrelationships.

The plasma calcium (normally 9–10.5 mg/100 ml) is partly bound to protein and partly free, ionized, diffusible calcium. (See Table 1.4) The latter is important for blood coagulation, cardiac and skeletal muscle contraction, and nerve function. Tetany is due to a decreased ionized calcium in the central nervous system. There is an increased ionized calcium in acidosis, and a decrease in alkalosis.

The calcium in bone is of two types: a readily exchangeable reservoir, and a larger pool of calcium that is slowly exchangeable. Plasma calcium is in equilbirium with the readily exchangeable bone calcium.

Plasma calcium levels control its rate of absorption from the gastrointestinal tract. Plasma calcium also controls the rate of excretion of

Table 1.4. Calcium and Phosphorus

Normal Calcium and Phosphorus	
Serum calcium	9−10.5 mg/100 ml
Serum phosphate	3−4 mg/100 ml
Calcium phosphate product (Ca × PO₄)	30−40 mg/100 ml

Calcium and Phosphorus in Hyperparathyroidism	
Serum calcium	8−12 mg/100 ml
Serum phosphate	4.5−8 mg/100 ml
Calcium phosphate product	70 mg/100 ml
Parathormone	Excessively elevated

parathyroid hormone (parathormone)—a low level of ionized calcium increases the production of the hormone and vice versa.

Vitamin D, which has recently been classified as a hormone, facilitates the intestinal absorption of calcium. Vitamin D precursors undergo a series of metabolic transformations to be converted to 1,25-dihydroxycholecalciferol (1,25-DHCC), the biologically active form of the steroid. Figure 1.5 summarizes the steps in the metabolism of cholecalciferol to 1,25-DHCC. Normal kidney function is necessary for the conversion of 25-HCC to 1,25-DHCC (16,30).

Almost all dietary phosphate is absorbed from the gastrointestinal tract into the blood and later excreted in the urine. When the plasma phosphate level is below 3.0 to 4.5 mg/100 ml, no phosphate is excreted by the kidneys; but above this concentration the rate of phosphate excretion is directly proportional to the increase. Thus, the kidneys are responsible for maintaining an extracellular phosphate concentration of 3.0–4.5 mg/100 ml. Phosphate excretion is also affected by the parathyroid hormone. Increased parathyroid hormone causes increased excretion of phosphate; decreased parathyroid hormone causes decreased excretion of phosphate.

Bone is a living tissue with a collagenous protein matrix that has been impregnated with mineral salts, especially calcium phosphate. Adequate amounts of protein and minerals must be available for the maintenance of normal bone structure. Throughout life, the mineral in the skeleton is being actively turned over, and bone is constantly being resorbed and reformed. New bone formation in adults is due to the activity of cells called osteoblasts that cause the formation of a network of collagen fibers. This matrix then calcifies. Also, the cartilage in the center of the

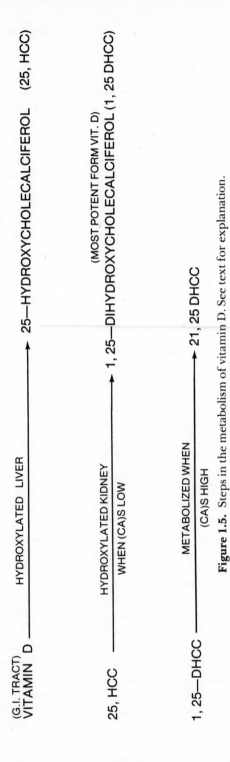

Figure 1.5. Steps in the metabolism of vitamin D. See text for explanation.

(G.I. TRACT)
VITAMIN D ——— HYDROXYLATED LIVER ———→ 25—HYDROXYCHOLECALCIFEROL (25, HCC)

25, HCC ——— HYDROXYLATED KIDNEY WHEN (CA)S LOW ———→ 1, 25—DIHYDROXYCHOLECALCIFEROL (1, 25 DHCC) (MOST POTENT FORM VIT. D)

1, 25—DHCC ——— METABOLIZED WHEN (CA)S HIGH ———→ 21, 25 DHCC

bone shaft is invaded by cells called osteoclasts, which erode previously formed bone. Osteoblasts are thus associated with bone formation and osteoclasts with bone resorption. The enzyme, alkaline phosphatase, is associated with osteoblast activity. The enzyme increases the concentration of phosphate in the vicinity of osteoblasts and causes calcium phosphate salts to precipitate in bone.

As mentioned earlier, parathyroid hormone (parathormone) is important in phosphate and calcium metabolism. Parathormone is produced when the free, ionized serum calcium decreases. Parathormone causes an increase in the activity of osteoclasts and a decrease in the activity of osteoblasts. This results in dissolution of bones to release more calcium and phosphorus. Also, parathormone decreases the tubular reabsorption of the phosphate ion from glomerular filtrate, which decreases the precipitation of calcium phosphate.

As long as the kidneys, parathyroid gland, bone, calcium, phosphorus, and vitamin D are working synchronously, the plasma levels of calcium and phosphate and calcium phosphate product (calcium × phosphate) are maintained in a normal range. In chronic renal failure a sequence of events occurs that, if untreated, leads to bone disease and soft-tissue calcification. This sequence of events and the related management are discussed in detail.

Figure 1.6 is a schematic representation of the events that cause calcium phosphate imbalances in renal failure.

Since the kidney is the chief means of excretion of phosphate, the decreased GFR in chronic renal failure (Figure 1.6A) results in a retention of phosphate and elevation of the serum phosphate level (Figure 1.6B). Elevation of serum phosphate disturbs the calcium phosphate ratio, and to compensate there is a decrease in ionized serum calcium (Figure 1.6C), because it is bound to phosphate to form the insoluble compound, calcium phosphate.

The parathyroid glands respond to a decreased serum calcium by producing parathormone (PTH) (Figure 1.6D), which affects the bone, gastrointestinal tract, and kidneys (Figure 1.6E). In the bone, parathormone causes a proliferation of osteoclasts and a degeneration of osteoblasts. The effect of the increased activity of osteoclasts is to cause resorption of calcium and phosphorus from bone to plasma, thus increasing the serum calcium level (Figure 1.6F). Depending on the GFR, parathormone may decrease the tubular reabsorption of phosphate and increase urinary excretion, thus controlling the serum phosphate level to some extent. When GFR falls below 10% of normal, the clearance of phosphate ceases, despite a high level of parathormone; and as resorption of calcium and phosphate from bone takes place, the plasma phos-

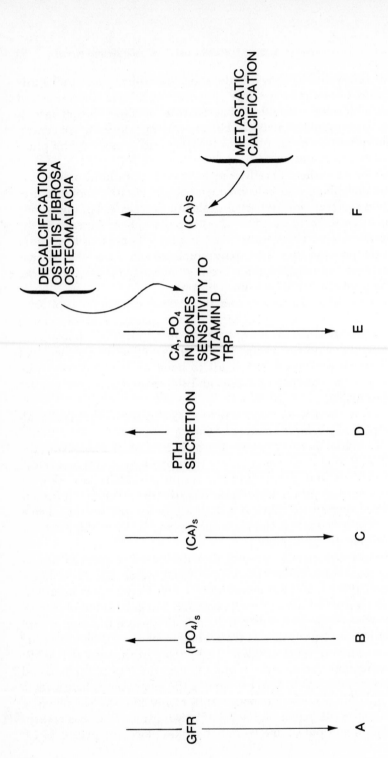

CALCIUM, PHOSPHORUS, BONE, KIDNEY, VITAMIN D, AND PARATHYROID GLANDS

Figure 1.6. Schema of events that cause calcium phosphate imbalances in renal failure. See text for explanation.

phate level also rises. Since the additional phosphate cannot be disposed of through the renal route, the serum calcium concentration cannot increase and remains a stimulus for increased parathyroid secretion. A secondary hyperparathyroidism develops and is one of the factors causing dissolution of the skeletal system (osteomalacia, osteitis fibrosa, and osteosclerosis). These conditions are manifested as bone pain, fractures, subperiosteal erosions, and periarticular calcifications. When the plasma calcium phosphate product exceeds 70 mg/100 ml, there is extensive precipitation of calcium phosphate crystals, and calcifications may occur in the brain, eyes, gums, joints, lungs, myocardium, blood vessels, and skin. Osteoblastic activity increases as an effort to repair bones; as a result, alkaline phosphatase levels also increase.

Another disturbance that aggravates the calcium phosphate imbalance is the acidosis associated with chronic renal failure. As skeletal calcium carbonate is used to buffer the acidosis, demineralization of bones increases.

To further complicate the problem, the diseased kidney is unable to convert vitamin D precursors to the active metabolite form (1,25-DHCC). There is decreased absorption of calcium from the gastrointestinal tract because of the lack of active vitamin D.

The outcome of these effects is demineralization of the skeleton. Some degree of demineralization is present in practically all instances of renal failure. The skeletal manifestations may not be clinically symptomatic in many patients, but often extreme skeletal disturbances develop that dominate the course of renal failure.

Lowering of serum phosphate is the most important therapeutic modality in the prevention and treatment of renal osteodystrophy. The usual method of accomplishing this is the administration of phosphate binding medications. Aluminum hydroxide gels are commonly used. The medication must be taken at mealtime so that food and phosphate binder will be present in the gastrointestinal tract at the same time. The aluminum in the gel binds with phosphates in the food to form the insoluble compound, aluminum phosphate. The aluminum phosphate is excreted in the feces, thus preventing absorption of phosphate from the gastrointestinal tract. The outcome of this therapy is a fall in serum phosphate and a rise in serum calcium. Aluminum gels are often constipating, so stool softeners such as Doxidan or Colace must be given concomitantly (15).

Examples of commonly used phosphate binding medications are Amphojel and Basajel. These medications are supplied in gel, tablet, capsule, and cookie form, so if the patient finds one form unpalatable another form may be substututed. Table 1.5 shows equivalent dosages of various phosphate binding medications.

Table 1.5. Equivalent Dosages of Phosphate Binding Medications

Preparation	Basic Dosage	Elemental Aluminum Content	Approximate Equivalent Dose to 30 ml Amphojel
Amphojel liquid	30 ml	665 mg	
Amphojel (5 gr tablet)	1	104 mg	6.4 tablets
Amphojel (10 gr tablet)	1	208 mg	3.2 tablets
Alucap	1	126 mg	5.3 capsules
Phos-Lo cookie	1	416 mg	1.6 cookies
Basaljel tablet	1	173 mg	4.0 tablets
Basaljel capsule	1	173 mg	4.0 capsules
Basaljel liquid	30 ml	852 mg	23.5 ml
Extra-Strength Basaljel liquid	30 ml	2080 mg	9.6 ml

Vitamin D supplements may be administered to increase the serum calcium level. The most commonly used form is dihydrotachysterol. Newer analogues of vitamin D, such as 1,25-dihydroxycholecalciferol (1,25-DHCC), 25-hydroxycholecalciferol (25-HCC), and 1,α-hydroxycholecalciferal, are currently available only for investigational use (30). Serum phosphate must be within a normal range before vitamin D is started; otherwise metastatic calcifications may occur. The patient should also be observed for hypercalcemia when vitamin D is administered.

When the serum phosphate level is in a normal range, oral calcium supplements may be used as a therapy for low serum calcium. Calcium may be administered as calcium lactate or calcium carbonate. Proprietary preparations of calcium include Titralac and Neo-Calglucon syrup.

A subtotal parathyroidectomy (seven of the eight glands removed) is indicated if the patient has severe bone disease. Reminieralization of bone occurs slowly after this operation.

Nursing Approach

Problem No. 15:   Limited mobility secondary to renal osteodystrophy.

SUBJECTIVE
  Bone pain.
  Muscle pain.
  Limited mobility.

OBJECTIVE
  Serum calcium 9–10 mg/100 ml.
  Elevated alkaline phosphatase levels indicate progression of renal osteodystrophy (1.5–4 BU or 3–13 K-A units).

ASSESSMENT

Impairment occurs in the ability of the kidney tubule to excrete phosphate, usually when the GFR decreases to 20 ml/min (normal 100 to 120 ml/min). The serum phosphorus concentration rises in patients with renal failure as the GFR falls.

Inspection

Gait.

Strength.

Range of motion.

Muscle atrophy.

Condition of surrounding tissues and skin.

Swelling.

Palpation

Palpate joints, noting enlargement, swelling, tenderness.

Test range of motion of each joint.

PLAN

Objective 15: Given supportive therapy, the patient will maintain a level of activity that is as safe and painless as possible.

Nursing orders

1. Administer analgesics when necessary.
2. Consult physical therapy for baseline assessment of mobility and development of a plan of exercises to maintain strength and mobility.
3. Assist patient with passive exercises.
4. Encourage patient to use active exercises.
5. Administer local heat for symptomatic relief of pain.
6. Avoid immobilization when possible (increases protein catabolism).
7. Encourage patient to engage in moderate physical exercise.
8. Assess impairments of function and complaints of pain.

Problem No. 16: Disturbances in calcium metabolism (calcium deficiency).

SUBJECTIVE

Tetany.

Carpopedal spasm.

Seizures.

Confusion.

Alopecia.

Coarse dry skin.

Numbness and tingling of fingertips, toes, nose, and ears.

Nausea.

Diarrhea.

Generalized weakness.

OBJECTIVE

Positive Chvostek's sign.

Positive Trousseau's signs.

EKG may show a prolonged Q-T internal despite unchanged T-wave shape and duration.

Decreased serum calcium (below 6.5 mg/100 ml).

Increased serum phosphate (above 5 mg/100 ml).

Acidosis (bicarbonate levels less than 15 mEq/L).

ASSESSMENT

The severity and extent of osteodystrophy does not correlate well with the type or severity of the renal disease present (26). It is important therefore to focus on the assessment of *1*) electrolyte imbalances, *2*) the extent of functional impairment, and *3*) the patient's complaints of pain and discomfort.

Additionally, prolonged hypocalcemia leads to hyperplasia and hypertrophy of the parathyroid glands. Though the glands are not usually palpable, they enlarge markedly in patients with chronic renal failure. There is some evidence that enlargement roughly correlates with the degree of bone disease and the level of parathyroid hormone in the serum (26).

Assessment of the effects of vitamin D and supplemental calcium rests upon the frequent measurement of the serum calcium level. Treatment is reduced or discontinued when the calcium level or alkaline phosphatase levels return to normal.

PLAN

Objective 16A: Given palliative treatment, the patient will be protected from the effects of altered calcium metabolism as long as possible. (Criteria determined by evaluation of serum electrolyte levels and radiographic changes in bone).

Nursing orders

1. Administer drugs when indicated:
    a. Calcium supplements.
    b. Phosphate binding agents.
    c. Sodium bicarbonate.
    d. Vitamin D.
2. Observe for signs of vitamin D toxicity: nausea, agitation, anorexia, increase in blood pressure, unexplained rise in BUN.

3. Monitor serum phosphate levels while patient is taking medications:
   a. Noncompliance indicated by elevated levels.
   b. Lowered levels may create a problem of hypercalcemia.
   c. Calcium supplements administered only when the phosphate level is within acceptable limits because of the danger of inducing hypercalcemia (31) and/or calcium phosphate precipitation.
4. Monitor calcium levels.
5. Request radiologic evaluations periodically.
6. Avoid state of metabolic acidosis.
7. Observe for signs of secondary hyperparathyroidism.
8. Observe for blood in stool or for hematemesis.
9. Monitor serum potassium levels (elevation may occur when serum calcium and sodium levels are low).
10. Administer aluminum hydroxide gels with meals (Amphojel and Basajel).
11. Instruct patient to avoid drugs containing magnesium, owing to the risk of intoxication (Gelusil, Maalox, Mylanta, Milk of Magnesia).

Objective 16B: Given an explanation of the manifestations of uremia, the patient will understand the symptoms expressed in the musculoskeletal system.

Nursing orders
1. Describe the influence of altered calcium metabolism upon the normal functioning of the body.
2. Explain the symptoms the patient is experiencing in terms of altered metabolism.
3. Prepare the patient for dialysis or for subtotal parathyroidectomy where indicated.
4. Answer patient's questions frankly, assessing level of understanding, acceptance of symptoms, and plans for the future.

REFERENCES

1. D V Brundage: *Nursing Management of Renal Problems.* St. Louis, Mosby, 1976.
2. J D Harrington, E R Brener: *Patient Care in Renal Failure,* Philadelphia, Saunders, 1973.
3. D W Smith, C P H Germain: The patient in renal failure, in *Care of the Adult Patient.* Philadelphia, Lippincott, 1975, pp 1149–1169.
4. F L Bower: *The Process of Planning Care: A Theoretical Model.* St Louis, Mosby, 1972.

5. S Carlson: *A Practical Approach to the Nursing Process in Practice.* New York, The American Journal of Nursing Co, 1974, pp 20–26.

6. H Yura, M B Walsh: *The Nursing Process: Assessing, Planning, Implementing, and Evaluating.* New York, Appleton-Century-Crofts, 1973.

7. C Campbell: *Nursing Diagnosis and Intervention in Nursing Practice.* New York, Wiley, 1978.

8. K Gebbie, M A Lavin: Classifying nursing diagnoses. *AJN* 74(2): 250–253, 1974.

9. L Lewis: The I believe . . . about the nursing process—key to care, in *The Nursing Process in Practice.* New York, The American Journal of Nursing Co, 1974, pp 12–19.

10. S Papper: *Clinical Nephrology.* Boston, Little, Brown, 1971.

11. L Tapia, J S Cheigh, D S David, et al.: Pruritis in dialysis patients treated with parenteral lidocaine. *N Eng J Med* 296(5): 261, 1977.

12. B Bates: *A Guide to the Physical Examination.* Philadelphia, Lippincott, 1974.

13. G L Hansen: *Caring for Patients with Chronic Renal Disease: A Reference Guide for Nurses.* Philadelphia, Lippincott, 1972.

14. A Golden, J F Maher: *The Kidney.* Baltimore, Williams & Wilkins, 1971.

15. W J Stone: Therapy of constipation in patients with chronic renal failure. *Dialysis and Transplantation* 6(7), 1977.

16. C Hampers, E Schupak, E Lowrie, et al.: *Long-Term Hemodialysis,* ed 2. New York, Grune & Stratton, 1973.

17. D L Makoff, J R DePalma: Electrolyte and acid-base abnormalities, in S G Massry and A L Sellers (eds): *Clinical Aspects of Uremia and Dialysis.* Springfield, Ill, Charles C Thomas, 1976, pp 284–303.

18. C Hudak, P M Redstone, et al.: *Clinical Protocols: A Guide for Nurses and Physicians.* Philadelphia, Lippincott, 1976.

19. P E Teschan, H E Ginn: The nervous system, in S G Massry and A L Sellers (eds): *Clinical Aspects of Uremia and Dialysis.* Springfield, Charles C Thomas, 1976, pp 3–33.

20. N Callaghan: Restless legs syndrome in uremic neuropathy. *Neurology* 16: 359, 1966.

21. P Wiedmann, M H Maxwell: Hypertension, in S G Massry and A L Sellers (eds): *Clinical Aspects of Uremia and Dialysis.* Springfield, Ill, Charles C Thomas, 1976, pp 100–145.

22. G Bailey: *Hemodialysis Principles and Practice.* New York, Academic, 1972.

23. E C Boedeker, J H Dauber (eds): *Manual of Medical Therapeutics,* ed 21. Boston, Little, Brown, 1974.

24. E Goldberger: *A Primer of Water, Electrolyte and Acid-Base Syndromes.* Philadelphia, Lea & Febiger, 1977.

25. R M Raga, M S Kramer, J L Rosenbaum: Long term use of nandrolone decanoate and iron in dialysis patients. *Dialysis and Transplantation* 6(4): 36, 1977.

26. J P Merrill, C L Hampers: *Uremia: Progress in Pathophysiology and Treatment.* New York, Grune & Stratton, 1971.

27. M P Fichman: Metabolic and endrocrine abnormalities, part IV, pituitary, gonadal and thyroid function, in S G Massry and A L Sellers (eds): *Clinical Aspects of Uremia and Dialysis.* Springfield, Ill, Charles C Thomas, 1976, pp 273–283.

28. H Feigenbaum: The dialysis nurse and psychosexual awareness. *Journal AANNT* 1(1).

29. B W Hickman: All about sex . . . despite dialysis. *AJN* 77(4): 606–607, 1977.

30. J W Coburn: Use of newer vitamin D analogues in renal osteodystrophy treatment. *Dialysis and Transplantation* 5(1): 28, 1976.

31. M O Fearing: Osteodystrophy in patients with chronic renal failure. *Nursing Clin North Am* 10(3): 461–468, 1975.

BIBLIOGRAPHY

Bagdale J D: Metabolic and endocrine abnormalities, part II, hyperlipidemia, in Massry S G, Sellers A L (eds): *Clinical Aspects of Uremia and Dialysis.* Springfield, Ill, Charles C Thomas, 1976, pp 230–240.

Bailey G: *Hemodialysis Principles and Practice.* New York, Academic, 1972.

Bates B: *A Guide to the Physical Examination.* Philadelphia, Lippincott, 1974.

Becknell E P, Smith D M: *System of Nursing Practice: A Clinical Nursing Assessment Tool.* Philadelphia, F A Davis, 1975.

Black D A K (ed): *Renal Disease,* ed 3. Oxford, Blackwell Scientific Pub, Ltd, 1972.

Brundage D V: *Nursing Management of Renal Problems.* St Louis, Mosby, 1976.

Del Greco F, Krumlovsky F A: Hypertension in chronic renal failure. *Dialysis and Transplantation* 4(5): 44, 1975.

Downing S R: Nursing support in early renal failure, *AJN* 69(6): 1212–1216, 1969.

Eschback J W: Anemia, in Massry S G, Sellers A L (eds): *Clinical Aspects of Uremia and Dialysis.* Springfield, Ill, Charles C Thomas, 1976, pp 146–178.

Fichman M P: Effect of uremia and dialysis on carbohydrate and lipid metabolism. *Dialysis and Transplantation* 5(4): 16, 1976.

Ganong W: *Review of Medical Physiology,* ed 4, Los Altos, Calif, Lange Medical Pub, 1969.

Golden A, Maher J F: *The Kidney.* Baltimore, Williams & Wilkins, 1971.

Hampers C, Schupak E, Lowrie E, et al.: *Long Term Hemodialysis,* ed 2. New York, Grune & Stratton, 1973.

Hansen G L: *Caring for Patients with Chronic Renal Disease: A Reference Guide for Nurses.* Philadelphia, Lippincott, 1972.

Harrington J D, Brener E R: *Patient Care in Renal Failure.* Philadelphia, Saunders, 1973.

Hekelman F P, Ostendorp C A: Nursing approaches to conservative management of renal disease. *Nursing Clin North Am* 10(3): 431–447, 1975.

Johnson D W, Mathog R H: Hearing loss in patients with chronic renal failure. *Dialysis and Transplantation* 5(5): 42, 1976.

Jones L: Hypertension: medical and nursing implications. *Nursing Clin North Am* 11(2): 283–295, 1976.

Kopple J D: Metabolic and endocrine abnormalities, part III, nitrogen metabolism, in Massry S G, Sellers A L (eds): *Clinical Aspects of Uremia and Dialysis.* Springfield, Ill, Charles C Thomas, 1976, pp 241–273.

Massry S G: An evaluation of hypocalcemia pathogenesis. *Dialysis and Transplantation* 5(1): 14, 1976.

Massry S G, Coburn J W: Divalent ion metabolism and renal osteodystrophy, in Massry S G, Sellers A L (eds): *Clinical Aspects of Uremia and Dialysis.* Springfield, Ill, Charles C Thomas, 1976, pp 304–387.

Merrill J P, Hampers C L: *Uremia: Progress in Pathophysiology and Treatment.* New York, Grune & Stratton, 1971.

Papper S: *Clinical Nephrology.* Boston, Little, Brown, 1971.

Parfitt A M: Soft tissue calcification in uremia. *Dialysis and Transplantation* 5(1): 17, 1976.

Pitts R: *Physiology of the Kidney and Body Fluids,* ed 3. Chicago, Year Book Medical Pub, 1974.

Potter D E: Renal osteodystrophy in children. *Dialysis and Transplatation* 5(1): 24, 1976.

Powell A H: Physical assessment of the patient with cardiac disease. *Nursing Clin North Am* 11(2): 251–257, 1976.

Schemmel R: Fluid intake and renal failure. *Dialysis and Transplantation* 4(5): 50, 1975.

Scribner B (ed): *University of Washington Teaching Syllabus on Fluid and Electrolyte Balance.* Seattle, Univ of Washington, 1953.

Sherrard D J: Bone disease in uremia. *Dialysis and Transplantation* 1(3), 1976.

Smith D M: Writing objectives as a nursing practice skill. *AJN* 71:319–320, 1971.

Strauss M B, Welt L G (eds): *Diseases of the Kidney,* ed 2. Boston, Little, Brown, 1971.

Valtin H: *Renal Function: Mechanisms Preserving Fluid and Solute Balance in Health.* Boston, Little, Brown, 1973.

Westervelt F B: Metabolic and endocrine abnormalities, part I, carbohydrate metabolism, in Massry S G, Sellers A L (eds): *Clinical Aspects of Uremia and Dialysis.* Springfield, Ill, Charles C Thomas, 1976, pp 212–230.

Yura H, Walsh M B: *The Nursing Process: Assessing, Planning, Implementing, and Evaluating.* New York, Appleton-Century-Crofts, 1973.

2
Psychosocial Aspects of End Stage Renal Disease

Mary Eccard, R.N., M.S.N.

No account of a disease process is complete without a review of the psychological implications of that disease and of the effects on the patient's total life style. End stage renal disease provides the nurse with an opportunity to study the effects of chronic illness not only on the patient but also on his family and other significant support network. An understanding of the process of adaptation to a chronic illness further assists the nurse in developing helpful intervention approaches and techniques.

While it is generally accepted that chronic illness affects all parameters of an individual patient's life, chronic renal failure and its treatment modality probably disrupt and reorganize more aspects of a patient's life than do other chronic illnesses. The patient's normal daily activity, leisure and work routines, family relationships, role relationships within the family, and intellectual "sharpness" are all affected, as are his general beliefs about himself as a healthy (physically) functioning person. Norman B. Levy supports this notion by pointing out that the center-based renal programs in the country offering two- to three-times-a-week treatments provide a unique opportunity to look at the patient's and his relatives' lives over a prolonged period and consequently to look at those issues unique to chronic illness and especially to the dialysis procedure (1). Nursing recognition of, support through, and intervention during this adaptation process is one of the most critical services the patient has available to him. The nurse's prolonged contact with the patient often makes her privy to patient communication that other health team members don't receive.

The purposes of this chapter are:

1. To review the adaptation process of the adult patient with end stage renal disease.
2. To delineate some patient and family responses to this process.
3. To suggest possible appropriate nursing interventions.
4. To support a collaborative approach to the care of the patient with end stage renal disease.

IMPACT OF CHRONIC ILLNESS

The impact of any chronic illness occurs when the patient begins to recognize that his symptoms have long-range meaning for his subsequent life. The manner in which the patient responds to his early symptoms and the knowledge of their meaning reveals something about his general coping patterns. The patient with end stage renal disease must adjust to the diagnosis and medical regimen that accompanies chronic disease and also to the expectations that he is dependent on the mechanical treatment of hemodialysis for several hours a week for the remainder of his life. Further, the physical well-being that can often be restored in a chronic disease such as diabetes, some forms of cancer, lung or heart disease cannot be restored to the patient with end stage renal disease. Indeed, his entire life style is affected, and, while the treatment makes him feel better, he will never be well. His diet, work pattern, finances, social activity, body appearance, family relations, and sexual activity are only some of the altered life events (1,3,4,5). The professional nurse must recognize the implications that these changes have for the patient and his family, planning her care and intervention to facilitate an orderly process of adjustment (6). These initial changes, as well as the progression of the disease process, precipitate repeated crises for the patient. The nurse must be able to recognize and deal with these crises in a constructive manner that allows maximum growth for the patient.

The adaptation process that the patient works through allows him at various stages to recognize and accept the parameters of his illness. It will be helpful if the nurse recognizes the stages described by Reichsman and Levy as part of the adaptation process. These are termed *1)* the "honeymoon" phase, *2)* disenchantment and discouragement, and *3)* long-term adaptation (7). These stages parallel the typical grief process that the nurse is familiar with in her practice. The nurse's interventions should be timed to permit the most productive outcomes for the patient.

Her interventions and approaches should meet individual patient needs and be consistent with the stage or period the patient is experiencing. Examples of interventions will be outlined below as the stages are described further.

Stages of Adaptation

In the early stages of renal failure the patient will experience signs and symptoms that are vague, conflicting, and unpredictable. Levy describes these types of experiences with slow setbacks and return to a reasonable level of well-being as continuing for a short time and the patient's mood vacillating with them (7). The realization of progressive disability will have an impact on the patient soon enough. The nurse must assist the patient in coping with these changes within his current life pattern but should not change that pattern for him (6). This "honeymoon" period may last from six weeks to six months and the patient's improvement may be very noticeable (7). It is important for the nurse to recognize that, although proper treatment will dispel the uremic symptoms the patient experiences, the patient will never feel perfectly well again (2). The patient's mood at this time may be particularly hopeful and happy with a tendency to overlook difficulty and inconvenience (1). The nurse must guard against suggesting to the patient in her action or communication that his previous state of health can be restored.

Dealing with these early symptomatic patterns may be confusing for both the nurse and the patient. The weakness, headaches, and nausea experienced by the patient may occur either before or after dialysis. Patterns or events that precede a feeling of sickness may not be identifiable by the patient or the medical staff. One element is predictable: the stresses the patient is undergoing are numerous and unending. Two examples of patients' reactions to the stress follow:

> A 26-year-old mother of two children stated after her third week on dialysis, "Every time I think things are going better I begin to feel sick all over again. How can I take care of my children and husband when I'm not sure I can take care of myself?"
>
> A 28-year-old man, after two months on dialysis, was frequenting the hospital with vague complaints of nausea and headache. His wife indicated that because of the unpredictability of *his* feeling sick they seldom did anything anymore. She said she felt that there was little left for them together.

A frequent occurrence during this early adjustment is the nurse's expectation that dialysis will allow the patient to feel physically well enough to adjust quickly to the treatment modality. Often the family believes that the treatment process will be a cure. The prospect of incorporating this treatment and all of its contingencies into a life style is overwhelming. Nurses may be inclined to tell both the patient and his family that he will be "like he was before," able to return to work and "normal" functions. The nurse may hold this expectation herself. The exception the nurse does include is that the patient will have to spend a significant portion of his day—up to three times a week—"on the machine." The inconsistency in the message that the patient will be normal (even though on dialysis) is confusing and difficult to understand. A patient may ask, "What will be normal?" The nurse needs to be willing to begin to explore the patient's feelings of disappointment and recognize the patient's perception of the events occurring.

> A 22-year-old woman was admitted with a diagnosis of lupus erythematosus and renal failure. She was initially eager to learn and cooperative. Her medical course required that she remain in ICU for a prolonged period. The nursing staff began teaching her about her disease, treatment, and self-care. After three weeks the psychiatric nurse consultant was asked to see the patient because "she just doesn't remember anything and she isn't trying to get well." The assessment interview revealed a woman who understood her disease but who was very afraid that because she felt weak all the time and had to go everywhere by cart, she would not be able to walk. She thought that if she could only walk around the room she would feel as if she would be normal again.

In this case it was important that the staff nurses assess the patient's perceptions and the goals she held for herself.

Helping the patient to work toward those goals that are realistic, one at a time, will decrease frustration and allow energies to be utilized for learning or for other activities. During the "honeymoon" phase it is important that the rapid changes the patient experiences be put into perspective for both the nurse and the patient. The nurse should recognize the importance of coordinating her goals with those of the patient.

The second stage defined by Reischman and Levy is disenchantment and discouragement. This may begin slowly or quickly and may last from three to twelve months. The nurse must be willing to recognize her own need to have the patient function independently and productively during this stage. While the goal of independence and productivity for the patient is not wrong in itself, the impatience that accompanies it may cause undue discomfort for the patient and his family. Levy states that at this stage the patient is most likely beginning to struggle with the idea of having to depend on the machine for the remainder of his life. The fear of rejection by the staff and family reinforces the patient's feelings of entrapment (8). A too vigorous pushing for independence may heighten this fear. The nurse's assessment of the patient's functioning before his illness can guide her in appraising realistic goals for the patient's return to any previous activity. It is helpful for the nurse to encourage the expression of feelings, such as anger, helplessness, or hopelessness, that the patient may be experiencing. Discussion of his feelings about the illness and dialysis can promote the patient's acceptance of his feelings and his current situation.

Another common display during this period is denial of the problem entirely. The patient may state that he doesn't need dialysis or he may forget his medication or dietary restrictions. If this occurs, the nurse should provide a noncritical, listening attitude. This attitude of acceptance of the patient's feelings is important. At the same time the nurse is communicating that she knows the facts of his disease process and will assist him in having his physical care completed. Recognition that instruction about the machine, shunt, and course of illness during this phase may be minimally retained by the patient can help the nurse pace her future teaching efforts. While the goal of hastening the patient's participation in self-care is not in itself inappropriate, the timing of instituting the teaching plans is an important consideration. Because the patient may retain only some material, the nurse needs to focus on identifying gaps in information. Her goals and interventions should be planned to bridge these gaps. Integration of the diagnosis of the illness must precede acceptance and integration of *new* facts and information about the illness.

The phase described by Reischman and Levy as long-term adaptation requires variable quantities of time, depending on the patient's own coping skills. This phase, as the others, may vary considerably from patient to patient. Once the patient has accepted his illness, he must continue to adapt to marked, continuous change. Acceptance of the sick role and its restrictions may be overwhelming. The patient may react with anger to questions about his management. He may continue to be unwilling to accept the care of and dependence on others and express this by uncooperativeness, derogation, or blame of others.

It is important that the nurse neither argue with the patient, nor insist that other professionals are right, nor agree that the patient is right in his assessment that his care is not adequate. Recognition that the patient's anxiety fluctuates and that his capacity to "think things through" rationally or to learn new material is compromised will assist the nurse in competently meeting needs for physical care. The patient then learns from this approach that feelings are acceptable, that some dependency on staff and some involvement in his own care are desirable in his adjustment.

An essential skill is the ability to assess how the patient and his family are coping and then support those coping patterns that are adequate. Identifying those events that are most stressful to the patient and the responses that allow him to maintain equilibrium is helpful. For example, the patient may experience dialysis as a very lonely time and desire to have a family member present who is supportive; or he may find the dialysis very anxiety provoking and desire to read or sleep in order to cope with this feeling. Allowing these activities without interruption may assist in the patient's healthy progressive adaptation to the procedure and the disease.

When the patient has further adapted to the sick role and the changes and restrictions this role places on his life style, it is appropriate to teach him about his disease and care in more detail. If he has received this instruction earlier in his treatment, it is important to assess his level of comprehension and retention of information about his disease. The patient's response to the information given or questions asked should guide the nurse in determining the quantity and quality of instruction needed. The nurse's energy and activity should be directed at maintaining the patient's present functions and participation in self-care and at preventing future problems.

When the patient reaches the stage described by Reischman and Levy as acceptance of his illness, he will to some degree turn his energies toward dealing with the reality of the loss of time from his life that his illness occasions. His attempts to adjust to the lasting changes that have occurred in a manner that is workable for him are important to note and support.

Although the renal patient may experience some relief from his nausea, fatigue, and fluctuation in mental alertness, these "remissions" are only temporary. A return to his level of function that existed before his disease is an impossibility. He must now deal with this reality. The patient is daily confronted with his "differentness" and his new circumstances. It is important that the patient establish his own goals that allow him a choice in his productivity level. More crucial, however, is the staff and family acceptance of his chosen level of productivity.

Discussion with the patient of these stages of adaptation gives the nurse a framework for looking at the reactions of the patient with end stage renal disease. Within the time period of each of these stages the nurse can further note defense mechanisms the patient uses. The nurse should not confront these adaptive mechanisms; rather she should recognize their importance in helping the patient maintain emotional equilibrium.

Defense Mechanisms

Defense mechanisms are unconscious maneuvers that a person uses in attempting to ward off anxiety that is produced by perceived threats. The defense mechanisms most commonly documented in connection with chronic renal patients are denial, displacement, projection, regression, intellectualization, isolation of affect, and reaction formation (8,9). Consideration of intervention with patients using those defenses must incorporate a careful understanding of the purposes the defenses have for each patient. The reader is referred to a basic psychiatric text for full description of the defense mechanisms mentioned. Some behavioral manifestations of these defenses in the chronic renal patient are described here.

The nurse's ability to work therapeutically with any patient is determined by her understanding of herself and the needs of the patient. Given the stresses encountered by the renal patient, it is particularly important that the nurse work to establish a firm basis for an ongoing relationship with her patients. This requires that she demonstrate a genuine interest in the patient and his condition. Establishing an understanding of how the patient coped with stress before the illness, as both he and the family see it, will allow the nurse the opportunity to see the effect of the current stresses on the patient. The defenses mentioned are adaptive for the patient, depending on the degree of their use and the effect they have on the patient's adaptation to his illness. Regardless of the value the nurse places on the defense the patient is using, she must not tamper with that mechanism until she has a clear understanding of the patient's ability to cope with the anxiety produced by the situation in a more healthy manner. Clearly, the mechanism the patient utilizes wards off anxiety that would otherwise affect his functioning and allows him a sense of equilibrium and the ability to function. Therefore recognition of the mechanisms, their usefulness to the patient and his family, and their effect on the treatment process are areas for the nurse's assessment and consideration. Working around these defenses rather than confronting them is probably the best approach.

Denial is documented in studies by Wright et al., De-Nour et al., Short and Wilson, and Reichsman and Levy as one of the most prominent and perhaps useful mechanisms utilized by the dialysis patient (10,9,11,7). The negative aspects of denial generally come to mind—such as overlooking obvious symptoms of the original disease process; ignoring cannula difficulty and precautions regarding physical activity; failing to follow the dietary regimen; abusing fluid restrictions; and, in its extreme, failing to come for scheduled dialysis. Levy asserts that denial may indeed serve a function that is essentially adaptive (8). Denial protects the patient from feelings of helplessness that are common with the disease process. If the denial affects the patient's compliance with the medical regimen or dialysis, the physician should consider the beneficial effects of his intervening with the patient. The nurse should work with those manifestations of denial in her encounters with the patient without punitive remarks or restrictions while at the same time communicating that she will care for his needs in a competent manner.

The use of *displacement* can be recognized by the patient's overzealous interest in a portion of his treatment or life that is more controllable than the disease process itself. De Nour et al. describe a group of patients' occupation with their shunts and care of their shunts as a displacement of the fear of death and bodily change (9). By meticulous care of their shunts the patients accomplished mastery over some part of their lives. It is useful to recognize that this may help the patient in his own care as well as decrease his anxiety about the disease.

Projection may be recognized in a number of behaviors. The most common among dialysis patients described by De Nour et al. is that of attributing fear of body change to others by stating that others "are disgusted by the shunt" and attributing demands for coping behavior to the family by stating that "they expect me to work as before" (9). Another manifestation of the patient's use of projection is his attribution of his own angry or aggressive feelings to the staff. For example, "The nurses are always angry at me when I'm on dialysis," or "That nurse is too rough when she sticks me, she must be trying to hurt me." These remarks must be weighed for their reality and then accepted as a means the patient uses to reduce his anxiety. By using projection the patient is spared the pain of his own feelings. Recognition of the utility of this defense mechanism for the patient at that moment can help the nurse deal with her own feelings about the accusations.

Regression is the adoption of previous behaviors that have resulted in a feeling of well-being. For the dialysis patient regression can be a helpful mechanism, since a certain amount of dependency on staff and equipment is a requirement for treatment. Buchanan and Abram describe the other extreme of this behavior in the patient who is extremely demanding and overdependent on staff for care. They observe that the family can perpetuate this behavior out of a need to be involved in the patient's care (12). The nurse can intervene by identifying the events that precipitate the behaviors. She can then manipulate the environment so that the regression is not reinforced.

Reaction formation and isolation of affect are two further defenses commonly used. The nurse can see *reaction formation* in the patient who deals with feelings of disgust, dislike, or aggression toward dialysis by expressing excitement about the procedure or affection for the staff. Showing no overt aggression and getting along extremely well with the staff also indicate use of this mechanism, as described by De Nour et al (9). Reaction formation is further used by the patient who expresses extreme autonomy and independence in response to his fear of his need to be cared for by the staff and to his fear of the procedure. *Isolation of affect* can be identified when the patient reports recurrence of symptoms or shunt difficulties with no affect or in an indifferent, shallow manner.

Intellectualization is seen in the patient who employs reason and logic to defend against uncomfortable feelings. This mechanism is usually the one that is most acceptable to the staff.

The use of defenses must always be understood as unconscious and unplanned by the patient. De Nour et al. document evidence that the defenses utilized in their group of dialysis patients were "labile and often brittle," breaking down under even slight stress. This breakdown of defenses can cause the patient to transiently experience "anxiety, depression, and paranoid trends" (9). The nurse's recognition of this process allows her the privilege of understanding the patient's responses, mood changes, and adaptations. She can then work with the behavioral outcomes in a constructive manner by using basic psychiatric knowledge and skills.

Mood Variations

The section on adaptation process has described the predominant reactions the staff nurse should be aware of in the dialysis patient. The defense mechanisms identified indicate some of the variation in moods the patient might manifest. Anxiety, depression, withdrawal, fear, and anger are but a few of the emotional states that can precipitate fluctuation in a patient's moods. Cummings has described the pressures on the dialysis patient in physiological, social, and interpersonal terms (13). Ample reasons for the reactions and variations mentioned are provided by his descriptions of *1)* decrease in intellectual functions due to waste accumulation, with less effective use of functions such as concentration, abstraction, and generalization; *2)* pressures on the patient's financial security and productivity, with resultant family role relationship readjustments (for example, the man as breadwinner and disciplinarian relinquishes these duties to his wife; the wife as organizer and housekeeper has half the time to do the same activities); and *3)* changes in one's self-concept and feelings of self-worth. De Nour et al. observe, "Surprising changes in combination and intensity of defenses over short periods of time were observed, resulting in ever-changing clinical pictures, changing behavior and facets of personality" (9). These investigators further report that the use of a great many defenses may take an undue toll on the personality. Although relationships may be maintained, they are generally shallow, and little energy is available for new relationships. It follows that the patient may become rigid, unable to adapt effectively to new situations or activities, and may display little or no interest in things outside his illness sphere.

The nurse's response to these variations in mood should be formulated after she has gained a thorough understanding of the patient's situation. She should communicate that anxiety and upset are acceptable; give information in a calm, reassuring manner; provide a climate of hope and helpfulness; recognize that patient reactions are not always personally intended; and provide the patient with self-care tasks that are easily accomplished to help build his self-esteem and restore his self-concept.

Family Involvement

The diagnosis and treatment of end stage renal disease definitely take a toll of the family members as well as of the patient. The patient's significant others, if relied on for caring and support before illness, will be called upon after diagnosis for more support but perhaps in a different way. It is important to understand the relationships that existed before the illness and the patient's ability to rely on family supports for assistance. While the nurse cannot take responsibility for mediating or building the relationships that exist, she can use her assessment to help plan intervention approaches and treatment schedules to add as little additional stress as possible to the current relationships. Understanding that even the best relationships will require new definition when a chronic illness affects one member allows the nurse to exercise foresight in putting resources and referral information at her diaposal. Cummings suggests that the nurse estimate the amount of communication that occurs between spouses and the degree of understanding that each member demonstrates about the illness and treatment modalities (13). These observations can give her cues about the level of involvement of the spouse and family and guide her in making decisions about teaching plans and other nursing care activities.

Communicating with the patient about plans for treatment that are nursing responsibility heightens the patient's sense of participation in his care. Communicating indications of patient progress to the patient and the person he identifies as his primary support may also heighten the patient's sense of not being alone with his illness. This approach further reduces the chance of misunderstanding of information, since the family member and the patient can check out their perceptions with the nurse and with each other.

The entire family structure may be in flux as a result of the illness, and more dysfunction than is necessary can occur if the family strengths aren't called forth. Among other reactions, the family may respond with quilt. Awareness of this possible dysfunction may give the nurse the impetus to approach the family members to assess their perceptions of the illness and their coping abilities. A careful exploring of any previous events that may have resembled this one for the family can assist them in mobilizing resources that may be forgotten. Support for the family to continue normal activity rather than devoting all time to the patient is helpful. Further, guiding the family to call on previous information and skills makes use of the nurse's crisis intervention skills to avert a breakdown of the strengths that exist in the family.

Community Support Systems

The psychological stresses the patient encounters, and the many losses that intensify these, can only be compounded by an excessive financial burden. The nurse needs to be aware not only of resources to provide psychological supports for the patient and family but also of the financial and community resources that might be of assistance in coping with the financial burden. In-center dialysis itself can cost in excess of $25,000 a year. Dialysis done in the home can cost up to $12,000 per year. Obviously few individuals or families can manage such amounts without assistance. Options open to the patient with end stage renal disease are "HR-1" (section 299-1 ESRD Medicare), state Medicaid, American Kidney Fund, Kidney Foundation, State Renal Programs, and private insurance providers. Private foundations and church or community groups may aid the renal patient in need of transient assistance. While this list is not exhaustive, each patient and family should know that such resources may help them meet their financial responsibilities. The patient and/or his family should be directed to the appropriate person adept in facilitating use of these resources.

ADJUSTMENT TO CHRONIC ILLNESS

Adjustment to chronic illness occurs as the patient integrates the experience of illness into a life style that is acceptable for him. The long-term adaptation that the patient accomplishes is highly individualistic. The nurse who enhances the patient's strengths during this phase will contribute generously to the patient's sense of handling his illness in an "acceptable" manner.

Personal Adjustments

The stresses the renal patient encounters are similar for every patient; however, the ability to withstand these and adjust to them depends on the individual's strengths and developed coping methods. Recognition of the commonality of the experience can help the nurse establish a strong basis from which to plan her interventions.

Wright, Sand, and Livingston categorize the many stresses that dialysis patients undergo in the following manner: 1) losses the individual encounters in physical health, social activities, and financial-community status; 2) injuries or threats of injuries to the body and the shunt area; and 3) frustrations experienced by individuals whose instincts and needs are affected by the medical regimen (10).

Some of the physical losses encountered by these patients are impairment of intellectual function, loss of a general sense of physical well-being with concomitant malaise and irritability, weight changes, and degenerative changes in bones and muscles with resultant gait difficulty and activity restrictions. Social losses include those of withdrawal from group and club memberships (volunteer, sports, activity) and a loss of support from extended family and friends if geographical relocation is necessary to obtain treatment. A loss of job and income, or an inability to maintain role expectations in the home or community, deprives the person of esteem that is derived from these activities. When such life-style modifications are forced on the patient in areas of planning, recreation, vocational goals, and financial security, their effect on his self-concept needs close attention. His reaction may be defensiveness, determination to overcome, passive acceptance, anger, use of any number of the defense mechanisms, or withdrawal from his family, friends, and the treatment staff.

The second category of stresses includes fear of injury to the shunt or fistula by normal activity such as walking or by infection or clotting that would prevent access for dialysis. Nephrectomy is also an insult to the body's integrity, and the patient may fear loss of the organs. Coping with injury or threat of injury may be manifested by the patient's overly meticulous care of the shunt, fear of new staff's doing a procedure for him, a refusal to have a nephrectomy done, or a generalized heightened anxiety about any scheduled or anticipated procedure.

Finally, the patient must learn to cope with the frustrations he encounters in his basic drives. Eating, sex, and aggressive impulses must be dealt with in different manners. Restrictions on diet allow the patient few of the pleasures others derive from eating. Horari et al. reported that most patients had considerable reduction in libido and sexual activity (3). Similar findings are documented by Levy (8). Halper describes the area of aggressive impulses as particularly problematic in patients where work or physical activity rather than intellectual activity are the primary outlets (5). The nurse must be prepared to be open to discussion of these frustrations.

All of these stresses may give the patient an inordinate sense of loss of control over his environment and himself. Interventions that allow him a feeling of regaining that control are most appropriate and useful. Gentry and Davis observe that the patients they studied "appeared similar in perceptions that their life was controlled by something or someone external to themselves" (4). They note that this reaction develops early in dialysis rather than over a long period.

Wright et al., Halper and Gentry, and Davis report the same basic psychological pattern of adaptation to prolonged dialysis. The longer the patient undergoes dialysis, the less the patient shows interest in his current life situation or new relationships. A tendency to respond in a socially acceptable manner increases, and affect becomes less (10,5,4). Therefore denial may be viewed as an uncontrollable consequence for the dialysis patient, and may, as Levy states, be a functional adaptation (8).

Support System

The areas of stress defined by Wright, Sand, and Livingston and outlined here as personal stressors have particular ramifications for the family. The physical changes require that the individual find new or different ways to maintain his/her status in the family unit. The man who can no longer work must find other ways to maintain his position and esteem in the family unit; the woman who can no longer do the housework must find new ways to keep the home running and maintain her esteem with her children and husband. The role reversals or realignments that occur as a result of the disease cause changes in responsibilities, decision making, and communication.

Family members may be unable to continue in their "normal" social activities because of new responsibilities shifted onto them. Relationships between spouses and their friends may deteriorate as the physical illness forces the couple to socialize less frequently.

The physical changes may also disrupt the companionship within the family unit itself. The children in a family may be forced to take on roles of mediators between the parents or of confidantes to one or the other of the parents. The children's efforts as negotiators may not be successful because they may not have the skills necessary for these roles.

The patient's shunt or fistula may be difficult for the family to accept. The restrictions placed on the limb where the shunt or fistula is located may cause the patient to favor that extremity and therefore keep a parent from displaying physical affection for a child. In a more general way, the physical changes in appearance may be frightening for a young child to see in his parent. The family must have available to them skilled people who can help them deal with these changes in a healthy, productive manner.

The nurse, with proper training, can offer this assistance or can refer the family to the psychiatric clinical nurse specialist or social worker available in the setting.

NURSING ASSESSMENT

The previous sections have defined some specific nursing interventions appropriate for family and patients at various stages in the adaptation process. This section reviews those assessment factors previously mentioned and develops a format of questions for the initial psychosocial assessment of the patient and family.

The nursing assessment of the patient and family experiencing end stage renal disease should include the following major areas:

1. How does the patient feel about himself? This inquiry should include questions that yield a clear picture of how the patient believed himself to function before his illness and how he sees that his function will change as a result of the illness. This information delineates the stresses the patient has encountered and how he sees himself working with them.

2. How does the patient perceive other's responses to him? Again the patient's previous perception of his function is just as important as his current assessment. The nurse should note if the patient sees others relating to him as a likable, capable individual. Knowledge of these responses may hint as to how the patient will relate to staff and his family now. The kind of support he receives from the family, the way he receives it, and his ideas of whether his illness will affect that support are also important areas.

3. How does he identify himself with others in similar circumstances? Knowledge of how the patient views other persons with chronic illness and his ability to identify the similarities or differences in their coping styles may assist him in pursuing a more productive pattern for his own life.

4. How does he identify and accept the attitudes of the staff caring for him? The patient who believes that the staff are capable and willing to work with him for his comfort and treatment will undoubtedly be the more desirable patient. The nurse must be aware of those defense mechanisms that the patient uses that would bias her perception of the patient. It is important to realize that the patient may not be able to express his true feelings because of fear of retaliation by the staff. This recognition will assist the nurse in understanding what may otherwise be viewed as uncooperativeness of the patient. Exploration of these aspects via communication about the patient's perception of staff attitudes will help the nurse work *with* the patient in delivering care.

Family assessment is equally important when working with chronic renal patients. The observation of the amount and kind of communication that occurs between the patient and family will allow the nurse the opportunity to see the strengths and supports available to the patient. The family should be viewed as a unit. The manner in which they have worked together in times of stress is important in assessing how they might continue to work together in the present situation. It is unrealistic to expect that a family who has not previously had strong relationships and worked together will now do so without assistance. The nurse needs to serve as an open listener and to suggest that the members discuss their feelings and issues as they arise. This facilitation of communication can offer the patient and family support and new problem-solving skills. Resources available that can offer formal counseling need to be offered to the family when the nurse deems this appropriate. A chaplain, psychiatric clinical nurse specialist, social worker, or psychiatrist versed in family treatment are a few of the possible resources.

Individual and family assessments help the nurse establish a baseline of information that can be expanded over the lengthy treatment period ahead. It cannot be stressed enough that the relationship the nurse forms with the patient in the early phases of treatment is critical for a continued helping relationship throughout the illness. As the patient experiences new stresses, his ability to ask for and accept assistance from the nurse will reflect the quality of the relationship the nurse has previously established with him.

TERMINATING THE TREATMENT

Discussion of the patient's decision to die also brings to the fore the feelings the staff may have relating to death. The literature reveals that dialysis as a life event is pervasive and stressful. Abram observes, "The assault on the patient's independence, self-esteem, body-image, and physical sense of well-being is significant to the point of intolerance" (2). The reactions of the staff to the patient's experiencing these life-stressful events are critical in assuring working relationships. It must be recognized that the staff's reactions may cloud or affect their ability to work with the patients at all. The leadership people in the unit must work out approaches with the staff so that the problems of dealing with patients' struggles with illness can be constructively encountered.

When dealing with a patient who has multiple physical system problems related to chronic renal disease, the question of quality of life becomes a concern of the treatment team. A case study is presented that raises some ethical questions for consideration:

1. Is suicide sometimes a rational decision?
2. Should a severely depressed patient be permitted to make decisions regarding life-and-death issues?
3. Is it not the health care givers, who valie life as a primary goal, who are defeated when the patient and family choose death as an alternative to treatment?

A 26-year-old married female with juvenile onset diabetes mellitus presented with severe multiorgan involvement and rapidly progressive renal failure. She had completed college but was forced to quit her job because of diabetic retinopathy resulting in total left-eye blindness and decreased right-eye vision. Her medical management was complicated by recurrent pleural effusions, recurrent fevers, pericarditis with effusions, congestive heart failure, profound episodes of hypoglycemia due to insulin sensitivity followed by episodes of respiratory arrest, and constant eye pain secondary to increased intraocular pressure in her left eye.

In order to receive treatment the patient and her husband were forced to relocate in a city about five hours drive from their home. They left their family supports and familiar belongings behind. The patient's husband assumed responsibility for almost all of her care because of her difficulty with sight and her weakness. The rapidity with which the changes occurred did not allow much time for adjustments. Both the patient and her husband, although aware of the difficulties in dialysis treatment of a diabetic, chose to begin maintenance dialysis and continued it for 18 months without question about continuing the procedure. Toward the end of the 18-month period the patient began to experience frequent severe headaches and eye pain. Close medical examination revealed that the alternative to the pain was enucleation. Fluid and diet management became increasingly difficult, and the patient decreased her weight by 25 pounds. Multiple changes occurred within the family unit during this period. The illness thrust drastic role changes on both persons. The patient could no longer attend to household duties, to work, or to the needs of her husband (physical or emotional). The patient's husband gave up his job and outside activities to care for his wife and their home. These losses, coupled with the environmental changes and resultant isolation from familiar people, compounded the couple's sense of hopelessness and helplessness. In the nineteenth month of illness the patient began to ask questions about what would happen if she chose to stop dialysis. The nursing staff answered her questions directly and explored some of the meaning behind the questions. Indeed, the patient stated that since she could no longer work, care for her husband's needs, be a sexual partner, walk, or eat, and since the financial burden was becoming greater, she wished to stop dialysis.

The staff called a psychiatric nurse clinical specialist to assist in dealing with this problem.

This case exemplifies one extreme of complexity that can evolve in treatment of a chronic renal failure patient. It also highlights the importance of an interdisciplinary approach to care of similar complex patient situations. The nurse's role in care and the facilitation of an interdisciplinary approach is discussed later.

The first essential is assessment on a continuing basis of the patient's and family's abilities to cope. Referral to an individual competent in dealing with the psychological impact of repeated discouragement in treatment is needed early in the patient's treatment course. Staff openness to asking for assistance at any point in the treatment course is very important.

Second, it is also essential that the nurse assume responsibility for keeping the primary physician aware of the patient's changing psychoemotional status. The physician has little prolonged contact with the patient on chronic dialysis. The nurse must assume a primary role in facilitating the patient's communication regarding adjustment problems and see that information is passed on to the physician and social worker.

Third, communication between the patient and family members must be encouraged. The discussion of feelings of mutual support should be prompted if and when the nurse hears cues from the patient or family in this area.

Fourth, family members who are seemingly overwhelmed by the demands of caring for the patient need opportunities to discuss their own frustrations and worries. If the staff nurse can't provide this time, appropriate referrals need to be made (for example, to a chaplain, psychiatrist, psychiatric nurse, social worker) for the family member alone.

Fifth, attempts to broaden an isolated family's contacts in a new community are important. Information about available community group resources for social as well as financial assistance may be needed.

Finally, persistence in establishing communication time and routes between the patient, family members, and physician to reevaluate and discuss alternatives to current treatment is crucial.

The nurse has the unique opportunity to collaborate with all members of the team in her daily activities with patients. Sharing her knowledge about the patient with other team members helps to create an atmosphere of working together for the patient's welfare. In the case presented above, the provision of consistent nursing personnel for the patient helped identify those issues that needed a broad approach. The patient's trust in one staff member allowed her the safety to express her feelings. The patient's decision to die is a difficult process to work through; concern for it is, however, a part of caring for that individual's life.

This case description does not answer the questions posed but rather raises issues for consideration when treating a patient with end stage renal disease. The nurse needs to consider the treatment of the whole patient and his family unit. Although she cannot provide the answers to such dilemmas as the question of death by choice, she can provide a climate to facilitate the human concern over such issues. She can thus assure that these issues are dealt with openly and with input from all pertinent people, including, especially, the patient and the family.

SUMMARY

The aspects of end stage renal disease discussed here are largely those observed as experiences in hospitalized patients. The impact of and adjustment to end stage renal disease has many ramifications for the patient and the family. While the reactions reported here may be incapacitating for some, some patients and their families with proper resources and support adjust strikingly well to end stage renal disease. This adjustment may be a function of the circumstances of the disease onset (longstanding vs. sudden) and of the age of the patient.

The patient and family responses delineated are probably those most commonly seen in the process of adjustment to end stage renal disease. The nursing interventions suggested aren't meant to be all-inclusive, rather they are possible approaches. The section on defense mechanisms covers only the most frequently observed defenses in a dialysis population. Other mechanisms may be used, and the nurse needs to be familiar with them as well. The importance of working with the defense is obvious if the staff recognize that the patient uses it to ward off overwhelming anxiety.

Finally, we have looked at a collaborative approach to a patient considering terminating dialysis. The collaborative aspects of delivering total patient care are extremely important. It is hoped that this type of approach will be facilitated from admission through discharge and into outpatient treatment.

REFERENCES

1. N B Levy: Coping with maintenance hemodialysis—psychological considerations in the care of patients, in S G Massry and A L Sellers (eds): *Clinical Aspects of Uremia and Dialysis.* Springfield, Ill, Charles C Thomas, 1976.

2. H S Abram, G L Moore, F B Westervelt, Jr: Suicidal behavior in chronic dialysis patients. *Amer J Psychiat* 127(9), 1971.

3. A Harari, H Munitz, H Wizsenbeck, et al: Psychological aspects of chronic hemodialysis. *Psychiat Neurol Neurochir* 74, 1971.

4. W D Gentry, G C Davis: Cross-sectional analysis of psychological adaptation to chronic hemodialysis. *Chron Dis* 25, 1972.

5. I S Halper: Psychiatric observations in a chronic hemodialysis program. *Med Clin North Am* 55(1), 1971.

6. M A Crate: Nursing functions in adaptation to chronic illness. *Am J Nurs* 65(10), 1965.

7. F Reischman, N B Levy: Problems in adaptation to maintenance hemodialysis: a four-year study of 25 patients. *Arch Intern Med* 130, 1972.

8. N B Levy: Psychological studies at the Downstate Medical Center of patients on hemodialysis. *Med Clin North Am* 61(4), 1977.

9. A Kaplan-De Nour, J Shaltiel, J W Czaczhes: Emotional reactions of patients on chronic hemodialysis. *Psychosom Med* 30(5), 1968.

10. R G Wright, P Sand, G Livingston: Psychological stress during hemodialysis for chronic renal failure. *Ann Intern Med* 64(3), 1968.

11. M J Short, W P Wilson: Roles of denial in chronic hemodialysis. *Arch Gen Psychiat* 20, 1969.

12. D C Buchanan, H S Abram: Psychological adaptation to hemodialysis. *Dialysis and Transplantation* Feb-March, 1976.

13. J W Cummings: Hemodialysis—feelings, facts, fantasies. *Am J Nurs* 70(1), 1970.

BIBLIOGRAPHY

Abram H S: The psychiatrist, the treatment of chronic renal failure and the prolongation of life: I. *Am J Psychiat* 124: 1351–58, 1968.

Abram H S: The psychiatrist, the treatment of chronic renal failure and the prolongation of life: II. *Am J Psychiat* 126: 157–67, 1969.

Abram H S: Psychotherapy in renal failure. *Curr Psychia Ther* 9: 86–92, 1969.

Abram H S: Survival by machine: the psychological stress of chronic hemodialysis. *Psychiat Med* 1: 37–51, 1970.

Anger D W, Anger D: Motivation and adjustment levels of hemodialysis patients. *Dialysis and Transplantation* 4(2), 1975.

Beard B H: Fear of death and fear of life: the dilemma in chronic renal failure, hemodialysis and kidney transplantation. *Arch Gen Psychiat* 21, 1969.

Brundage D J: *Nursing Management of Renal Problems.* St. Louis, C V Mosby Co, 1976.

Cramond W A, Knight P R, Lawrence J R: The psychiatric contribution to a renal unit undertaking chronic hemodialysis and renal homotransplantation. *Br J Psychiat* 113, 1967.

Dansak D A: Secondary gain in long-term hemodialysis patients. *Am J Psychiat* 129, 1972.

Fishman D B, Schneider C J: Predicting emotional adjustment in home dialysis patients and their relatives. *J Chronic Dis* 25, 1972.

Fox R G, Swazey J P: *The Courage to Fail—A Social View of Organ Transplants and Dialysis.* Chicago, Univ of Chicago, 1974.

Foy A L: Dreams of patients and staff. *Am J Nurs* 70, 1972.

Friedman E A: Psychosocial adjustment to maintenance hemodialysis. *New York State J Med* March, 1970.

Glassman B M, Siegel A: Personality correlates of survival in a long-term hemodialysis program. *Arch Gen Psychiat* 22, 1970.

Hickman B W: All about sex . . . despite dialysis. *Am J Nurs* 77(4), 1977.

Hollon T H: Modified group therapy in the treatment of patients on chronic hemodialysis. *Am J Psychother* 26, 1972.

Kaplan-De Nour A: Psychotherapy with patients on chronic hemodialysis. *Br J Psychiat* 116, 1970.

Kaplan-De Nour A, Czaczkes J W: Emotional problems and reactions of the medical team in a chronic hemodialysis unit. *Lancet* 2, 1968.

Kaplan-De Nour A, Czaczkes J W: Team-patient interaction in chronic hemodialysis units. *Psychother Psychosom* 24, 1974.

Kaplan-De Nour A, Schaltier J, Czaczkes J W: Emotional reactions of patients on chronic hemodialysis. *Psychosom Med* 30, 1968.

Kaye R, Leigh H, Strauch B: The role of liaison psychiatrist in a hemodialysis program: a case study. *Psychiat Med* 4, 1973.

Kossoris P: Family therapy: an adjunct to hemodialysis and transplantation. *Am J Nurs* 70, 1970.

Levy N B (ed): *Living or Dying—Adaptation to Hemodialysis.* Springfield, Ill, Charles C Thomas, 1974.

Marshall J R: Effective use of a psychiatric consultant on a dialysis unit. *Postgrad Med* 55, 1974.

Moore G L: Nursing response to the long-term dialysis patient. *Nephron* 9, 1972.

Raimbault G: Psychological aspects of chronic renal failure and hemodialysis. *Nephron* 11, 1973.

Schowalter J E: The adolescent patient's decision to die. *Pediatrics* 51(1), 1973.

Short M J, Wilson W P: Roles of denial in chronic hemodialysis. *Arch Gen Psychiat* 20, 1969.

Sorensen E T: Group therapy in a community hospital dialysis unit. *JAMA* 221, 1972.

Sullivan M F: The dialysis patient and attitudes toward work. *Psychiat Med* 4, 1973.

Viederman M: Adaptive and maladaptive regression in hemodialysis. *Psychiatry* 37, 1974.

3
Learning to Live with Dialysis: A Personal Perspective

Edith T. Oberley, M.A.

Terry D. Oberley, M.D., Ph.D.

PART I

The recent growth of renal dialysis into a full-scale industry complete with its own bureaucratic maze, corporate monopoly, and big money concerns has spawned a question asked with increasing persistende: "Is it worth it? Should we be pouring millions into the renal program to prolong the lives of a few thousand people who will only be miserable anyway?"

As a dialysis patient since 1972, my answer to that question might be subject to some bias. However, I would like to do my part to counteract the prevailing public image of the dialysis patient as a pathetic creature tied to a machine from which the only release is imminent death or new life with a transplanted kidney.

Being on dialysis can be not only a satisfactory, but a fulfilling and productive way of life, depending on the patient's personal philosophy and the fabric of circumstances surrounding him/her. In fact, I have found the home dialysis routine to be so successful and stable that only serious dialysis-related complications or a dramatic advance in transplantation immunology could induce me to alter my choice of treatment.

Part of this success is due to luck. I have been fortunate, and I am grateful. Part of the success depends also, however, on other factors that have been within the realm of my own control. Within the set of restricting circumstances imposed by kidney failure, there are still a number of options remaining in a patient's life. Among the options available, I have chosen to: do home dialysis . . . become an active participant in my own care . . . learn everything possible about the limitations and possibilities of my treatment . . . remain physically stable through dietary regulation . . . accept the slower pace of life and more limited activity . . . yet continue an active working and social life. And most important, I have chosen to *commit* myself to dialysis as a way of life.

My wife and I have concluded that a patient needs three essential factors for success in dialysis: *1*) stable physical and mental health, *2*) the opportunity to pursue one's most cherished goals, and *3*) hope for the future. All these are interrelated; achievement of one ideal may mean automatic fulfillment of another, and vice versa: loss of one may lead to loss of all.

These are, of course, desirable ideals for anyone, but the point is they are difficult but not impossible for the dialysis patient to achieve. Attaining them simply requires a little more ingenuity, consistency, and careful analysis than if the patient were free to live in the usual haphazard way.

How to mold these ideals into reality? Good physical and mental health is at best an elusive abstraction, even for the person who is free of disease. There are specific programs, however, which patient and staff *together* can undertake to foster good health in the dialysis patient.

One is sound education about kidney failure, its treatments, their limitations and their potential. To gain some control over his/her present and future life, the dialysis patient must learn to understand and solve some of his own dialysis problems himself. For example, I had to learn for myself the beneficial effects of exercise in reducing the insomnia that used to plague me.

A cardinal rule: *the patient has the right to know.* The patient educated in the reasons for diet, medications, adequate dialysis, and their relationship to complications will be more alert to any potential problems. Until a patient learns *why* he is dizzy, has headaches, feels nauseous, feels thirsty, he is in no position to remedy these problems through intelligent dietary regulation. Following the diet through *understanding* is much better than following the diet by *rote.* I feel I regulate myself much better because I understand the relationship between, for example, a fluid overload and disequilibrium. Another advantage to education about the treatment: the patient can make intelligent choices about such vital matters as dialysis versus transplantation.

Education about dialysis should take place throughout the whole course of the treatment, rather than being concentrated into a single onslaught of information in an orientation course. Patients at the start of dialysis are confused, fearful, and overwhelmed—hardly an auspicious state of mind to absorb the mountain of psychosocial, dietary, medical, and technical information about a process that looms threatening to change every aspect of life.

Understanding of dialysis is an ongoing, evolving process. I am still learning about the ways my own metabolism and cardiovascular system respond to various durations and degrees of dialysis runs.

After the formal orientation course, effort should be made to keep patients abreast of recent developments and events in the field. This is one way to foster that essential hope for the future needed to spark faith in a life with dialysis. Staff can distribute brochures from major nephrology meetings showing directions for the future in renal technology. Anticipation of major advances such as the suitcase kidney are most encouraging for a dialysis patient.

Books, magazines, and newsletters for patients should be readily available. A patient library is a fine idea. Regular conferences with a dietitian and other support personnel will add to the patient's store of understanding.

Education need not be confined to information provided by the staff. In our experience, the most encouraging events of the early dialysis days were the opportunities to talk to successful patients who had strong and positive attitudes toward life with dialysis. Some units, recognizing the value of such an encounter between a new and an experienced patient, have appointed a stable, successful patient as "patient coordinator," a person who visits all new patients and helps them become acquainted with their new way of life.

For the dialysis patient, knowledge is truly power, whereas ignorance is the surest path to abject dependence. To a patient, an understanding of the machine that sustains his life also means mastery over a technology that otherwise would subjugate him.

Education is only one step to physical and mental health. Without education, a patient has no rationale for understanding the strict dialysis regimen. A vital corollary to education is *exercise,* without which the patient cannot regain the physical strength necessary to meet life's daily demands. It seems to me that exercise should be a strongly stressed element of a patient's rehabilitation program.

If a sedentary life is bad for the health of the general population, consider its effects on the dialysis patient. Given the prevalent tendencies toward cardiovascular disease and bone demineralization, regular, moderate exercise should be doubly beneficial to the dialysis patient.

The correlation between exercise and cardiovascular strength is common knowledge, and much has been written about the reduction of osteoporosis in the elderly through the maintenance of physical activity.

The anemia of ESRD is a great deterrent to physical activity, but regular exercise, I have found, is essential for my own stability. As a patient I need much rest, but I also need activity to heighten mental alertness and speed reequilibration postdialysis. A program to regain strength can have the same beneficial effects as a program of education: it is a motivator, a starter, an ongoing accomplishment in which the patient can take pride.

A third specific ingredient in the factors leading to physical health is *individualized treatment.* When away from home, I have dialyzed in units where the standard assumption is that all the patients are overweight and the standard treatment is to ultrafiltrate until they are gasping and cramping. What chance does the patient who carefully watches his fluid have in such surroundings?

A setting in which each patient is carefully monitored and treated according to his/her individual needs is essential for good health. It seems obvious to belabor the point that each patient's needs are different—even to the point that each separate dialysis for one patient must be handled differently. The patient without the benefit of self-dialysis training or without a staff sensitive to his/her dialysis needs is at the mercy of anyone who may accidentally leave the venous pressure turned up too high.

Individualized treatment also involves careful monitoring of chemistries and vital signs and discussions with the patient about changes in treatment. Making the patient a *partner* in the medical treatment is an excellent way to foster independence and interest. Such an approach requires a philosophical commitment on the staff's part to move away from the autocratic or paternalistic "good patient–bad patient" dichotomy.

To me, a "good patient" is not one who just unquestioningly accepts and mechanically performs every detail of the doctor's orders, but one who seeks to learn, who strives for independence within the necessary limitations of dialysis.

Factors relating to physical health are specific and measurable; those relating to mental health are more subtle and elusive. One important aspect of mental health is the continuation of strong ties with family and friends. Studies have shown that those who make the best adjustment to dialysis are those who have strong relationships to support them in times of stress. This certainly has been true in my own case. I was able to finish medical school partly because my family believed so strongly in me and made sacrifices in their own lives to create an optimum situation for me, the newly initiated dialysis patient whose continuous hypotension literally prevented me from knowing for many months which way was up!

An important point: my family regards me as a *person,* not a patient, and the distinction between these two views has a great influence on any patient's self-image. Another way dialysis patients can fall into that pit of dependency is to have everyone around treat them as chronically ill people. This view is devastating for the self-image.

What else affects the dialysis patient's self-image, another important aspect of mental health? Body image seems to play a role in lowered self-esteem. Some patients are very self-conscious about their "disfigured" fistula or cannula arm or their unhealthy complexion. I have noticed, however, that the healthiest patients who have made a conscious and determined effort to make dialysis work have no visible signs of illness in their countenances. The positive attitude that leads to self-knowledge and physical and mental health puts a sparkle in the eye and color in the cheek, proving again how interrelated all the factors for success in dialysis are.

Another important element leading to good mental health in the dialysis patient is a good relationship with the staff. Volumes could be written on this topic; it must suffice to say here that a mutual staff/patient discussion of everyone's rights and responsibilities is a useful foundation for building positive relationships. Also, the staff attitude I mentioned before toward a *partnership* with patients is most valuable. Patients need to find staff accessible for questions, for counselling, and other help. By the same token, patients should be encouraged not to take for granted the help they do receive; they need to understand that the responsibilities that accompany their "partnership" are essential.

Staff members can be helpful in the sort of situation where a patient must reorganize his/her schedule and priorities in order to keep his/her most important life's goals in sight. This is the third essential ingredient I mentioned for success in dialysis: the opportunity to pursue one's most cherished goals. For example, because of dialysis, I am able to perform the things I care about most: do medical research and have a family. These are what give my life meaning. But if either were curtailed through scheduling problems or medical complications, great frustration would result.

As it is, I am grateful to dialysis for the new lease on life. Other patients ought to be able to feel the same way, and staff can be a great help by examining the facets of the patient's life that could be improved. Here are some basic questions that should be asked about every patient:

Job—Can he/she work? If not, why not? Daytime treatment? Could he/she be transferred to a later shift? Not physically able to resume former job? Could vocational counselling provide an alternative?

Family—Are they supportive? How could they be counselled and helped to become even more so?

Recreation—Is the patient free to travel? Could he/she benefit from our help in arranging dialysis in another city for vacation? Could he/she obtain a portable machine?

Social life—Has it been curtailed? Is there a local kidney patient's group? Could new patients be introduced to other patients their own age? Does patient have access to kidney magazines to establish contact with others in his/her situation?

Mode of dialysis—If in-center, would home dialysis make the schedule more flexible? If home dialysis, are stresses present that we could alleviate?

One other factor that has enabled me to lead a fulfilling vocational and family life is the flexibility afforded by home dialysis. Feelings of dependence generated by being tied to a machine leads some patients to feel they have lost control over their daily lives as well as their overall future. In my own case, home dialysis has enabled me to overcome such dependency. Being in charge of my own treatment has given me the same sense of independence that I felt *before* ESRD.

Not only is my schedule more flexible with home dialysis, but I can take care of any problems that require extra dialysis at my own convenience. An extra measure of the home patient's independence comes with the necessity to rely on his own judgment when routine problems—mechanical, technical, or physical—arise.

A patient on home or self dialysis analyzes and monitors his own symptoms day by day to find answers to his problems. Trained to be alert to any physical malfunctions, the self-care patient pays careful attention to sleep patterns, appetite, thirst, blood pressure, and sexual function. Fluctuations in these areas give important clues as to the success of the dialysis regimen without any clinical evaluation.

Home dialysis, run in a stable setting, can contribute to all essential ingredients for dialysis success: better physical health through factors just mentioned; better psychological health through convenience of scheduling, fewer hospital visits, greater independence; flexibility and convenience of scheduling offer the patient a chance to be more productive (pursue cherished goals); and lastly, introduction of portable or continuous dialyzers into general home use would certainly keep alive that spark of hope for a better future for kidney patients.

No matter how much we may juggle schedules, hematocrits, and exercise programs around, dialysis remains an imperfect therapy; its limitations are apparent. That is why we kidney patients are sustained in large part by a hope for the future. We've seen dialysis become faster and more streamlined . . . seen conditions like bone disease and neuropathy viewed with growing understanding . . . seen dialysis patients reenter the world of "normalcy" with resounding success. This encourages us; but we await the day when: synthesized erythropoeitin vanquishes that dragging anemia . . . intelligent use of the gastrointestinal tract allows greater absorption of uremic toxins . . . the etiology of cardiovascular disease in renal patients is fully understood and preventive measures taken . . . portable machines allow us full mobility. Without these prospects for the future, the present routine would be rather stultifying. Patients should be invited to view the panorama of renal research that will one day affect their lives.

Ultimately, the touchstone of failure or success in dialysis is the patient's own philosophy of life. In coming to terms with dialysis, a patient must accept the fact that every aspect of life must now be lived with moderation. For people whose pleasures and fulfillment are linked to physical activity, this is very hard to accept. No more prolonged, strenuous sports, no more carefree eating and drinking, no more freedom to travel, and for some, no more job and/or no more sexual activity. These losses can be unsupportable, especially the latter two.

The goals and self-image of some people like a physical education teacher I once met may be destroyed by renal failure and dialysis. Such patients should probably be placed on the transplant list. There are others, though, who can accept the necessary moderations and limitations *if* dialysis still allows them the chance to pursue their most cherished goals. I know many patients—artists, teachers, homemakers, farmers, journalists, students, technicians—who have had the flexibility to accommodate to dialysis and still continue pursuing their goals.

The human spirit is really remarkably resilient. That quality, along with an awareness of the variety of choices available to one seemingly trapped by kidney failure, gives life its meaning.

TERRY D. OBERLEY, M.D., PH.D.

PART II

Events in the life of a family first encountering kidney failure may take on the speed and suddenness of a whirlpool, as everything begins to revolve around a central, all-consuming problem. To stay afloat at the whirlpool's edge and resist the strong undertow that threatens to pull everyone into a vortex of confusion and despair can require uncommon physical and mental stamina.

Elements of family life that were once predictable, stable, and orderly may become a chaotic jumble. The family may have to contend with changes in income, residence, mobility, diet, social life, and general expectations of the future. One example among many would be the young couple who were forced deeply into debt to buy a house when their landlord refused to allow a home dialysis machine in their apartment.

These external pressures may intensify the internal emotional maelstrom that accompanies an event like kidney failure. Aside from the changes in day-to-day living, there is the strain of seeing the steady deterioration of a loved one's health, of accepting the concept of life prolonged artifically, of coping with new responsibilities and uncertainty about the future.

Kidney failure happens not just to a renal patient but to his/her family as well. Both patient *and* family members need rehabilitation; both have sustained severe emotional stress and basic life changes. My message: *family members could help the dialysis staff in the patient's rehabilitation if they themselves could receive guidance and counsel on coming to terms with their situation.*

On the basis of our own and other's experience, Terry and I have concluded that strong, sensitive family support is one of the greatest factors in a dialysis patient's ultimate rehabilitation and success with the treatment. A family's love, commitment, and dedication to the success of the dialysis venture is a heartening, invigorating presence in a patient's life. As Terry pointed out, it is one of the things a patient has to live for.

Such support, essential as it may be, must be proffered in the right way. Family members must be educated and counselled on how to provide a healthy foundation on which the patient can rebuild his physical and psychological self. Family members, particularly spouses with no guidance through the confusing scene surrounding the beginning of dialysis, can be a hindrance rather than a help. Their demonstrated love and concern can take the form of excessive solicitude, fearfulness, grief, or overreaction to every problem. Or perhaps, unable to cope with the stresses and changes, they may withdraw into detachment, leaving the patient to fend for himself. Such attitudes, if prolonged, can lead to trouble, establishing patterns of dependency or resentment.

A family's emotional adjustment will take some time, even with the presence of sympathetic help. Aside from the necessity of adjusting to the reality of chronic illness, a spouse may have a number of new responsibilities. In the first adjustment to dialysis, the patient is drained of energy, unable to perform activities we all take for granted: mowing the lawn, shopping for groceries, balancing the checkbook. In our own case, Terry did not gain much strength or stability until he had been on dialysis a year; there was always the uncertainty of wondering whether he *would* be able to resume normal activity.

Taking over household tasks may lead to confusion about roles within the family. While the patient is adjusting to dialysis, the spouse may also be responsible for major decisions formerly handled by the patient. The spouse may become the breadwinner if the patient is no longer able to work. The spouse's fulfillment of these responsibilities may have a negative effect on the patient, who may feel despondent, resentful, or guilty about placing extra burdens on the family.

The spouse may have conflicting emotions in response to the growing complexity of family life: fear for the patient and for their future together . . . fear that a mistake in home dialysis might cause a fatal accident . . . resentment toward the patient or toward the entire situation . . . a sense of helplessness that the family's fate is in the hands of the medical staff, the government, and other outside agencies. Feelings of guilt about these negative reactions can compound the whole problem.

And there are also mixed feelings about dialysis in general: gratitude for its powers and frustration at its limitations. It is also very hard to accept the fact that one's husband or wife is now being kept alive by artificial means.

The home dialysis partner is in a unique position. Here is a person who is not stricken with kidney disease, but who has nonetheless chosen to become intimately involved with this complex treatment for renal failure. The commitment in terms of time, space, scheduling, and the psychic stress of performing a lifesaving medical treatment becomes the same for the family as for the patient.

The home dialysis partner has also been thrust into the totally unfamiliar role of a quasi-nurse, partially responsible for sustaining the life and health of a loved one. The balance in the relationship between patient and partner may shift; questions may arise: "Am I a wife (husband) or a nurse?" the spouse may wonder.

How then, under these difficult circumstances, can a spouse or other family member be expected to provide intelligent, valuable support to the patient? Here is where the staff's support is invaluable. Immeasurable help can be given through education and guidance by a trained dialysis staff, not only to families of home patients, but to all dialysis family members. Many adverse reactions, such as extreme fear or grief, are born of ignorance about dialysis.

Family members, along with patients, need to learn the nuts and bolts of dialysis. Knowledge reduces fear, and an understanding of the basic chemistry of dialysis, of the reasons for symptoms and complications, of the rationale behind the medications and diet, provide motivation to succeed. Such knowledge wards off family members' extreme reactions to the typical unpleasant symptoms of vomiting, headaches, and hypotension in the early dialyses. Those with no medical knowledge have many misconceptions about dialysis; my own assumption on seeing these symptoms was that Terry would never be able to tolerate the treatment. Basic information on such matters would have been very reassuring.

Family members do need reassurance. They can see for themselves that the patient's health is terrible; they need to know that good physical and psychological adjustment is possible, that improvement, a slow process lasting perhaps as long as a year, will indeed occur.

Patients and their families attach intense importance to every word of the dialysis staff, particularly the doctor, in these early months. Hungry for information, anxious for encouragement, they are totally dependent for a time on the physical and moral sustenance of those who are saving their lives. It is a period when the fostering of trust between patient, family, and staff is crucial to the ultimate success of the dialysis experience.

Family members also need help in developing an overall, long-term perspective of their situation. They need to understand first that they are not responsible for the patient's disease: that despite whatever technical assistance they may provide with food preparation or with the dialysis treatment, proper adherence to the treatment by dialysis, diet, and medication is the patient's choice and responsibility. Families should be encouraged to lead full, active lives apart from dialysis concerns; sacrificing all other interests to the domination of dialysis can only lead to resentment.

Fostering independence and responsibility on the patient's part is a delicate proposition. Families need help in finding the right balance between two extremes: treating the patient always as a sick, dependent person or burdening the patient with expectations that are beyond his capacity to fulfill. They need to understand the importance of helping the patient when necessary without taking over vital functions he could perform himself.

Speaking of vital functions, what about sexual counselling? Spouses should know that it is available, but should never be told that sexual dysfunction is inevitable, because it is not.

These are just a few of the ways staff can help in that difficult transition of early dialysis. Family members, armed with necessary knowledge and given guidance and positive ways to cope, can ease the staff's task of helping the patient toward rehabilitation.

With the passage of time and the help of experienced, compassionate people, these early dialysis problems ease. The patient gains in physical strength and confidence, and the family gains enough experience to realize that life with dialysis will not be intolerable after all. Much adjustment evolves simply with the passage of time, which heals the rawest of frustrations.

Though that whirlpool with its threatening vortex is still there, its velocity has slowed, and those who survived the whirlpool's initial impelling force find themselves at its outer edges, in far less turbulent waters. In this more placid setting one may find acceptance, serenity, and an appreciation of life more poignant than ever before. Passing through such an experience may be a trial, but it has its rewards as well.

One reward may be stronger family relationships, rooted in a mutual commitment and sense of common purpose. In a sense, dialysis families are pioneers on a medical frontier much like the homesteaders of a century ago, who were drawn together by their struggle for very subsistence. We ourselves have found that kidney failure has taught us an abiding appreciation of family life and simple shared enjoyments like the sight of a birch tree against a blue sky.

It took some time to arrive at this point, however; in 1972, we felt submerged in a sea of uncontrollable circumstances. Terry was in the middle of an M.D.-Ph.D. program at Northwestern University when he began dialysis, and we had a new baby just two months old. Terry's physical adjustment was slow and the effects of uremia and wide blood pressure fluctuations plagued him constantly as he struggled to rotate through the clinical services during his medical training.

We were hopelessly clumsy at learning home dialysis procedures. Our inability to distinguish between a venous and arterial line seems ridiculous now, but at the time loomed as a major obstacle in our path.

The first six months of life with dialysis was a limbo of questions: Will Terry ever feel well again? Will he be able to finish medical school? Can we hope to offer our baby a normal upbringing with a kidney machine in our home? Will we ever travel to visit our family? Will we ever feel serene and at peace again?

The answer to each is a resounding *yes*. What helped bring us out of our limbo? A strong relationship (essential) . . . a caring home dialysis nurse, Sue Hansen . . . the chance to do home dialysis . . . the blessing of restored health . . . a faith in our future.

As far as my own feeling now about home dialysis is concerned, in the past years we have traveled a long road. The initial extreme solicitude, the sympathy pangs for each dialysis symptom, the nervousness before and during treatment, the resentment at its intrusion into our life, have diminished almost completely. Even fear of the future, a difficult problem to overcome when one is aware of the formidable array of complications that beset kidney patients, diminishes as stability continues and acceptance grows.

I was given the impression when we started that some psychological deterioration would take place; that the stresses would erode our relationship. The opposite has occurred; dialysis, now almost as routine as washing the dishes, is actually a pleasant time of sharing and communicating well. Terry and I are more grateful than we can say to have the opportunity to thus pursue our lives together.

The dialysis partnership is teamwork, not just technical and physical, but moral and spiritual, which can be a growing experience for everyone involved.

EDITH T. OBERLEY, M.A.

4

Teaching the Patient About End Stage Renal Disease

Carolyn J. Bess, R.N., M.S.N.

End stage renal disease is a devastating illness that affects both the patient and his family. The ability of the patient to live with this illness centers on his understanding of a complicated treatment regimen and his ability to adapt his life style to fit it. Understanding and adaptation are required of not only the patient but also of his family unit. In many patient situations a family is not present or does not hold the key role in a patient's life. Other nonrelated persons become the "significant others" and serve as "family members." From the point when a patient's family and/or significant others are identified, their educational needs become the same as the patient's. For the sake of clarity in this chapter, the word "patient" includes the patient per se, the family, and/or significant others.

The patient's need to understand his disease and his treatment regimen is based on several factors. End stage renal disease is a permanent condition. The chronic nature of the patient's illness does not allow him the opportunity to receive a reward of normality or health in the future. The best reward offered is "feeling better" but never again "normal." The chronic nature of the illness presents a tremendous problem for the patient, family, and health care team. Teaching is a desirable method for heightening the patient's ability to understand his physical condition and to accept the changes in his life style. To successfully control the chronic nature of the problem, the quality of life established by a treatment regimen must be acceptable to the patient. Compliance problems inherent with these patients are centered around factors adversely affecting life style. The strain on family roles and the ever-present financial burdens are two examples. The complicated nature of the treatment regimen is a very obvious reason why a knowledgeable patient is essential.

No other chronic illness in today's society requires as many diet restrictions, as many medications, or as large a volume of technical knowledge as is required for the patient with end stage renal disease. The complexity of dialysis alone prompts many patients to elect an in-center dialysis program rather than a home dialysis program. This choice may negatively affect the patient's adjustment to his new life style. The time and financial demands are greater for in-center dialysis patients than home dialysis patients.

The three terms used frequently when referring to dialysis are in-center dialysis, self-care dialysis, and home dialysis. These terms are defined here for the sake of clarity. *In-center dialysis* is dialysis performed within a clinic-type setting. Renal patients come to a center for a specific period of time, usually three times a week. Nurses and dialysis technicians dialyze these patients at their appointment times. There is little if any patient involvement in the dialysis treatment.

Self-care dialysis occurs in that same center and at that same appointed time. The significant difference is the amount of involvement of the patient in his own dialysis treatment. The nurse and/or technician offer assistance only as needed. The patient is in control of his treatment, but when he needs help it is present. In some situations self-care dialysis may allow patients to have more flexibility in appointment times. Evening shifts may be developed by using less personnel on evenings. This flexibility might allow a patient to work during the day and dialyze in the evening.

Home dialysis is dialysis performed in the patient's home and conducted by the patient and his assistant (significant other). The travel time required and the general lack of flexibility of time when having in-center dialysis decrease a patient's chances of maintaining a normal life style. Time for normal activities such as work and recreation is greatly reduced. In addition to time problems, the patient loses a degree of independence when choosing in-center dialysis. The cost of each dialysis is greater for in-center dialysis than home dialysis. Home dialysis does entail a greater initial cost than in-center dialysis. Self-care dialysis is one attempt to respond to the dilemma of in-center versus home dialysis. Although self-care dialysis is still more expensive than home dialysis, there is no initial cost and more independence is allowed. However, many time constraints remain. All-important is the requirement of patient involvement in his own care. Treaching the patient about the dialysis procedure thus becomes an essential element of a teaching program.

The degree of danger related to a lack of patient's knowledge reinforces the need for his understanding of his treatment regimen. An understanding of his disease and its treatment regimen decreases fear related to the unknown and improves the patient's motivation to follow a regimen. In order to sustain this motivation it is important that the patient receives benefits from learning. These benefits vary from patient to patient.

RESPONSIBILITY AND ACCOUNTABILITY

The nurse is responsible and accountable for a well-informed patient. In the nursing profession patient rehabilitation has several definitions. The essential component of those definitions is to return the patient to as near normal functioning as is possible within his physical, psychological, and sociological limitations. The overall objective of teaching is to return the patient to independent functioning. Therefore teaching is one very effective method of rehabilitation.

The nurse and patient share the responsibility for patient learning. *Responsibility* is defined as an expectation of an individual to perform in a certain way. The nurse and patient are expected to teach and to learn, respectively. Provision for learning is the nurse's responsibility. *Accountability* is defined as an obligation to perform at a certain level. The nurse is accountable for the content and the quality of teaching that occurs. The patient accepts the responsibility for understanding his care as long as the content is presented on a reasonable level. An assessment of the patient's readiness to learn, ability to communicate, and learning needs identifies that reasonable level of understanding. The teaching plan and its evaluation and modification document the accomplishment of that reasonable level of understanding. For example, patients with special learning disabilities require some alterations in the method of teaching. For various reasons, there are patients who cannot learn. The teacher identifies these patients and documents the problems. The health team including the patient discusses these problems and alternative approaches.

PRINCIPLES OF TEACHING
Readiness to Learn

As health care providers, nurses have the knowledge and skills to teach patients about renal disease and its treatment regimen. Although principles of teaching can be applied to all chronically ill patients, the patient with end stage renal disease presents special problems. These problems become apparent at the initiation of the teaching-learning process. The first step in teaching is to evaluate the patient's readiness to learn. Readiness involves both physical and psychological components. Evaluation of readiness requires that the health teacher be skilled in obtaining and validating information by use of a nursing history and other health records. Readiness to learn is the beginning of a successful teaching-learning process. Readiness cannot be measured in time. Therefore, the nurse working in a hospital acute dialysis setting and the nurse working in a long-term dialysis center are equally responsible for initiating the teaching process. The evaluation process is basically the same in both settings.

Physical Readiness

Careful consideration of the patient's current physical state is essential. A patient whose physiological survival is being threatened cannot comprehend complex or lengthy explanations. Simple and short directions with repetition is the desired approach. When a patient's physiological state is unstable, there is a real discrepancy between what he needs to know and what he is capable of understanding. As the nurse observes such physiological parameters stabilizing, she should repeat her initial patient interview. During this interview she is reviewing the patient's present physical state and his understanding of his present condition.

The formal nursing history and the informal conversation with the patient provide valuable data concerning physical readiness. The physical examination portion of the history is absolutely vital to assessing a patient's physical readiness to learn. During the acute stage of renal disease the body experiences tremendous physical stresses. Presence of uremia and equally persistent anemia physically alters the patient's ability to comprehend. As the patient is medically treated for renal disease, there may be concomitant disabilities or illnesses to be considered. The new threat to his homeostasis, renal disease, does not decrease the importance of other chronic threats such as diabetes mellitus or heart disease. The astute nurse uses the patient's past knowledge and experience to his advantage. Knowledge of patient disabilities is equally important to the nurse in evaluating the patient's readiness to learn. Poor eyesight or deafness are examples of physical disabilities that have special meaning to the nurse planning a teaching program.

Psychological Readiness

Psychological readiness includes the patient's current mental status and his previous knowledge and experience. The patient interview is a means to obtain data related to psychological readiness.

The patient's emotional status, his motivation for learning, and his general attitude toward health care are the main components of mental readiness. Initially the emotional climate is one of apprehension and anxiety. The uremia may cause mental alterations such as forgetfulness and shortened attention span, which increase the anxiety already present. In order to cope with his anxiety a patient may use any of several coping behaviors. The degree to which a patient can use denial does not directly relate to the seriousness of his illness. Patients ignore symptoms or minimize their importance. Denial can be in relation to time. An example is the patient who clings to the hope that kidney function will return any day. Until the patient accepts his diagnosis and the indicated treatment regimen, teaching is of minimal value. Depending on the extent of his denial, a patient can learn to accept his illness through the use of a teaching program. This acceptance through teaching occurs less frequently than nurses would like to think.

Another patient coping behavior is anger. It is not unusual for a patient to be angry. Renal patients contend with physical symptoms that serve to reinforce ill-humor. A patient's ill-humor does not preclude his learning, but free-floating anger is a definite block to learning. The aggressively angry patient, if not handled appropriately, can destroy a group teaching program. A nurse must have the ability to set limits on the patient's behavior.

Depression is a very prevalent coping behavior in response to chronic illness. Passive, withdrawn behavior is characteristic of depression. Patients are overwhelmed by their illness and are unable to deal with the stress by their usual mechanisms. Also, depression can entail anger that is internalized. Different from the aggressive patient, the depressed patient does not affect group learning but does affect his individual ability to learn. Patient education can be a very effective means to help the patient cope with slight to moderate depression. The patient learns to resume control of his life and his surroundings. Severe depression blocks patient learning and is a pathological state. The nurse who identifies such a patient should discuss that patient with the physician.

These coping behaviors are not all-inclusive but make up the major responses to anxiety. It is this complex emotional climate with which the nurse deals.

Another component of mental readiness is a patient's motivation to learn. The difficulty patients have in adjusting to their illness is one cause of lack of motivation. The lack of motivation can also derive from a patient's value system; an example is the patient who because of religious beliefs is very specific about his dietary requirements. Another example is the patient who values enjoying his life today in the fullest without regard for tomorrow, whereas health is a future-oriented goal. Variations in values are also observed between cultural groups and socioeconomic classes. The nurse attempts to reconcile these values by reordering and altering them.

For motivation to be successfully reinforced, the patient must receive benefits from his learning. The use of incentives for learning improves motivation. Motivation can be external or internal. External incentives are praise or concrete rewards. Internal motivation is based on a patient's believing that his learning is useful to him (1).

The third component of mental readiness is a patient's general attitude toward health care—more specifically, his attitude toward who should be responsible for his health care. For example, if the patient believes that no one but the physician should tell him how to care for himself, the nurse finds being his teacher very difficult. Another example is the patient who firmly believes that the doctor and nurse are responsible for his health care and he is merely a passive observer. This patient sees no benefits to his learning. A final example is the patient who has no confidence in health care givers in general and strongly believes that he will be the judge of what is good or bad for him. These situations are not all that uncommon, and therefore the challenge to the health teacher is even more profound. The examples given reinforce the need for a total team effort in establishing and implementing a patient's teaching program.

In addition to mental readiness, psychological readiness to learn is based on a patient's previous knowledge and experiences. Basic indicators of general knowledge are a patient's formal education level and his ability to read. As educators have learned, an individual's high school diploma does not mean that he can read. Although the level of education is essential information, the nurse finds that a patient's ability to learn is not limited by little formal education. The nurse must know the educational level to individualize the teaching program to the patient's method of learning. Age is one indicator of the patient's developmental level. Life experiences can expand or limit that level. Some individuals are limited in their experience within the world. Their vocabulary is greatly restricted, and their ability to solve problems is limited. On interview the nurse observes a slow, careful individual who is oriented to short-term, action goals. This less mature individual must see, hear, feel, smell, and taste in deference to reading (1).

The patient's past experience related to health education plays an important role. His past medical record offers some data related to his response to health teaching. The likelihood of similar problems' occurring along with the current health crisis is high. Preconceived ideas concerning health education can be significant blocks for the learner. Positive learning situations related to past health teaching can be a valuable stimulus to learning.

COMMUNICATION

In order to accomplish effective teaching the nurse needs to promote effective communication and to maintain an environment conducive to learning. Communication is divided into two categories, verbal and nonverbal.

Verbal Communication

Verbal communication includes the spoken word. Effective verbal communication demands two components. First, the nurse must use a vocabulary consistent with the patient's vocabulary. She evaluates vocabulary usage during the initial interview. Careful consideration is given to everyday language usage versus medical terminology. Another consideration is the patient's ability to speak and understand English. Special attention is given to evaluating the special language problems. Second, the nurse must obtain feedback from the patient as to his understanding. Verbal feedback sometimes is deceiving. The nurse must not assume the patient understands just because he says, "I understand." The nurse asks questions specific to the communication required. Repetition of the verbal communication given is the basic method used for feedback.

Nonverbal Communication

Nonverbal communication assumes written and behavioral forms. The written form is used frequently in the teaching-learning setting. At this point the nurse uses the evaluation of the patient's ability to read and write. To communicate concerning renal disease and its treatment she establishes a glossary of commonly used terms. This list of definitions, along with all other written educational material, must be supplemented with verbal communication. Evaluation of the renal patient's understanding of instructions (verbal and written) can be accomplished by use of written tests.

Nonverbal behavior by the nurse and patient affects communication. The nurse, for example, can indicate interest or boredom by nonverbal behavior. Much nonverbal behavior is unconscious. In order to offer the patient that extra incentive to learn, the nurse needs to make a conscious effort to nod her head and smile. Impatient or disinterested behavior by the nurse can be a serious block to learning. The patient's nonverbal behavior gives the nurse clues about readiness to learn and ability to understand verbal communication. Such clues alone are not conclusive, but they can be indicators of success or failure.

Physical Environment

The learner's physical surroundings are important to his ability to concentrate. Physical discomfort of any kind, especially discomfort related to temperature and seating arrangements, is undesirable. Distraction due to noise and equipment failure reduces the patient's ability to take in all the material presented. The nurse's responsibility is to control the environment to the best of her ability.

ASSESSMENT OF LEARNING NEEDS

The process used in assessing learning needs depends on the method of teaching to be used. When a single patient is to be taught, the learning needs of that patient are assessed. When a group of patients is to be taught, their learning needs are assessed to be those of the average renal patient. The group classes should retain some flexibility to serve the needs of specific membership, but the classes must ultimately remain structured. Within the assessment phase the nurse identifies those patients who can only learn in a one-to-one teaching relationship. In order to make that determination, the nurse ascertains the patient's readiness to learn, his ability to communicate, and his specific learning needs. If there are patients who are having significant problems with their readiness to learn and their ability to communicate, these problems prevent these specific patients from benefiting from group classes. In some situations the patient and nurse are able to resolve or lessen the blocks to group instruction. A group allows the patient to have contact with patients with similar adjustment problems.

Assessment of Individual Patient Learning Needs

In order to effectively assess learning needs, the nurse must interview the patient. She asks him questions about his knowledge of renal disease and its treatment regimen. This questioning session provides the data needed for establishing the patient's individualized teaching plan. A significant part is played by the nurse's ability to listen and observe.

Listening involves receiving and accurately interpreting information. When listening, the nurse may receive direct and/or indirect requests for knowledge. Responding to the patient's requests by including them in the teaching plan gives significant motivation for the patient to learn.

Observation of the patient entails correctly identifying patient behavior. The patient expresses needs verbally and nonverbally. Assessing learning needs requires that a nurse be trained in interviewing and teaching techniques and that she possesses a thorough knowledge of renal disease and its treatment regimen.

Structured Classes: Assessment of Patient Learning Needs

For structured classes to be effective the participants must have common learning needs. To identify those commonalities is the nurse's responsibility.

IMPLEMENTATION OF A STRUCTURED TEACHING PROGRAM
Development of a Content Outline

To develop a content outline the nurse reviews the current literature on end stage renal disease and its treatment regimen. She further defines the relevant body of knowledge by using certain resources. Those resources are the nurse's knowledge and experience, the physicians' input, the renal patients' responses, and the opinions of other health team professionals. Usually a nurse has some experience in teaching patients on a one-to-one basis; this experience in teaching provides the basis for developing and implementing a structured teaching program.

Physicians' input is sought in order to take full advantage of their medical knowledge and experience. It is extremely important to include the physicians not only in the planning phase, but also in the teaching phase. The well-informed physician is an excellent source for patient referrals to the teaching program.

Another way of determining the reasonable body of knowledge is by interviewing renal patients. Prior renal patients can offer valuable suggestions for setting up positive learning experiences. The patients' experiences in trying to understand their disease and its treatment regimen give the nurse some insights into the initial and long-term adjustment problems they encounter. An example of patient input is the type of questions that patients most frequently ask during individual instructions.

Consultations with other health team professionals add additional expertise to the resources. Professional persons such as dietitians and social workers are those called on most frequently. After processing all this information, the nurse develops a content outline. An example of a content outline can be found at the end of this chapter just before the teaching program.

Development of Teaching Objectives

Teaching objectives are statements of expectations as a result of the teaching-learning process. Teaching objectives should be written as clearly as possible. Since learning is the important concept, objectives are stated in relationship to what the patient is to learn. In this chapter the difference between the teaching and behavioral objectives is in the degree of preciseness of the objectives. The teaching objective states what the patient learns at the end of the entire session. The behavioral objective specifies the exact behavior expected within the delineated subject areas. Behavioral objectives are discussed in more detail later in this chapter.

Classification of Objectives

In order to classify objectives in health teaching, it is necessary to review the three domains developed by educators and psychologists. These domains are used to define behaviors in relationship to objectives.

The *psychomotor domain* deals with motor skills and includes perception of a stimulus, preparation, guided response, mechanism (habit), complex overt response, adaptation, and origination of motor skills (1). Mastering of motor skills is necessary in a great portion of health teaching. The simple skills are mastered first. The more complex skills are left for later.

The *cognitive domain* deals with intellectual abilities and includes knowledge, comprehension, application, analysis, synthesis, and evaluation (2). Cognitive learning occurs in all health teaching. The process entails starting with concrete concepts, then progressing to the more abstract ones. A concept is an idea, not a word or an object (1).

The *affective domain* deals with expression of feeling and includes attentiveness, responsiveness, acceptance of values, organization of values, and characterization by a value (2). This domain requires increasing commitment to a feeling. The hierarchy develops from simple awareness to a complex system of values (1).

Development of Class Content

After determining the teaching objectives, the nurse develops the teaching program further by listing the class content devoted to each objective. Within an extended program such as the one that renal patients must attend, the nurse begins with content that requires simple skills, thoughts, and feelings. An example is seen in the order of content within the psychomotor domain. The nurse begins with skills such as shunt care and progresses to the more complex dialysis procedure. Within the cognitive domain the content begins with the patient's disease process and progresses to the more complex complications of renal disease. Within the affective domain the patient is first expected to be willing to try. Hopefully, he progresses to a commitment to adhere to his treatment regimen.

The class content must be detailed and include all content to be covered. When behavioral objectives are utilized in the teaching plan, the expected behaviors specifically define the class content. Behavioral objectives are a method of stating class content in learning terms.

Development of Behavioral Objectives

Behavioral objectives are statements of specific patient behaviors that are expected after a teaching-learning process. The behavioral objective specifies one behavior in one subject area. The most frequent error made in writing behavioral objectives is a lack of clarity. In describing patient behavior, the nurse uses verbs that can be interpreted precisely. For example, the verbs such as identify, state, describe, and demonstrate are specific and can be evaluated. On the other hand the verbs such as feel, believe, and think are easily misunderstood and cannot be evaluated adequately (1). Within the teaching program presented at the end of this chapter, the behavioral objectives are categorized in their appropriate domains.

Teaching and Learning Activities

After the behavioral objectives are completed, the teaching and learning activities are stated. Teaching and learning activities include methods and materials to be used by the nurse. For example, lecturing, question-and-answer sessions, and demonstrations are standard types of activities. It is important to make the activities suit the behavioral objectives. The nurse must remember that teaching and learning activities that add any degree of complexity to the content is undesirable. Learning made simple provides a patient with a much broader knowledge base from which he can build more complex concepts.

Activities should make the learning process pleasant and interesting. The nurse's originality and creativity are exhibited at this stage of implementation. The methods and materials should be suited to the age and educational level of the patients. Clarity, neatness, and eye appeal are very important. Teaching and learning activities should demonstrate organization and accuracy in content. Other areas that should be considered are the class size and the time required for the planned activities.

Class Size and Time Requirements

There is always a desirable class size and duration. Problems arise when pressures make that size or duration infeasible. It is still very important to set maximum class sizes and minimum time commitments, so that the program remains flexible enough to allow for some individual patient instruction. It is best to plan for that flexibility early.

EVALUATION

Evaluation is performed to determine if learning has occurred. Evaluation of the teaching-learning process, whether individualized or group, is essential. Methods used vary from patient interviews, to questionnaires, to written tests. Whatever evaluation method is used, the end product of the teaching-learning process must be stated clearly before the teaching occurs. As we noted earlier, the use of behavioral objectives allows the nurse and patient to understand what is expected of the patient. The more precise the behaviors, the more specific the evaluation.

Another type of evaluation that should occur in a structured teaching program is the patient's individual evaluation of each instructor. This evaluation process can provide the instructor with valuable information. The instructor may find a need to improve her teaching style and techniques or find that a new teaching approach was well received by the patients. The purpose of evaluation is to improve the patient learning process.

Nurses as teachers must remember that patient education is a continuous process. A patient who completes a formal educational program such as outlined in this chapter has the opportunity to acquire a large volume of knowledge and skills. For various reasons patients may fail to learn and/or retain much of the material presented. This humanistic factor reiterates the need for the entire health team to review, clarify, and reinforce all important points regarding the patient's treatment regimen. During a patient's regular health check-up or clinic visit, the nurse and/or patient can then expand his control of his health and his life by increasing his knowledge of his treatment regimen.

PATIENT TEACHING PROGRAM

The remainder of this chapter presents certain parts of a patient teaching program. Examples are given of enough of the teaching program to offer the reader assistance in planning, implementing, and evaluating a teaching program.

Special attention should be given to the teaching and behavioral objectives. Because of space limitations, all of the teaching objectives listed are not developed here into individual teaching sessions. The sessions chosen demonstrate typical teaching situations. The behavioral objectives are placed in their appropriate domain. An example is given for each domain to clarify this technique.

The teaching and learning activities listed are not exhaustive. The nurse should experiment with different activities in order to develop the best possible for the individual patient's learning experience.

End Stage Renal Disease Patient Teaching Program Content Outline

    I. Introduction
        A. Purpose of program
        B. Expectations of the patients
        C. Discussion of patient's feelings regarding his renal failure and
           its treatment
   II. The Normal Kidney
        A. Structure
        B. Function
        C. Structure and function of the normal urinary tract
  III. Kidney Failure
        A. Types
        B. Causes
  IV. Medication Regimen
        A. Purpose of each prescribed drug
        B. Side effects of each prescribed drug
        C. Times for medication administration
        D. Financial resources

V. Dietary Regimen
  A. Protein
  B. Potassium
  C. Sodium
  D. Fluids
  E. Calories
  F. Discussion of individual dietary plans
VI. Access to Circulation
  A. External shunt
  B. Internal arteriovenous fistula
  C. Arterial graft
VII. Dialysis
  A. Types
  B. Principles
  C. Procedure
  D. Complications
  E. Interpretation of lab values related to dialysis
VIII. Complications of Chronic Renal Failure
  A Causes
  B. Signs and symptoms
  C. Diagnostic methods
  D. Medical management
  E. Prevention
IX. Transplantantation
  A. Principles
  B. Operative procedure
  C. Postoperative stage including complications
  D. Long-term care
X. Resources for Patients with Renal Disease
  A. Health care
  B. Community
  C. Financial
XI. Evaluation of the program

End Stage Renal Disease Patient Teaching Program Teaching Objectives

1. To be familiar with the purpose of the teaching program and to demonstrate an interest in learning about end stage renal disease and the treatment regimen.
2. To understand the structure and function of the normal kidney.
3. To understand types and causes of kidney failure, with emphasis on the patient's specific diagnosis.

4. To understand the basis of the medication regimen and to implement the prescribed regimen.
5. To understand the basis of the prescribed dietary plan and to implement the individualized plan.
6. To be familiar with the various types of circulatory access for hemodialysis with specific information regarding the patient's circulatory access.
7. To demonstrate the ability to perform the required care of the patient's selected circulatory access.
8. To understand the principles of dialysis.
9. To be familiar with the various aspects of the dialysis procedure.
10. To demonstrate the ability to initiate, monitor, and discontinue the dialysis procedure.
11. To understand the specific complications of dialysis in relation to cause, prevention, and management.
12. To demonstrate the ability to perform measures regarding prevention and/or management of complications during the dialysis procedure.
13. To be able to relate lab values to the signs and symptoms of uremia.
14. To be able to make necessary adjustments in the dialysis procedure in relationship to lab values.
15. To understand the causes, signs, symptoms, diagnostic methods, prevention, and management of complications of end stage renal disease.
16. To understand principles of renal transplantation.
17. To be made aware of health care, community, and financial resources for patients with end stage renal disease.

End Stage Renal Disease Patient Teaching Program Lesson Plans

Lesson I

OBJECTIVE: To be familiar with the purpose of the teaching program and to demonstrate an interest in learning about end stage renal disease and the treatment regimen.

Class Content
  1. Introductions
  2. Overview of the teaching program including:
     a. The purpose of the course
     b. Reasons why the program is important to the patient.

  c. The written material to be utilized.

  d. The expectations that the instructor has of the patient.

3. Patient discussion of feelings regarding his renal failure and its treatment.

Teaching and Learning Activities*

- Introductions to instructors and other class members.
- Hand out booklets containing objectives and behavioral objectives.
- Group discussion.

Behavioral Objectives

Upon completion of this lesson the patient will be able to:

Cognitive Domain

1. State the purpose of the teaching program: To learn about renal failure and the treatment regimen.

Affective Domain

2. Express a willingness to try to understand renal failure and the treatment regimen.
3. Be aware that instructors are available to answer questions.
4. Be aware that the written information received is important.
5. Be aware that much of the program will be individualized to his needs.
6. Be aware that by learning more about his disease and the treatment regimen he will have more opportunities for making decisions that affect his life and his health.
7. Be aware that he will be exposed to the ideas of other patients.
8. Be aware that other patients are facing some of the same problems that he faces.
9. Be aware that he can expect to regain strength; therefore, he should begin to make plans for his future.

Lesson II

OBJECTIVE: To understand the structure and function of the normal kidney.

Class Content

1. Structure and function of the normal kidney.
2. Structure and function of the normal urinary tract.

Teaching and Learning Activities

- Lecture

*The teaching and learning activities are suggestions and are not limitations.

- Slides of the structure of the kidney, nephron, and urinary tract.
- Glossary of most commonly used terms.

Behavioral Objectives
Upon completion of this lesson the patient will be able to:

Cognitive Domain
1. Describe the kidneys in regard to size and number.
2. State the location of the kidneys.
3. Explain that one healthy kidney is adequate for normal functioning.
4. State major functions of the kidney:
    a. Regulate the amount of fluid in the body.
    b. Remove waste products from the blood.
    c. Maintain proper balance of chemicals.
    d. Regulate blood pressure.
    e. Help control the production of red blood cells.
5. Describe the pathway of urine from the kidney pelvis to the outside as follows:
    a. Ureters, long thin tubes, carry the urine from the kidney pelvis to the bladder
    b. The bladder is a reservoir for urine and is located in the lower abdomen
    c. The urethra, a tube, carries the urine from the bladder to the outside of the body
6. Define the terms:
    a. Urea.
    b. Nitrogen.
    c. Creatinine.
    d. Electrolyte.

Lesson III

OBJECTIVE: To understand types and causes of kidney failure, with emphasis on the patient's specific diagnosis.

Class Content
1. Types and causes of kidney failure.

Teaching and Learning Activities
- Lecture
- Slides
- Discussion

Behavioral Objectives
Upon completion of this lesson the patient will be able to:

Cognitive Domain

1. Describe the types of renal failure:
    a. Acute renal failure develops rapidly and may be reversible or irreversible.
    b. Chronic renal failure develops more gradually and may be partial or complete.
2. State what type of renal failure he is experiencing.
3. State that renal failure is caused by many different diseases and conditions.
4. Identify that the causes can be divided into two areas: abnormalities inside and outside the kidneys.
5. State the cause (if known) of his renal failure.

Affective Domain

6. Verify that the kidneys are unlikely to improve after a chronic disease once they have failed to the point that dialysis is required.

Cognitive Domain

7. State that people with renal failure can usually manage to maintain a reasonable state of health by following the three principles of treatment:
    a. Taking *drugs or medications* exactly as prescribed.
    b. Following the *diet*.
    c. Regular *dialysis*.

Affective Domain

8. Verify that the treatment for renal failure is complicated.

Class Content
2. Patient's specific diagnosis.

Teaching and Learning Activities
• Individual or small group discussion.

Behavioral Objectives
Upon completion of the specific lesson relating to the individual's diagnosis,* the patient will be able to:

Cognitive Domain

Chronic Glomerulonephritis
1. Identify that chronic glomerulonephritis is one of the most common causes of kidney failure.
2. State that the disease is not inherited.
3. State that chronic glomerulonephritis is a chronic inflammation that affects the glomerulus.

*The diseases listed are examples of common causes of renal failure.

4. Define inflammation as the irritation that surrounds an injured tissue.
5. Identify that streptococcal infections are the most frequent cause of glomerulonephritis.
6. State that the inflammation eventually destroys all of the glomeruli in both kidneys.
7. Identify that the destruction of the glomeruli leads to loss of the entire nephron and decreased renal function.

Systemic Lupus Erythematosus (SLE)
1. State that SLE is not inherited.
2. State that SLE involves a type of inflammation of the glomeruli.
3. Define inflammation as the irritation that surrounds an injured tissue.
4. State that the cause of SLE is unknown.
5. Identify that SLE can affect many other organs in the body.
6. Explain that it is essential to watch for development of complications in addition to kidney failure.
7. Identify some of the additional complications of SLE:
   a. Pleurisy (pain in the chest on breathing).
   b. Pericarditis (inflammation around the heart).
   c. Arthritis (pain and swelling of the joints).
   d. Skin rash.

Chronic Hypertension (high blood pressure)
1. State that high blood pressure (HBP) is one of the most common causes of kidney damage.
2. Identify that HBP has few warning symptoms.
3. Describe the cycle developed by the HBP damaging the kidney and the increasing kidney damage causing the blood pressure to go even higher.
4. Identify that HBP leads to kidney damage called nephrosclerosis or chronic scarring of the kidney.
5. Explain that if the blood pressure is not controlled, the blood vessels become thickened, circulation to the kidney gradually fails, and kidney function eventually decreases to the point that dialysis is required.
6. Identify that HBP may be controlled.

Malignant Hypertension
1. State that malignant hypertension is a very severe form of HBP.
2. Identify that the extremely high levels of blood pressure quickly destroy the kidneys to the point that dialysis is required permanently.

3. State that malignant hypertension can complicate any kidney disease that causes hypertension.
4. Identify that some patients who have had malignant hypertension require bilateral nephrectomy after they begin dialysis because the blood pressure is so severely elevated.

Chronic Pyelonephritis
1. Define chronic pylonephritis as a chronic infection of the kidneys.
2. State that the infection must be widespread and serious in order to destroy both kidneys.
3. Identify that there are usually some structural abnormalities (problems) with the urinary tract that make infection more likely.
4. State that with chronic pyelonephritis the kidney becomes a mass of scar tissue with very little normal tissue.
5. Identify hypertension as a frequent complication.
6. Explain that patients with this disease can receive a kidney transplant but their own kidneys must be removed in order to prevent infection from damaging the transplant.
7. Identify that urinary tract studies with x-rays and other tests are necessary so that any abnormalities (problems) may be corrected.

Diabetic Nephropathy
1. State that diabetes mellitus damages blood vessels throughout the body after a number of years by causing thickening of the walls of the smaller blood vessels.
2. Define diabetic nephropathy as a thickening of the blood vessels in the kidney.
3. Identify the other organ systems adversely affected by the thickening of vessels: eyes, brain, and heart.
4. State that the additional kidney complication of diabetes mellitus is frequent infections.

Polycystic Kidney Disease
1. State that polycystic kidney disease is an inherited condition.
2. Explain that on the average half the children will develop the disease.
3. State that the disease does not usually appear before the age of 20.
4. Explain the disease process as one in which the kidney gradually becomes a mass of cysts displacing and destroying normal kidney tissue.
5. Identify that the kidneys become quite large.
6. Identify the large size of the polycystic kidneys as one cause of pain.

7. State the common complications:
    a. Urinary tract infections.
    b. Bleeding from the polycystic kidneys.
    c. Kidney stones.
8. Identify that the polycystic kidneys must be removed before a kidney transplantation is performed.
9. State that removal of polysystic kidneys is a major operation.

Lesson IV

OBJECTIVE: To understand the basis of the medication regimen and to implement the prescribed regimen.

Class Content
1. Basis of medication administration.
2. Discussion of medications that patients must take, including the purpose, the side effects, and the times when the medications should be taken.
3. Discussion of financial resources for drug costs.

Teaching and Learning Activities
• Lecture
• Slides.
• Charts with samples of medications and the current cost.

Behavioral Objectives
Upon completion of this lesson the patient will be able to:

Cognitive Domain
1. Identify that an important part of treatment of kidney failure is medications (drugs).
2. List the names of the drugs he should take.
3. List the drugs he should not take.
4. State the specific purpose of each prescribed drug.
5. List the times when he should take his medications.
6. Describe the major side effects of prescribed drugs.
7. Identify the importance of discussing the occurrence of drug side effects with a member of the health team.
8. Identify the importance of reviewing the list of prescribed medications with a member of the health team at regular intervals.
9. State that he should carry a list of all his prescribed medications with him at all times.
10. Identify the need to have all medication bottles labeled with the name and instructions for taking the drug.

11. State that medications can differ in size and color depending on brands.
12. State the importance of verifying medications with his druggist when he questions the size or color.
13. Identify method for financial support for the cost of drugs.

Lesson V

OBJECTIVE: To understand the basis of the prescribed dietary plan and to implement the individualized plan.

Class Content
1. Purposes of the dietary regimen.
2. Results of dietary noncompliance.
3. Requirements and limitations of the dietary regimen.
4. Provision of prescribed dietary regimen for each participant.
5. Sample menus of the dietary regimen.
6. Ways to apply the dietary regimen to social situations.

Teaching and Learning Activities
• Lecture.
• Slides.
• Food models.
• Sample menus.
• Individualized planning sessions.

Behavioral Objectives
Upon completion of this lesson the patient will be able to:

Cognitive Domain
1. Identify that the maintenance of health depends upon eating the proper foods in the proper amounts.
2. Define nutrients as substances in food that the body needs.
3. State that proper nutritional balance requires that nutrients are added to the body in the same amounts in which they were lost.
4. Identify that patients with kidney failure develop serious disturbances in the balance of many of the body's important nutrients and chemicals.
5. Define chemicals as substances in food and other ingestible material that the normal body can use or excrete as needed.
6. State that the prescribed diet can help restore and maintain a proper balance of these important nutrients and chemicals within the body.
7. State that the purposes of the prescribed diet are to control the

intake of fluid, to decrease the production of protein waste products, and to control the intake of the chemicals that are dangerous to the dialysis patient.

8. State that the results of too much sodium and fluid in the diet are hypertension, edema, and shortness of breath.

9. State that the results of excess amounts of protein in the diet *may* include pericarditis, neuropathy, nausea, vomiting, and other symptoms of uremia.

10. State that the result of too much potassium in the diet is hyperkalemia, which *may* cause serious problems with the heart.

11. State that the result of less than the proper number of calories in the diet is the utilization of protein for energy and thus an increase in uremic signs and symptoms.

12. Identify that eating an improper diet causes a deterioration of his medical condition and produces a need for more dialysis.

13. Describe the requirements and limitations of the fluid restriction.

14. Describe the requirements and limitations of the sodium restriction.

15. Describe the requirements and limitations of the potassium restriction.

16. Describe the requirements and limitations of the calcium restriction.

17. Describe the requirements and limitations of the phosphorus restriction.

18. Describe the calorie requirements of the diet.

19. State the reasons for the calorie requirements.

20. Identify the importance of reading all package labels.

21. Identify the importance of weighing and measuring all foods and liquids that are ingested.

Affective Domain

22. Identify the diet as an important part of the treatment regimen.

23. Verbalize a willingness to follow the prescribed diet.

24. Identify the need to apply the prescribed dietary regimen to social situations outside the home.

Psychomotor Domain

25. Plan menus that are within his prescribed dietary requirements and limitations.

26. Prepare meals that are within his prescribed dietary requirements and limitations.

27. Follow the prescribed dietary regimen.

Lesson VI

OBJECTIVE: To be familiar with the various types of circulatory access for hemodialysis with specific information regarding the patient's selected circulatory access.

Class Content
1. Purposes of circulatory access.
2. Discussion of the three types of circulatory access including:
   a. Surgery.
   b. Appearance.
   c. Advantages.
   d. Disadvantages.
   e. Possible problems.
   f. Care of the access.

Teaching and Learning Activities
• Lecture.
• Slides.
• Models of external cannula.
• Demonstrations.

Behavioral Objectives
Upon completion of this lesson the patient will be able to:

Cognitive Domain
1. State the purposes of the circulatory access.
2. Describe the blood flow from the body to the artificial kidney and back to the body.
3. List the three types of circulatory access:
   a. External cannula.
   b. Internal fistula.
   c. Arterial graft.
4. Recognize the three types of access.
5. State the advantages of each access.
6. State the disadvantages of each access.
7. Describe the surgery required for his selected circulatory access.
8. List the possible problems of his selected circulatory access.
9. List the signs and symptoms of shunt problems that should be reported immediately to the physician.
10. State the shunt problems that can wait until a regularly scheduled visit to the physician.
11. Describe the care of his selected access.
12. State the purpose of Coumadin therapy for external shunts.
13. State the purpose of antibiotic therapy for external shunts.

Lesson VII

OBJECTIVE: To demonstrate the ability to perform the required care of the patient's selected circulatory access.

Class Content
1. Procedure for the following:
   a. Cleaning the external shunt.
   b. Checking for the patency of the shunt.
   c. Checking for infection of the shunt.
   d. Protecting the shunt against injury.

Teaching and Learning Activities
   • Demonstration.
   • Return demonstration.

Behavioral Objectives*
Upon completion of this lesson the patient will be able to demonstrate the ability to:

External Cannula

Psychomotor Domain
1. Clean his shunt every day following the procedure correctly.
2. Observe for skin rash that can develop as a reaction to the cleansing agents or an antibiotic ointment.
3. Apply a sterile dressing to the shunt as demonstrated.
4. Check for patency of the shunt by feeling for the thrill or listening for the bruit.
5. Observe for the signs of a clotted shunt at least three times a day:
   a. Dark bluish or black blood noted in the tubing.
   b. Areas of clear fluid (serum) mixed with particles of visible blood clot.
   c. Coolness of the shunt.
   d. Pain in the shunt area.
6. Observe for signs of infection, including pain, tenderness, drainage, redness, and swelling around the shunt.
7. Place a piece of tape around the connection to prevent accidental disconnection.
8. Keep two cannula clamps (bulldog clamps) on the dressing at all times.
9. Use the cannula clamps as demonstrated.

*The patient will only be required to complete the part of the lesson that involves his selected circulatory access.

Cognitive Domain

10. List the precautions to be taken to prevent decreased blood flow to the shunt.
11. List the precautions to be taken to prevent contamination of the shunt site.
12. List the precautions to be taken to prevent injury to the shunt and/or the shunt extremity.
13. List the main reasons for revising or replacing a shunt.
14. Define a shuntogram.

Internal Fistula

Psychomotor Domain

1. Perform fistula exercises as demonstrated.
2. Rotate the needle puncture sites.
3. Apply firm pressure to needle puncture sites after dialysis.
4. Apply sterile bandages after needles are removed.
5. Observe for a hematoma or bleeding after venipuncture.
6. Observe for patency of the fistula.

Cognitive Domain

7. List the precautions to be taken to prevent clotting of the fistula.

Arterial Graft

Psychomotor Domain

1. Rotate the needle puncture sites.
2. Apply firm pressure to needle puncture sites after dialysis.
3. Apply sterile bandages after needles are removed.
4. Observe for a hematoma or bleeding after venipuncture.
5. Observe for patency of the graft.
6. Observe for infection of the graft.

Cognitive Domain

7. List the precautions to be taken to prevent clotting of the graft.

Lesson VIII

OBJECTIVE: To understand the principles of dialysis.

Class Content

1. Purpose of dialysis.
2. Principles of dialysis involving the following areas:
   a. Preparation for dialysis.
   b. Process of dialysis.
   c. Machinery used.

Teaching and Learning Activities
- Lecture.
- Slides.
- Demonstrations.

Behavioral Objectives
Upon completion of this lesson the patient will be able to:

Cognitive Domain
1. State the purpose of dialysis.
2. Identify the main principle of the dialysis system.
3. Identify that waste products are produced when the body uses food.
4. State that urea and creatinine are two of these waste products.
5. Explain the process of diffusion.
6. Define a semipermeable membrane.
7. Explain the process of osmosis.
8. List the contents of dialysate.
9. State that weight gain should be kept to a pound to one and one-half pounds a day.
10. State that dialysis is used to remove a reasonable amount of fluid.
11. Describe how fluid is forced across the semipermeable membrane.
12. Define negative pressure.
13. Define positive (venous) pressure.
14. Define total transmembrane pressure.
15. Define dry weight.
16. Describe how to calculate the amount of fluid to be removed during dialysis.
17. State how to calculate the total transmembrane pressure.
18. Identify that dialyzers vary considerably in design, ultrafiltration rate, clearance, and priming volume.
19. Identify the purposes of the delivery system.
20. State the purpose of each monitor and alarm of the delivery system.
21. List the requirements of the water supply for the delivery system.
22. Describe the path of blood through the dialyzer.
23. State that the blood path is a completely sterile system.
24. State that the dialyzer and tubing are primed with saline before dialysis is started.
25. State the three major reasons saline is used during dialysis:
    a. To remove air from the blood lines and dialyzer.
    b. To replace fluid lost during dialysis when necessary.
    c. To flush blood from the dialyzer at the end of the dialysis.

26. State the purpose of heparin during dialysis.
27. State the reason for determining the clotting time during dialysis.
28. State the purpose of determining the rate of blood flow during dialysis.

REFERENCES

1. Barbara K Redman: *The Process of Patient Teaching in Nursing.* St. Louis, Mosby, 1976.
2. Benjamin S Bloom. *Taxonomy of Educational Objectives: The Classification of Educational Goals, Handbook 1 and 2: Cognitive and Affective Domain.* New York, David McKay, 1974.

BIBLIOGRAPHY

Anger D: The psychologic stress of chronic renal failure and long-term hemodialysis. *Nursing Clin North Am* 10(3): 449–460, 1975.

Bille D: A study of patients' knowledge in relation to teaching format and compliance. *Supervisor Nurse* 8(3): 55–62, 1977.

Bloom B (ed): *Taxonomy of Educational Objectives: The Classification of Educational Goals, Handbook 1: Cognitive Domain and Handbook 2: Affective Domain.* New York, David McKay, 1974.

Bryant D, Sullivan M: In-center self care dialysis. *JAANNT* 4: 36–38, 1977.

Caldarola D: Consequences of patient education in self care. *JAANNT* 4: 52–53, 1977.

Casper B: How well do patients understand hospital jargon? *AJN* 77(12): 1932–1934, 1977.

Corea AL: Current trends in diet and drug therapy for dialysis patients. *Nursing Clin-North Am* 10(3): 469–479, 1975.

Flegle JM: Teaching self-dialysis to adults in a hospital. *AJN* 77(2): 270–272, 1977.

Harrington J, Brener E: *Patient Care in Renal Failure.* Philadelphia, Saunders, 1973.

Hassett M: Teaching hemodialysis to the family unit. *Nursing Clin-North Am* 7(2): 349–362, 1972

Hekelman FP, Ostendarp C: Development and standardization of core curriculum for home dialysis. *Heart and Lung* 3(1): 117–121, 1974.

Jones P: Patient education—yes or no. *Supervisor Nurse* 8(5): 35–43, 1977.

Kesler AR: Pitfalls to avoid in interviewing outpatients. *Nursing '77* 7(9): 70–73, 1977.

Klausmeier HJ, Goodwin W: *Learning and Human Abilities: Educational Psychology.* New York, Harper & Row, 1971.

Kratzer JB: What does your patient need to know? *Nursing '77* 7(12): 82–84, 1977.

Kucha D: The health education of patients: assessing their needs. *Supervisor Nurse* 5(4): 26–29, 1974.

Kucha D: The health education of patients: development of a system (part 1). *Supervisor Nurse* 5(5): 8–21, 1974.

Kucha D: The health education of patients: development of a system (part 2). *Supervisor Nurse* 5(6): 8–11, 1974.

Mager RF: *Preparing Instructional Objectives.* Palo Alto, Calif, Fearon Pub, 1962.

Murray R, Zentner J: Guidelines for more effective health teaching. *Nursing '76* 6(2): 44–53, 1976.

O'Neill M: Guidelines for teaching home dialysis. *Nursing Clin-North Am* 6(4): 641–654, 1971.

_____ : *Patient Teaching Manual.* Nashville, Dialysis Clinic, Inc, 1977.

Pearson B: Learning tool selection. *Supervisor Nurse* 6(3): 30–31, 1975.

Pohl ML: *The Teaching Function of the Nursing Practitioner.* Dubuque, Iowa, Wm C Brown, 1973.

Redman B: *The Process of Patient Teaching in Nursing.* St. Louis, Mosby, 1976.

Smith EC: Are you really communicating? *AJN* 77(12): 1966–1968, 1977.

Strauss AL: *Chronic Illness and the Quality of Life.* St. Louis, Mosby, 1975.

Sturdevant B: Why don't adult patients learn? *Supervisor Nurse* 8(5): 44–46, 1977.

5
Nutrition for the Patient with End Stage Renal Disease

Victoria R. Liddle, R.D.

Since the introduction of dialysis in the 1950s the changes in the management of chronic renal failure have been very dramatic. The dialysis procedure has had many improvements in both equipment and techniques; mediations have been improved; and the diet has gone from one with almost no protein to one in which, under certain circumstances, the patient is encouraged to eat more protein.

Loss of renal function can now be compensated for by management of medications and diet until the creatinine clearance has decreased to 5 ml/min or until the patient has become acidotic. Long-term hemodialysis or peritoneal dialysis therapy can then be added to the treatment along with a change in medications and diet, and the patient can be managed for an indefinite period or until a transplant becomes available. Good medical and dietetic management of the recipient of a transplant prolongs life and improves its quality.

Kidney function is necessary for the elimination of excess fluid, for removal of end products of protein metabolism, and for maintaining a chemical balance of the body. The "artificial kidney" is limited in replacing normal kidney function because it removes an inexact amount of fluid; it removes wastes by particle size; it cannot remove large amounts of uremic toxins because the dialyzer's time of use and efficiency are limited; and too rapid removal of wastes and fluid has adverse effects on the patient.

Good dietary management provides caloric adequacy to achieve ideal body weight; protein adequacy to maintain positive nitrogen balance with emphasis on provision of high-biological-value protein and/or essential amino acids; sodium control to prevent hypotension, hypertension, or excessive thirst; potassium control to prevent hypokalemia or

123

hyperkalemia; phosphorus control to augment the phosphorus-binding gels; fluid control to prevent hypertension and/or edema; and vitamin and mineral supplementation as needed. Importantly, too, the diet should be practical, palatable, and acceptable to the patient.

Common diet prescriptions are summarized in Table 5.1. The dietary exchange lists (see Appendix A) used for patients with initial renal failure should be identical to those used when he is started on dialysis. The diet pattern should be based on the patient's "normal" pattern as much as possible; however, he should be encouraged to divide the meals so that protein and calories are distributed throughout the day. It is important to have protein and calories available as the body requires them, rather than having the body break down its tissues and then try to rebuild them.

Once the diet pattern has been established for initial renal failure and the patient has learned to use the exchange lists, the change in diet prescription required after the implementation of hemodialysis will be a simple adjustment of the pattern and amounts of each exchange allowed.

The patient should be taught to relate his blood chemistry values to his dietary intake so that he can make changes in his selections to keep his chemistry values within an acceptable range. He may find a chart such as Table 5.2 useful. This enables him to see what is normal for him and gives him a guide to help monitor his blood chemistry values.

The remainder of this chapter discusses specific aspects of nutrition for the patient with end stage renal disease.

PROTEIN

Before the work published by Giordano (1) in 1963, dietary intake of protein was restricted in patients with chronic renal failure, but no studies had been done to determine the exact amounts or the type of protein to be allowed. Vomiting, nausea, anorexia, hiccupping, and diarrhea were common symptoms in patients with chronic renal failure. Giordano found that by feeding uremic patients 2 gm of essential amino acid nitrogen per day as a sole source of nitrogen, and by providing adequate calories, vitamins, and minerals, a positive nitrogen balance was achieved and many of the uremic symptoms disappeared. This was the first work to indicate that high-biological-value protein was necessary in the diet. Giovanetti and Maggiore (2), using a powdered essential amino acid mixture of eggs, found similar results. Other investigators began using this type of regimen to decrease the severity of uremia (3).

Twenty-two different amino acids ordinarily are required for synth-

Table 5.1. Suggested Diet Prescriptions

Nutrients and Ions	Initial Renal Failure	Hemodialysis	Transplantation
HBV protein	20−40 gm	1 gm/kg; adult 1.5 gm/kg; child	2 gm/kg
LBV protein	10 gm or less	15 gm or less	Limited by CHO
CHO	Unrestricted	Unrestricted	1−1.5 gm/kg
Fat	Unrestricted	Unrestricted	Unrestricted
Calories	45−50 kcal/kg/day; child 80 kcal	45−50 kcal/kg/day; child 80 kcal	To maintain ideal weight
Sodium	Individualized	Individualized (500−2000 mg)	Usually 2000 mg
Potassium	Individualized (40−70 mEq)	Individualized (40−70 mEq)	Usually unrestricted
Calcium	RDA (800−1200 mg)	RDA (800−1200 mg)	Individualized (no less than RDA)
Phosphorus	Unrestricted	Unrestricted	Individualized

esis of tissue proteins, and the absence of any one of them can prevent the formation of protein. The body can synthesize and mobilize the majority of these amino acids from dietary sources, but the classic studies of Rose in 1949 (4) demonstrated that some of the amino acids cannot be synthesized in amounts adequate for metabolic needs. These so-called "essential amino acids" must be provided every day in the diet in proper amounts and proportions together with an adequate supply of nonessential amino acids and calories if protein synthesis and other metabolic functions are to take place normally. The essential amino acids are leucine, threonine, methionine, valine, phenylalanine, lysine, isoleucine, tryptophan, and histidine. Bergstrom et al. (5) have shown that the requirements for essential amino acids in patients with chronic renal failure are about twice those of normal individuals.

The amount of nitrogen retained in the body is correlated with the pattern of essential amino acids provided by the dietary protein. Theoretically, if a protein had a pattern that was perfect for synthesis, then it would be used entirely to build body protein, and no urea would be formed. If the protein in food is deficient in one or more of the essential amino acids, the efficiency of tissue protein formation is restricted, and some of the dietary amino acids are used for the formation of urea.

Table 5.2. Guide for Monitoring Blood Laboratory Values

Substance	Normal Values	Dialysis Patients*	What to Do if Abnormal
BUN	10–20 mg	80–100	High: Eat less protein and more carbohydrates.
			Low: Eat more HBV protein.
Creatinine	0.3–2.0 mg	Males, 10–18	High: More dialysis or higher blood flow rate.
		Females, 10–15	
Calcium	8.5–10.5 mg	Same	Low: Eat more dairy products or take calcium supplements if serum phosphorus is normal.
			High: Omit dairy products.
Phosphorus	2.5–4.5 mg	Same	High: Take Amphojel or Basaljel with every meal.
			Low: Consult physician about decreasing dosage.
Albumin	3.8–5.0 gm	Same	Low: Eat more eggs and meat.
Sodium	136–146 mg	Same	High: Eat less foods and/or products containing sodium.
			Low: Be sure to include allowed sodium in daily diet.
Potassium	3.8–5.1 mEq	Same	High: Soak vegetables in water before cooking. Consult dietitian.
Hematocrit	Males, 45±5% Females, 42±5%	Usually lower	Low: Don't take iron supplement with phosphate binding medication, but take 30–60 minutes before meal time.

*After longest interdialytic intervals.

The biological value or nitrogen balance index of a protein is determined by the pattern of essential amino acids that it contains. An egg white is the dietary food that most nearly approximates the ideal pattern. Milk is second; meats, fish, and poultry follow. Plant proteins are "low-biological-value proteins" because of their poor patterns of essential amino acids.

The diets resulting from the work of Giordano (1), Giovanetti (2), and Berlyne and Shaw (3) were widely used during the middle 1960s for the management of renal failure. The diet was restricted to about 20 gm of high-biological-value protein with supplemental calories, vitamins, and minerals. Wheat-starch food stuffs and high-carbohydrate, high-fat desserts were the major sources of calories that were essentially free of nitrogen.

In 1968, Shinaberger and Ginn (6) reported findings for protein requirements in anephric patients on twice-weekly dialysis. They found that an intake of 0.8 gm of protein per kilogram of ideal body weight was adequate to achieve positive nitrogen balance during dialysis when all of the protein intake was of high biological value. They reported that 1.2 gm of low-biological-value protein per kilogram of body weight failed to maintain nitrogen balance.

In 1970, Rubini and Kopple (7) published results on more than 70 dietary studies of nondialyzed uremic patients. They compared isocaloric diets of 20 gm protein (Giordano-Giovanetti type), 40 gm mixed protein, and 1 gm/kg protein intake. The results showed that patients taking the 20 gm and 40 gm protein diets did well, but those taking 1 gm/kg protein quickly deteriorated and developed uremic symptoms. They also confirmed Ginn's nitrogen balance studies in patients receiving twice weekly dialysis. A high-caloric, 0.63 gm/kg of high-biological-value protein and 15 gm of low-biological-value protein diet was found to be most acceptable.

Most patients on maintenance hemodialysis do well on a protein intake of 1 gm/kg of ideal body weight with 80% of this protein coming from high-biological-value sources. This is adequate protein to maintain a positive nitrogen balance and a palatable diet and to keep the patient relatively free of uremic symptoms. Patients on chronic peritoneal dialysis lose considerable amounts of protein into the dialysate fluid and may require more protein in the diet than patients on maintenance hemodialysis.

Gotch et al. (8) have recently developed a computerized system that allows one to determine the actual protein intake of a patient, once he has been instructed about his dietary prescription and has stabilized on dialysis. This system allows the dietitian to work closely with the patient to help him with his daily protein requirements. It takes into consideration the patient's current renal function, the amount of dialysis he is receiving, and the amount of protein required for his lean body mass, and then calculates the amount of protein he is actually consuming between dialysis treatments.

Special Dietary Considerations

Occasionally a patient will not be able to tolerate a renal diet, and total parenteral alimentation (TPA) or a liquid dietary replacement may be necessary.

Dudrick (9) and Abel (10) used with good results a TPA treatment for patients with acute renal failure that was patterned after the Giordano-Giovanetti diet (essential amino acids and glucose).

Meng et al. (11) used a TPA preparation of essential amino acids, glucose, vitamins, and electrolytes, which they found effective in improving the nutritional status of patients with acute and chronic renal failure.

In the United States an oral supplement (Amin-Aid) is commercially available that is based on the same principle; and in Sweden amino acid tablets (Aminess) are available. Amin-Aid is a high-caloric essential amino acid dietary supplement with histadine added that is useful for patients who are extremely anemic or who cannot tolerate solid food.

There are new developments in the use of a low-protein diet supplemented with essential amino acids or a combination of α-keto or α-hydroxy analogues of essential amino acids for patients with advanced chronic renal failure. Mitch and Walser (12) have shown that the use of such a regimen can defer the need for dialysis.

Protein Intake for Children

Most pediatric nephrologists use the Recommended Daily Allowance (RDA) of protein for the child's height as long as it is possible to do so and prevent uremic symptoms. After hemodialysis is initiated, the protein intake should be 1.5 gm per kilogram of body weight with sufficient calories to promote a nutritional environment conducive to growth.

Aronson (13) and Holliday (14) have used infusions of essential amino acids in children with arrested growth from renal failure and found an improvement in the child's growth.

It is essential that the daily protein requirements be met for both adults and children. This is often impossible to accomplish unless each patient uses a food scale to weigh the lean cooked meat for a few weeks when he begins the renal diet. It is helpful for the patient to use food exchange lists for both high- and low-biological-value proteins. Using such a list, the patient doesn't have to calculate his diet every day; instead he establishes a pattern and makes appropriate selections from the exchange lists.

When the patient is ill and has loss of appetite, it is desirable to have him take his protein and calories in the form of a milkshake for each meal that he misses. The following recipe for such a milkshake is acceptable: 1 egg, 1 teaspoon of vanilla, 2 tablespoons of sugar, ½ cup of whipping cream, and ½ cup of ice cream. Liquid Amphojel may be added if desired.

SODIUM

Dietary sodium requirements vary with different types of renal disease. Before the initiation of dialysis, some patients with renal failure lose excessive amounts of sodium while others retain sodium and fluid. Each patient's sodium intake depends on his kidneys' ability to excrete sodium.

Sodium is necessary for the regulation of blood pressure and for the control of body fluid volumes (15). Sodium deficiency causes hypotension, dehydration, and weakness; hypernatremia results in hypertension, excessive thirst, edema, and shortness of breath. Sodium is found naturally in most foods, but the chief dietary sources are table salt, sodium preservatives, and taste enhancers. Sodium is also a component of medications such as sodium bicarbonate, which is sometimes given to treat the acidosis of renal failure.

The sodium requirement may be determined by actual measurement of the 24-hour urinary sodium excretion; follow-up methods include measuring weight gain and observing for edema and hypertension.

When a patient with renal failure has stabilized on maintenance hemodialysis, a 2-gm sodium diet is usually sufficient to maintain his sodium equilibrium and to provide a palatable diet. This restriction can be achieved by using a small amount of salt in cooking, by avoiding salty foods, cured or processed meats, and by avoiding adding salt to food at the table. When eating away from home, a renal patient can restrict his sodim intake by avoiding casseroles, gravy, or mixed dishes, instead selecting fried meats that can have the outside coating removed and vegetables that look as though they were originally frozen rather than canned. Giving the patient a list of foods that contain large amounts of sodium preservatives or taste enhancers and advising him to read labels will usually suffice to help him prevent excessive thirst, edema, and hypertension.

A note of caution is in order about excessive restriction of dietary sodium during chronic hemodialysis. If the patient does not have enough sodium in his diet, he will develop hypotension during and/or after dialysis and may develop shock and require large amounts of sodium and fluid replacement. Severe muscle cramps may also occur. How unfair to the patient if he is asked to follow an unpalatable low-sodium diet and strict fluid restriction and then he requires large amounts of normal saline during dialysis!

POTASSIUM

Potassium is necessary for proper function of the body. It is a component of all cells, and it functions in the control of reflexes and muscles. Its most important function is the control of heart strength and rhythm. Hypokalemia results in premature ventricular contractions, muscular weakness, breathing difficulty, and paralysis; hyperkalemia results in weakness, generalized muscular twitching, and cardiac arrest.

Potassium excretion by the kidneys is usually adequate as long as the patient has a creatinine clearance above 15 ml/min. Once kidney function has decreased to the point of requiring maintenance dialysis, potassium restriction is mandatory. A daily intake of 50 to 70 mEq potassium is usually optimal if the dialysate contains less than 3 mEq/liter.

Potassium occurs naturally in most foods, especially milk, meats, vegetables, and fruits. It is also used in salt substitutes and is added in place of sodium to special low-sodium dietary foods such as low-sodium baking powder and some low-sodium cheeses.

The high-biological-value protein in the renal diet provides most of the allowed dietary potassium. To keep the remainder of the diet low in potassium, nuts, chocolate, legumes, and vegetables and fruits that are high in potassium are usually avoided. About half the potassium can be leached out of vegetables if they are peeled, cut into small pieces, and soaked in water for 4 to 5 hours (16).

When a patient is being instructed on his potassium intake, the fruits and vegetables should be shown in exchange lists that group the foods according to potassium content. When the patient can see at a glance which foods are higher in potassium, he can make frequent selections from those with a lower potassium content and very occasionally select fruits or vegetables with a higher potassium content.

Patients who develop hyperkalemia because of noncompliance with potassium restriction can be instructed to take Kayexalate, a cation-exchange resin, with their meals. One gram of Kayexalate will bind approximately 1 mEq of potassium; one teaspoon of Kayexalate weighs

3.5 gm. Recipes have been developed for a Kayexalate candy, which is quite palatable (17).

VITAMINS

Vitamin intake for the patient on a renal diet may not meet the Recommended Daily Allowances (18,19) because of the protein and potassium restrictions and because the process of soaking vegetables in water to remove potassium also removes the water-soluble vitamins. In addition, the diaysis process removes water-soluble vitamins, particularly B₆.

Many vitamins and their metabolites are excreted by the kidney; therefore, in chronic renal failure some of the intake deficiencies may be offset by the lack of excretion.

Vitamin D is important in regulating calcium balance; it promotes the intestinal absorption of calcium and probably directly influences the process of bone mineralization. It is considered to be deficient in anephric patients and those with renal failure. Recent developments in the metabolism of vitamin D, namely its conversion to its active form 1,25-dihydroxycholecalciferol (20,21) by the kidney, have clarified the reasons for deficiency of this vitamin.

Kopple and Swenseid (22) have reviewed the complex problem of determining optimal dietary intake of vitamins for patients with renal failure. They determined that a supplement to meet RDA for thiamine, niacin, pantothenic acid, flavin, and biotin is probably adequate. Folic acid, vitamin B₆, and ascorbic acid are even more necessary for normal functioning, and they have recommended supplements of approximately 1 mg/day of folic acid and 100 mg/day of vitamin C. In addition to deficient intake of vitamin B₆, Dobbelstein et al. (23) have suggested that there might be an inhibitor of vitamin B₆ in uremic patients that requires an intake of vitamin B₆ greater than the RDA for normal persons. The appropriate daily dose for vitamin B₆ in renal failure is yet to be determined.

The fat-soluble vitamins A, E, and K do not require supplementation; in fact, cases of vitamin A toxicity have been reported in uremic patients.

IRON

Iron deficiency in patients with chronic renal failure is quite common as the result of several factors:

1. A decrease in the production of erythropoietin, the renal hormone responsible for stimulating red cell production by the bone marrow.

2. Blood loss from frequent diagnostic tests.
3. Blood loss during each dialysis from the blood remaining in the dialyzer at the end of dialysis.
4. Decreased intestinal absorption of iron.

Iron deficiency can be treated with oral iron supplements in the form of iron salts or with parenteral (intramuscular or intravenous) injections of Imferon. Iron requires an acidic environment for absorption, so oral iron preparations should not be given with aluminum hydroxide gels, which neutralize the acidity of the stomach and inhibit iron absorption (24). Imferon can result in inadvertent iron overload and hemosiderosis unless carefully monitored (25). Androgen therapy has been used to stimulate red blood cell production, but it may have virilizing effects and may also cause elevation of serum cholesterol levels.

Eschback et al. (26) have evaluated iron balance in hemodialysis patients. They concluded that by using serial serum ferritin determinations, iron stores can be quantified and the emergence of iron deficiency predicted.

CALCIUM AND PHOSPHORUS

In chronic renal failure, intestinal absorption and renal excretion of calcium and phosphorus are decreased. Phosphate excretion by the kidneys is directly related to the number of functioning nephrons. As kidney function decreases, phosphorus retention occurs and hyperphosphatemia develops. This, along with the hypocalcemia seen in renal failure, causes hypersecretion of the parathyroid hormone and results in bone disease. (See Chapter 1 for more detail.) One of the major complications of end stage renal disease is the development of bone diseases such as osteomalacia and osteitis fibrosa. This complication can be improved by correction of the calcium and phosphorus imbalance.

Vitamin D, the major factor promoting calcium absorption from the intestines, is converted to its active form 1,25-DHCC by the kidneys (20,21). In chronic renal failure there is deficient synthesis of the active metabolite of vitamin D, thus calcium deficiency and hypocalcemia develop. Brickman et al. (27) have shown experimentally that therapeutic administration of the synthetic active metabolite of vitamin D_3 will reverse the bone disease seen in patients with chronic renal failure.

Goldsmith et al. (28) have shown that, by controlling the retention of phosphate and by preventing depression of serum calcium, it is possible to prevent or reverse hyperparathyroidism and osteitis fibrosa. They have used phosphate binding medications (aluminum hydroxide gels) to correct the hyperphosphatemia and have used a dialysate calcium concentration of 7 to 8 mg/100 ml to correct the hypocalcemia. The patients responded to this treatment by showing a decrease in bone resorption and a decrease in serum immunoreactive parathyroid hormone levels.

Dietary control of calcium and phosphorus is not sufficient to prevent the hyperphosphatemia and hypocalcemia that occur in chronic renal failure. The chief dietary sources of calcium are dairy products, which are also high in phosphorus. If the serum calcium and phosphorus were controlled by diet alone, the diet would be very unpalatable.

Phosphate binding medications in the form of tablets, capsules, or liquid are taken with meals to control the absorption of phosphorus from the intestine. The phosphate binding medication may also be incorporated into a vehicle such as cookies, if the patient finds the other forms distasteful. The dietitian should work with the patient to find an acceptable form for taking the phosphate binding medication.

Unless a high-calcium dialysate is to be used, it is usually necessary to supplement the diet with some form of vitamin D and/or calcium. It is dangerous to use a high-calcium dialysate or a calcium supplement for patients who are not complying with the phosphate binding medication regimen; because with a high serum phosphorus *and* a high serum calcium the patient would develop calcification of soft tissues, including the walls of the arteries and electrical conducting tissue of the myocardium (29,20). This calcification has been shown to be reduced when the serum phosphorus is controlled (29,31).

CALORIES

The intake of calories for the patient with chronic renal failure is important as a means of achieving ideal body weight and preventing the utilization of protein for energy. It is difficult for an obese patient with renal failure to lose weight without becoming anemic and wasting protein. The activity level may be below that of a normal individual, so that the recommended intake of calories may be below the RDA for normal persons, but it should not be less than 20 to 50 calories per kilogram of body weight. The protein-sparing action of carbohydrates is essential for the patient with renal failure who is on a restricted protein intake.

Good sources of concentrated calories are jellies, jams, honey, sugar, hard candies, gum drops, and marshmallows. Many special products commercially available are caloric supplements without protein or electrolytes. These include: Wheatstarch products, Cal-Powder, Controlyte, Hycal, and Polycose.

Hypertriglyceridemia is a common finding in patients with chronic renal failure (32, 33). This is important in view of the fact that cardiovascular disease is the primary cause of death in patients with chronic renal failure (34,35). This factor must be considered when the calories are to be supplemented on a renal diet, as it may make a difference in the type of foods used for calories.

Sanfelippo et al. (36) have shown that triglyceride levels in patients with chronic renal failure can be reduced by reducing carbohydrates to 35% of total daily caloric intake and increasing the ratio of polyunsaturated to saturated fat to 2.0. This suggests that a calorie supplement of polyunsaturated fat is preferable to a high-carbohydrate source of calories.

FLUIDS

Before the initiation of dialysis fluid restriction is not always necessary. If the patient with chronic renal failure weighs daily, he can monitor his own intake by limiting the amount of fluid if he gains weight. Occasionally a patient will have cardiac involvement in association with renal failure; these patients should limit their daily fluid intake to the amount of urinary output each 24 hours.

Once hemodialysis is initiated, the daily fluid allowance should be 500 ml plus the amount of the previous 24 hours' urinary output. This corresponds to a fluid weight gain of approximately 1 pound per 24 hours, which can be easily removed during dialysis.

Patients who have difficulty adhering to their fluid restriction may find it useful to place an amount equal to their daily allowance in one container. Each time the patient consumes fluid he pours an equal amount from the container, thus he can easily see the amount he has remaining for the day, which should help him space his fluid intake during the day.

If a patient is unable to control his thirst, his sodium intake should be reviewed to be sure he is not exceeding his allowance. He should be taught that all foods that are liquid at room temperature should be counted as 100% fluid. It is also helpful to show him the amount of fluid contained in the foods allowed in his diet. The total of the water in the foods will be 500 to 800 ml that is not counted toward the daily fluid limit, since it only compensates for the insensible water loss of the body. Thirst and fluid intake can also be controlled by measures such as sucking on a lemon or hard candy or by taking medications with applesauce instead of water. It is also helpful for the patient to understand that the leg cramps often experienced during dialysis when considerable fluid has to be removed may be eliminated by adherence to the fliid restriction.

NUTRITION AFTER RENAL TRANSPLANTATION

After a patient receives a renal transplant, his diet is changed from the diet during dialysis (37). As soon as the transplanted kidney begins to function, the protein and potassium restrictions are no longer necessary, but the sodium restriction is maintained, since the transplanted kidney's ability to excrete sodium is variable. The glucocorticoids used for immunosuppression exert metabolic effects that can be partially corrected by dietary manipulation. Figure 5.1 is a schematic drawing of the metabolic effects of steroids.

Proteins

High doses of steroids tend to increase protein catabolism and decrease protein anabolism. The protein wasting that results may be prevented by a high-protein diet of a least 2 gm per kilogram of body weight per day.

Carbohydrates

Carbohydrate metabolism is also affected by high doses of steroids. There tends to be a resistance to the action of insulin, and glucose tolerance is impaired. The use of a low-carbohydrate diet of 1.0 to 1.5 gm/kg per day minimizes the hyperglycemia and hyperinsulinism and decreases the tendency toward fat deposition in a Cushingoid pattern.

Calcium and Phosphorus

Serum calcium and phosphorus levels are monitored frequently after renal transplantation. Because of the secondary hyperparathyroidism and bone disease common to chronic renal failure/dialysis patients, the calcium and phosphorus in the diet should meet the RDA of 800 to 1200 mg/day if blood levels permit.

When a patient is begun on maintenance doses of steroids (usually four to six months after transplantation), the protein and carbohydrate intake may be adjusted to maintain ideal body weight. The sodium allowance varies for each patient.

136

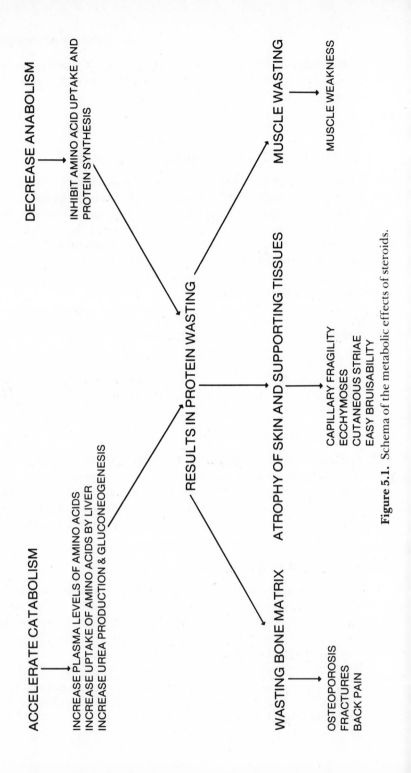

Figure 5.1. Schema of the metabolic effects of steroids.

REFERENCES

1. C Giordano: Use of exogenous and endogenous urea for protein synthesis in normal and uremic subjects. *J Lab Clin Med* 62: 231, 1963.

2. S Giovanetti, Q Maggiore: A low nitrogen diet with proteins of high biological value for severe chronic uremia. *Lancet* 1: 1000, 1964.

3. G M Berlyne, A B Shaw: Giordano-Giovanetti diet in terminal renal failure. *Lancet* 2: 7, 1965.

4. W C Rose: Amino acid requirements of man. *Fed Proc* 8: 546, 1949.

5. J Bergström, P Furst, L O Noree, et al.: Intracellular free amino acids in uremic patients as influenced by amino acid supply. *Kidney Int* 7: 8–345, 1975.

6. J H Shinaberger, H E Ginn: Low protein, high essential amino acid diet for nitrogen equilibrium in chronic dialysis. *Amer J Clin Nutr* 21: 618, 1968.

7. M E Rubini, J D Kopple: Dietary management of end stage uremia. *Bull New York Acad Med* 46: 950, 1970.

8. F A Gotch, J A Sargent, M Kein, et al: Clinical results of intermittent dialysis therapy (IDT) guided by ongoing kinetic analysis of urea metabolism. *Trans Amer Soc Artif Int Organs* 22: 175, 1976.

9. S J Dudrick, E Steiger, J M Long: Renal failure in surgical patients: treatment with intravenous essential amino acids and hypertonic glucose. *Surgery* 68: 180, 1970.

10. R M Abel, C H Beck Jr, W M Abbott: Improved survival from acute renal failure after treatment with intravenous essential L-amino acids and glucose. *N Eng J Med* 288: 695, 1973.

11. H C Meng, H H Sandstead, P J Walker, et al: The use of essential amino acids for parenteral nutrition in patients with chronic and acute renal failure. *Acta Chir Scand S* 466: 94, 1976.

12. W E Mitch, M Walser: Effect of nutritional therapy of chronic renal failure: quantitative assessment *Clin Res* 24: 407A, 1976.

13. A S Aronson, P Fürst, B Kuylenstierna: Essential amino acids in the treatment of advanced uremia: twenty-two months experience in a 5-year-old girl. *Pediatrics* 56: 538, 1975.

14. M A Holliday: Management of the child with renal insufficiency, in Lieberman (ed): *Clinical Pediatric Nephrology*. Philadelphia, Lippincott, 1976, p. 395.

15. F del Greco, W A Davies, N M Simon, et al: Hypertension of chronic renal failure: role of sodium and the renal pressor system. *Kidney Int* 7: *(1–2)* 176, 1975.

16. T T Tsaltas: Dietetic management of uremic patients: I. Extraction of potassium from foods for uremic patients. *Amer J Clin Nutr* 22: 490, 1969.

17. K Johnson, C Cazee, C Gooch, et al.: Sodium polystyrene sulfonate resin candy for control of potassium in chronic dialysis patients. *Clin Nephr* 5: 266, 1976.

18. J F Sullivan, A B Eisenstein: Ascorbic acid depletion in patients undergoing chronic hemodialysis. *Amer J Clin Nutr* 23: 1339, 1970.

19. J P Pendras, R V Erickson: Hemodialysis: a successful therapy for chronic uremia. *Ann Intern Med* 64: 293, 1966.

20. H F DeLuca: Recent advances in the metabolism and function of vitamin D. *Fed Proc* 28: 1678, 1969.

21. A W Norman: Evidence for a new kidney-produced hormone, 1,25-dihydroxycholecalciferol, the proposed biologically active form of vitamin D. *Amer J Clin Nutr* 24: 1346, 1971.

22. J D Kopple, M E Swendseid: Vitamin nutrition in patients undergoing maintenance hemodialysis. *Kidney Int* 7: (S–2) 79, 1975.

23. H Dobbelstein, W F Körner, W Mempel, et al: Vitamin B6 deficiency in uremia and its implications for the depression of immune responses. *Kidney Int* 5: 233, 1974.

24. S P Rastogi, F Padilla, C M Boyd: Effect of aluminum hydroxide on iron absorption. (abstract) Meeting of the American Society of Nephrology, Washington, D C, 1975, p. 21.

25. L R I Baker, M D Barnett, B Brozonic, et al.: Hemosiderosis in a patient on regular hemodialysis: treatment by desferrioxamine. *Clin Nephr* 6: 326, 1976.

26. J W Eschback, J D Cook, B H Schribner, et al.: Iron balance in hemodialysis patients. *Ann Intern Med* 87: 710, 1977.

27. A S Brickman, J W Coburn, A W Norman: Action of 1,25-di-OH-cholecalciferol, a potent kidney-produced metabolite of vitamin D3 in uremic man. *N Eng J Med* 287: 891, 1972.

28. R S Goldsmith, C D Arnaud, W J Johnson: Effects of calcium and phosphorus on patients maintained on dialysis. *Kidney Int* 7: (S–2) 118, 1975.

29. R Porter, A L Crombie: Corneal and conjunctival calcification in chronic renal failure. *Br J Opthalmol* 57: 339, 1973.

30. B Kolton, J Pedersen: Calcinosis cutis and renal failure. *Arch Dermatol* 110: 256, 1974.

31. R Verberckmoes, R Bouillon, B Krempien: Disappearance of vascular calcifications during treatment of renal osteodystrophy. Two patients treated with high doses of vitamin D and aluminum hydroxide. *Ann Intern Med* 82: 529, 1975.

32. J D Bagdale, D Porte Jr, E L Bierman: Hypertriglyceridemia: A metabolic consequence of chronic renal failure. *N Eng J Med* 279: 181, 1968.

33. R A Gutman, A Uy, R J Shalhoub, et al.: Hypertriglyceridemia in chronic non-nephrotic renal failure. *Amer J Clin Nutr* 26: 165, 1973.

34. E G Lowrie, J M Lazarus, C L Hampers, et al.: Cardiovascular disease in dialysis patients. *N Eng J Med* 290: 737, 1974.

35. J M Lazarus, E G Lowrie, C L Hampers, et al.: Cardiovascular disease in uremic patients on hemodialysis. *Kidney Int* 7: (S–2) 167, 1975.

36. M L Sanfelippo, R S Swanson, G M Reaven: Reduction of plasma trig-lycerides by diet in subjects with chronic renal failure. *Kidney Int* 11: 54, 1977.
37. V R Liddle, P J Walker, H K Johnson, et al.: Diet in transplantation. *Dialysis and Transplantation* 6: 9, 1977.

6
The Patient Receiving Hemodialysis

Larry E. Lancaster, R.N., M.S.N.

Hemodialysis is one treatment modality for patients with end stage renal disease. It is a relatively safe procedure that involves circulating the patient's blood through a semipermeable tubing that is surrounded by a dialysate solution in an "artificial kidney" (dialyzer). The purpose is to remove the waste products of metabolism from the blood and return the patient to a nearly normal fluid and electrolyte balance. Like other methods of managing chronic renal failure—conservative management, peritoneal dialysis, and renal transplantation—hemodialysis has advantages, disadvantages, and complications. Table 6.1 compares the advantages and disadvantages of hemodialysis and peritoneal dialysis.

The terms *chronic hemodialysis, intermittent hemodialysis,* and *maintenance hemodialysis* are used synonymously in this book to indicate hemodialysis that is performed on a regular, continuing basis to maintain life in persons with end stage renal disease. *Home dialysis* is carried out by the patient and an assistant in a home setting. *In-hospital hemodialysis* is performed in a hospital-based unit. Satellite centers or limited care facilities are out-of-hospital clinics that perform hemodialysis for one or several patients.

The purposes of this chapter are:

1. To outline the history of dialysis.
2. To review indications for initiation of hemodialysis.
3. To examine criteria for patient selection.
4. To compare and contrast advantages and disadvantages of hemodialysis and peritoneal dialysis.
5. To present a synopsis of some of the more important physical principles and technical aspects of hemodialysis.

Table 6.1. Advantages and Disadvantages of Hemodialysis and Peritoneal Dialysis

	Hemodialysis	*Peritoneal Dialysis*
Advantages	Highly efficient	More liberal diet
	May be used as chronic intermittent maintenance treatment	Dialysis Disequilibrium Syndrome rarely occurs
	Rapid treatment	Easily, quickly instituted
		Requires no special equipment or highly trained staff
		Heparin not required
		May be used for patients with unstable cardiovascular status
		Does not require circulatory access
		Venipuncture not required
		Safe for unattended overnight dialysis
Disadvantages	Permanent circulatory access required	Danger of peritonitis
	Special equipment and highly trained staff needed	Slow treatment—time consuming
	Heparin required	Less efficient than hemodialysis
	Expensive	Large protein loss
	Greater chance of Dialysis Disequilibrium Syndrome than with peritoneal dialysis	Less satisfactory for chronic intermittent maintenance treatment for certain categories of patients

6. To discuss patient assessment before, during, and after hemodialysis.
7. To discuss complications of hemodialysis.

HISTORY OF DIALYSIS

Significant dates and events in the history of dialysis are:

1890   Bicarbonate peritoneal lavage was used to treat cholera in Europe.

1913   The term "artificial kidney" was coined by Abel, Rowntree, and Turner at Johns Hopkins in Baltimore. They devised a "kidney" using celloidin tubing for membranes and used crushed leech heads (hirudin) for anticoagulation. The "kidney" worked inefficiently, but the experimental animals died from hypersensitivity to hirudin.

1923   Nicheles, in Germany, used the peritoneal membrane from an ox to make an "artifical kidney."

1935	Heparin was purified, and regenerated cellulose tubing was developed.
1942–43	Willem Kolff designed the "rotating drum artificial kidney." It was used successfully in Holland to treat patients with kidney failure. Kolff published his design in 1946.
1947	Kolff compared the effectiveness of peritoneal and intestinal lavage to hemodialysis and found hemodialysis superior for urea removal.
1947	VonGarretts, in Copenhagen, made a hand-wound "coil" kidney and used it successfully in humans.
1950–53	Teschan and colleagues used artificial kidneys to treat battle injuries with acute renal failure in Korean M.A.S.H. units. The survival of battle injuries with acute renal failure was improved.
1956	Kolff developed a "disposable coil" dialyzer and *gave* it to Travenol. No other company thought it had any application.
1957	Kiil developed the flat plate parallel flow dialyzer.
1959	After the design of the Quinton-Scribner external shunt, Scribner started the first two patients on chronic dialysis, using the Kiil dialyzer.
1964	Home dialysis was started by Curtis and Scribner in Seattle; Shaldon in London; and Merrill, Schupak, and Hampers in Boston.
1965	The subcutaneous arteriovenous fistula was developed by Brescia and Cimino.
1973	Federal support for dialysis through Medicare became available.
1974	Large-surface-area dialyzers became available that allowed a decrease in dialysis time.

INDICATIONS AND SELECTION
OF PATIENTS FOR HEMODIALYSIS

When chronic renal failure can no longer be controlled by conservative management (diet, medications, and fluid control) chronic maintenance dialysis is begun. Indications for initiation of chronic maintenance dialysis include a GFR less than 5 ml/min; serum creatinine levels greater than 10 mgm/100 ml; and uremic complications associated with end stage renal disease—anemia, bone disease, peripheral neuropathy, uncontrollable hypertension, and congestive heart failure (1).

Before the patient reaches end stage (the GFR is in the 10–30 ml/min range), the patient and family should be introduced to the concepts of dialysis and transplantation. (Principles of patient-family education are discussed in Chapter 4.) A visit to a dialysis unit and a conference with a dialysis nurse and a well-rehabilitated patient are often helpful. A conference with the social worker to ascertain the method of payment is advised at this time. Once the patient understands and accepts the necessity for dialysis, a circulatory access should be created in preparation for dialysis. This gives time for maturing of an arteriovenous fistula and may help the patient accept the undeniable fact that dialysis will be necessary. The patient must receive careful instruction regarding shunt care or fistula exercises. (See Chapter 7.)

There are no absolute contraindications for accepting patients for chronic maintenance hemodialysis and there are no age limits. The patient's understanding of the disease and its treatment and a willingness and ability to adhere to a strict regimen are essential for success. Other general guidelines for patient selection include:

1. The presence of terminal, irreversible renal failure for which conservative management is not effective.
2. The absence of other chronic and/or incapacitating illnesses.
3. An expectation for reasonable rehabilitation.
4. The patient's own desires regarding treatment.

PRINCIPLES OF HEMODIALYSIS

The physical principles involved in hemodialysis are discussed in two broad categories: 1) solute removal (mass transfer) and 2) fluid removal.

Solute Removal (Mass Transfer)

Solutes are removed from the blood during hemodialysis by the process of diffusion across a semipermeable membrane that separates the blood compartment from the dialysate compartment of a dialyzer. *Diffusion* is the movement of molecules from a region of higher to a region of lower concentration. The difference in the regions of concentration that causes movement of molecules is called the *concentration gradient*. Rate of diffusion depends on molecule size, size of the pores in the membrane, surface area of the membrane, temperature of the solutions, and the concentration of solute on the two sides of the membrane. If the molecule is too large to pass through the pores in the membrane, then that molecule is *nondiffusible*. The larger the surface area of the membrane, the more rapidly diffusion occurs. The higher the temperature of the solutions on either side of the membrane, the more rapidly diffusion occurs. Also, the greater the difference in the concentration gradient for a given solute, the more rapid the movement of molecules. When equilibrium is reached, diffusion ceases.

The general scheme for all hemodialyzers is the same. Blood and dialysate are pumped on opposite sides of a semipermeable membrane contained in a closed compartment. The blood contains excess quantities of metabolic waste products and some electrolytes. The dialysate on the other side of the semipermeable membrane contains the ideal concentration of electrolytes in the extracellular fluid (plasma) and is relatively free of waste products. Metabolic waste products (such as urea and creatinine) move from the blood to the dialysate because of the difference in concentration. Electrolytes move in both directions, and equilibrium is maintained. Red blood cells, white blood cells, and proteins are too large to pass through the pores in the semipermeable membrane into the dialysate. Bacteria and viruses, if present in the dialysate, are too large to pass through the semipermeable membrane into the blood. *Solute drag* (where solutes cross the membrane with water) is a minor source of solute removal during dialysis.

Figure 6.1 is a schematic representation of a typical hemodialysis system. Table 6.2 explains the symbols used in the figure. Reference is made to this diagram in explaining concepts of hemodialysis (1,3).

1. The amount of solute entering the blood side of the dialyzer in a specified time interval is the product of the *blood flow rate* (Q_{bi}) and the concentration of solute in the blood (C_{bi}) entering the dialyzer. ($Q_{bi} \times C_{bi}$)
2. Likewise, the amount of solute in the blood leaving the dialyzer in a specified time interval is the product of the blood flow rate (Q_{bo}) and

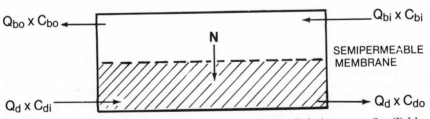

Figure 6.1. Schematic representation of a typical hemodialysis system. See Table 6.2 for definition of symbols. See text for explanation of drawing.

Table 6.2. Definition of Symbols

Symbol	Definition	Unit of Measurement
C	Concentration	mg/ml
Cl	Clearance	ml/minute
D	Dialysance	ml/minute
ER	Solute extraction ratio	percent
N	Solute flux	mg/minute
P	Pressure	minute/cm
Q	Flow rate	ml/minute
R	Resistance	minute/cm
U	Ultrafiltration	ml/minute
Subscripts		
b	Blood	
d	Dialysate	
i	Inlet	
m	Membrane	
o	Outlet	

the concentration of solute in the blood (C_{bo}) leaving the dialyzer. ($Q_{bo} \times C_{bo}$)

3. The amount of solute leaving the blood and entering the dialysate during a specified time interval is called *net flux* (N). Net flux is determined for a given quantity of blood by subtracting the concentration of solute in the blood leaving the dialyzer from the concentration in the blood entering the dialyzer. $N = Q_b(C_{bi} - C_{bo})$

4. Net flux may also be determined by measuring the difference in the concentration of dialysate entering the dialyzer and dialysate leaving the dialyzer. $N = Q_d(C_{do} - C_{di})$

5. Net flux is dependent on the surface area, the permeability of the membrane for a specific solute, and the mean concentration gradient between the blood and dialysate. Net flux increases as the surface area increases. Membrane permeability for a specific solute is related to the molecular size—higher for small molecules and lower for large molecules. Net flux is more rapid with high blood-dialysate concentration gradients. If blood and dialysate were flowing in the same direction from dialyzer inlet to outlet, the concentration gradient and net flux would decrease as the blood and dialysate approached the outlet. This problem is overcome and greater efficiency achieved by pumping blood and dialysate in opposite directions (countercurrent flow) through the dialyzer to maintain a similar blood-dialysate concentration gradient throughout the dialysis pathway. Other blood-dialysate pathways that are used include completely mixed (no

measurable difference at any point on the membrane); cocurrent flow (inefficient and not used clinically); and a crossflow dialysate pattern (involving a summing of concentration gradients along the membrane).

6. Clearance and dialysance are similar and are discussed together below.

Clearance (Cl), used to express the performance of the dialyzing process (4), is defined as the amount of solute removed from the blood as it flows through the dialyzer. The formula for solute clearance is:

$$Cl = \left(\frac{C_{bi} - C_{bo}}{C_{bi}} \right) Q_b$$

Clearance deals only with the solute concentration in the blood and does not consider the solute concentration in the dialysate. Dialysate solute concentration does, however, affect the clearance of solutes from the blood.

Dialysance (D), used to express the performance of a dialyzer (4), refers to the rate of solute removal from the blood by dialysis in relation to the transdialyzer and transmembrane solute concentrations. The formula for dialysance is:

$$D = \left(\frac{C_{bi} - C_{bo}}{C_{bi} - C_{di}} \right) Q_b$$

This formula shows that dialysance is related to blood flow, concentration of blood entering and leaving the dialyzer, and the concentration gradient between the blood and dialysate entering the dialyzer. Clearance decreases as the blood and dialysate pass through the dialyzer, because the mean concentration gradient decreases, owing to solute flux. The formula for dialysance partly eliminates the dependency on gradient and is used for expressing dialyzer performance. Dialysance rises rapidly as the blood flow through the dialyzer increases but levels off at high rates. The relationship between blood flow rate and dialysance is shown in Figure 6.2. Dialysance is also dependent on the surface area and permeability of the dialyzer membrane.

If the concentration of dialysate entering the dialyzer (C_{di}) is zero, as in the single-pass systems, the formula for dialysance is the same as that for clearance. In systems using recirculating dialysate, the deceasing blood/dialysate gradient must be considered, so the formula for dialysance is used.

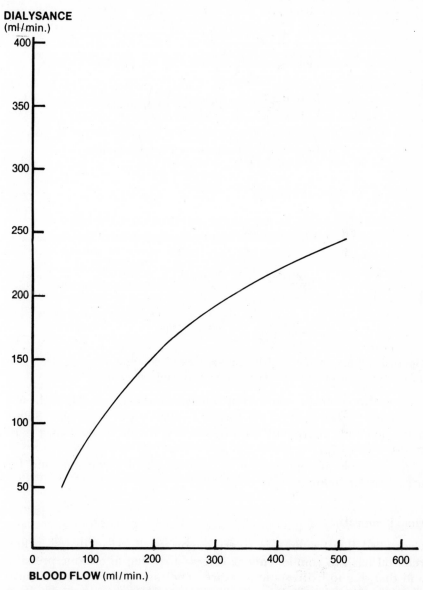

DIALYSANCE (ml/min.)

BLOOD FLOW (ml/min.)

Figure 6.2. The relationship between blood flow (ml/min) and dialysance (ml/min). Dialysance rises rapidly as the blood flow through the dialyzer increases but levels off at high blood flow rates.

$$C_{bi} = 140 \text{ mg\%} \qquad\qquad Q_b = 150 \text{ ml/min}$$
$$C_{bo} = 70 \text{ mg\%} \qquad\qquad C_{di} = 40 \text{ mg\%}$$

$$D = \left(\frac{C_{bi} - C_{bo}}{C_{bi} - C_{di}}\right) Q_b$$

$$= \left(\frac{140 \text{ mg\%} - 70 \text{ mg\%}}{140 \text{ mg\%} - 40 \text{ mg\%}}\right) 150 \text{ ml/min}$$

$$= \left(\frac{70 \text{ mg\%}}{100 \text{ mg\%}}\right) 150 \text{ ml/min} = 0.7 \times 150 \text{ ml/min}$$

$$= 105 \text{ ml/min}$$

$$ER = \frac{C_{bi} - C_{bo}}{C_{bi}} \quad {}_{di}$$

$$= \frac{140 \text{ mg\%} - 70 \text{ mg\%}}{140 \text{ mg\%} - 40 \text{ mg\%}}$$

$$= \frac{70 \text{ mg\%}}{100 \text{ mg\%}} = 0.7 = 70\%$$

Figure 6.3. Computation of dialysance and extraction ratio for urea. See Table 6.2 for definition of symbols. See text for further information.

The *solute extraction ratio (ER)* of a dialyzer is the term used for the $(C_{bi} - C_{bo})/(C_{bi} - C_{di})$ part of the formula expressed as a percent. Solute extraction ratio represents the effectiveness of the dialyzer as a mass transfer device (5).

An example of computation of dialysance and extraction ratio for urea is shown in Figure 6.3.

Fluid Removal

Controlled fluid removal is a very important aspect of dialysis. Fluid removal has two components or forces—that due to osmotic pressure and that due to hydrostatic pressure. The rate of fluid removal measured in ml/min is called the *ultrafiltration rate*.

Figure 6.4 depicts the principle of osmosis. *Osmosis* is the passage of a solvent (water) across a semipermeable membrane from an area of lesser solute concentration to an area of greater solute concentration. In Fig-

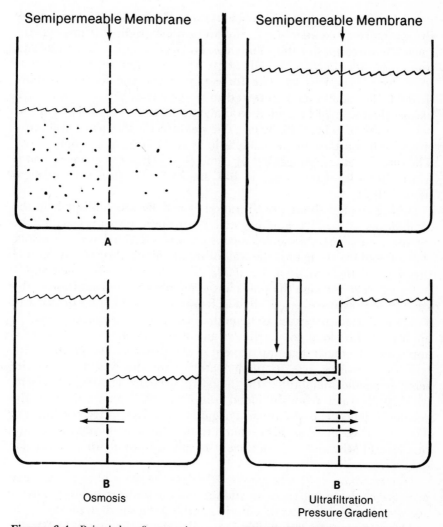

Semipermeable Membrane

A

B
Osmosis

Semipermeable Membrane

A

B
Ultrafiltration
Pressure Gradient

Figure 6.4. Principle of osmosis. There is an unequal concentration of solute on the two sides of the semipermeable membrane, and an osmotic gradient is present. Because the molecules of the solute are too large to cross the membrane, water molecules move to the side of greater concentration until a state of solute equilibrium exists.

Figure 6.5. Hydrostatic pressure. Water moves across the semipermeable membrane from a region of higher pressure to a region of lesser pressure.

ure 6.4A there is an unequal concentration of solute on the two sides of the semipermeable membrane, and an osmotic gradient is present. Because the molecules of the solute are too large to cross the membrane, water molecules move to the side of greater concentration until a state of solute equilibrium exists. The force that causes the solvent to move through the membrane is referred to as the *osmotic pressure*. In dialysis excess glucose may be added to dialysate to cause an *osmotic gradient* between the blood and dialysate. The net effect is that water will move from the blood into the dialysate as long as the osmotic gradient exists. The ultrafiltration rate caused by osmosis is difficult to estimate and is unpredictable; therefore, it has limited usefulness in clinical hemodialysis.

During hemodialysis, ultrafiltration is usually accomplished by the application of positive and negative hydrostatic pressures across the semipermeable membrane. *Hydrostatic pressure* is defined as the pressure that a liquid exerts against the wall of its container. (See Figure 6.5.) If the walls of the container are made of a semipermeable membrane, water will seep through the pores in the membrane in proportion to the amount of pressure exerted—that is, from a region of higher pressure to a region of lesser pressure. In hemodialysis a *positive hydrostatic pressure* is applied to the blood compartment and a *negative hydrostatic pressure* is applied to the dialysate compartment of the dialyzer. The positive hydrostatic pressure acts to push water from the blood across the semipermeable membrane; the negative pressure creates a vacuum, which pulls water from the blood compartment. Figure 6.6 shows the relationship between positive and negative pressures and water removal. The rate of water removal is related to the transmembrane hydrostatic pressure (TMP) and the coefficient of ultrafiltration for a particular dialyzer.

Transmembrane hydrostatic pressure (TMP) is the net sum of the average pressure of the blood entering and leaving the dialyzer minus the average pressure of the dialysate entering and leaving the dialyzer (6).

The *coefficent of ultrafiltration* for a dialyzer is the amount of water removed from the blood during a given period and at a specified pressure and is expressed in milliliters per hour per millimeter of mercury of transmembrane pressure (ml/hr/mmHgTMP) (6). The coefficient of ultrafiltration is related to the surface area of the membrane and permeability of the membrane to water. For example, if the coefficient of ultrafiltration of a dyalyzer is stated as 3.0 ml/hr/mmHgTMP, this means that for each mm Hg of transmembrane hydrostatic pressure exerted, 3.0 ml of water will be removed from the blood each hour of dialysis.

Applying the formula in Figure 6.7 to the situation in Figure 6.8:

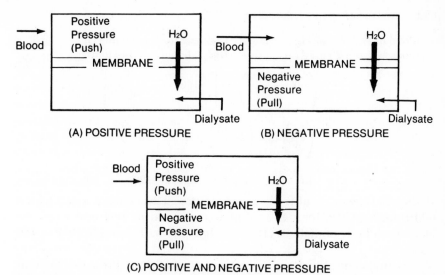

(A) POSITIVE PRESSURE **(B) NEGATIVE PRESSURE**

(C) POSITIVE AND NEGATIVE PRESSURE

Figure 6.6. Positive and negative hydrostatic pressures and water removal. The positive pressure in the blood compartment pushes water across the membrane; the negative pressure in the dialysate compartment creates a vacuum, which pulls water across the membrane from the blood compartment. The combination of positive and negative pressures is called the transmembrane pressure.

$$TMP = \left(\frac{\text{blood pressure in} + \text{blood pressure out}}{2}\right) minus$$

$$\left(\frac{\text{dialysate pressure in} + \text{dialysate pressure out}}{2}\right)$$

Figure 6.7. Formula for computing transmembrane hydrostatic pressure. See text for explanation.

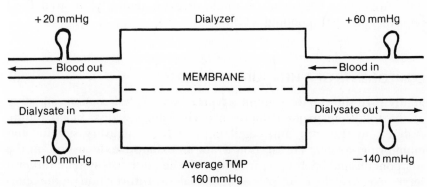

Figure 6.8. Application of negative and positive hydrostatic pressures to a typical hemodialysis system. See text for explanation.

151

Blood in = +60 mmHg   Dialysate in = −100 mmHg
Blood out = +20 mmHg   Dialysate out = −140 mmHg

$$TMP = \left(\frac{60 + 20}{2}\right) - \left[\frac{-100 + (-140)}{2}\right]$$

$$= \left(\frac{80}{2}\right) - \left(\frac{-240}{2}\right)$$

$$= 40 - (-120) = 40 + 120 = 160 \text{ mmHg}$$

If the coefficient of ultrafiltrration of the dialyzer were given as 3.0 ml/hr/mmHgTMP, then 480 ml of water would be removed from the blood each hour of dialysis. (160 mmHg × 3.0 ml/hr/mmHgTMP = 480 ml/hr)

In actual clinical dialysis, measurement of all four pressures to compute the TMP for desired ultrafiltration is not necessary. When using a coil dialyzer, the positive pressure on the blood side is of primary importance. When using a parallel flow plate dialyzer, the negative pressure on the dialysate side is of primary importance, but the positive pressure must be considered in computing the TMP.

The following factors must be considered when computing ultrafiltration:

1. Predialysis weight compared to dry weight of the patient.
2. Length (hours of dialysis treatment.
3. Intake during dialysis.
4. Changes in positive and negative pressures during dialysis.
5. The coefficient of ultrafiltration of the dialyzer.

Refer to Figure 6.9 for an example of computation of desired fluid removal and corresponding TMP.

COMPONENTS OF A HEMODIALYSIS SYSTEM

Figure 6.10 shows a diagram of a typical hemodialysis system consisting of the following major components: circulatory access, blood pump, dialyzer, method for anticoagulation, dialysate delivery system, and monitoring system. This section is not an exhaustive discussion on the components and operation procedure of a hemodialysis system; rather it serves to clarify the principles of hemodialysis. Information on the operation of specific hemodialysis equipment may be obtained from the manufacturer's literature.

Predialysis weight	155 lb		
Dry weight	150 lb		
Excess weight (500 ml = 1 lb)	5 lb	=	2500 ml

Plus:

Saline prime at beginning of dialysis	200 ml
Oral intake during dialysis	400 ml
Saline rinse at end of dialysis	150 ml
Total weight to be removed	3250 ml
Hours of dialysis	6 hr
Coefficient of ultrafiltration of dialyzer	3.0 ml/hr/mmHg

$$\frac{\text{Total weight to remove}}{\text{Hours of dialysis}} = \frac{3250 \text{ ml}}{6 \text{ hr}} = 542 \text{ ml/hr to remove}$$

$$\frac{\text{Weight to be removed per hour}}{\text{Coefficient of ultrafiltration of dialyzer}} = \frac{542 \text{ ml/hr}}{3.0 \text{ ml/hr/mm Hg}} = 180 \text{ mmHgTMP}$$

Figure 6.9. Computation of desired fluid removal and corresponding transmembrane pressure.

Circulatory Access

Circulatory access for hemodialysis is discussed in detail in Chapter 7 and is not considered in this section.

Blood Pump

Blood pumps are used to assist heart action in propelling the blood through the tubing and dialyzer. A blood pump is essential when the patient has an arteriovenous fistula to overcome the resistance of the fistula needles. The roller pump is one of the most commonly used types of blood pump. (See Figure 6.11.) The pump has two or more rollers that rotate in a closed compartment and squeeze the blood tubing against a semicircular wall. The roller is calibrated to give the proper blood flow rate when the correct size of tubing is used. When a blood pump is used, there must be no obstruction to the flow of blood through the tubing and dialyzer. If an obstruction exists inside the dialyzer or between the blood outlet of the dialyzer and the patient, pressure will build inside the dialyzer and could cause the membranes to rupture. If

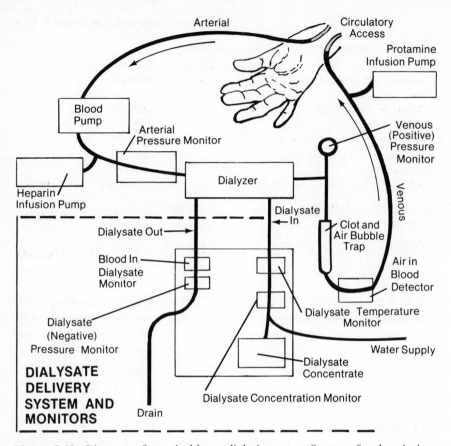

Figure 6.10. Diagram of a typical hemodialysis system. See text for description and explanation of components.

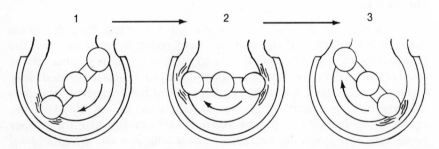

Figure 6.11. Diagram of a roller type blood pump. See text for description and explanation.

an obstruction exists between the circulatory access site and the pump, the arterial blood line will collapse from an insufficient supply of blood. In either case, the blood pump must be stopped until the problem is corrected.

Dialyzers

Currently three general designs of dialyzers are available: the coil, the parallel flow plate, and capillary (hollow fiber). There are advantages and disadvantages to each type. This section does not catalogue or compare currently available dialyzers, since the rapidity with which new dialyzers are being manufactured would make such a discussion quickly out of date. Rather, the general dialyzer types are described and factors related to dialyzer performance are considered to assist the operator in understanding the reason(s) for selection of a particular dialyzer for a given patient.

Coil Dialyzer

The coil dialyzer consists of tubes of semipermeable membrane (cellophane or cuprophan) held together by a mesh support. The cellophane and mesh supports are rolled into a compact coil. (See Figure 6.12A.) Blood is pumped through the tubes, and dialysate is pumped between the layers of the coil. The resistance to blood flow is high, and a blood pump is required. Ultrafiltration is accomplished by increasing the pressure in the blood channel to force water across the membrane.

Parallel Flow Plate Dialyzer

The parallel flow plate dialyzer consists of two layers of semipermeable membrane (such as cellophane or cuprophan) held together by semirigid and/or rigid supporting structures. (See Figure 6.12B.) Blood flows inside the two membrane layers, and dialysate flows countercurrent to the blood between the outside of the membranes and the adjacent supporting structure. To increase the dialyzing surface area, several layers of this module are contained inside one dialyzer.

There is a low resistance to blood flow, and a blood pump is not required to propel blood through the circuit; however, a blood pump is necessary if the patient has an arteriovenous fistula and may be used with any type of access to maintain uniformity of blood flow. Ultrafiltration is achieved by controlling the negative pressure via a pump to the dialysate circuit and by controlling the positive pressure within the blood compartment.

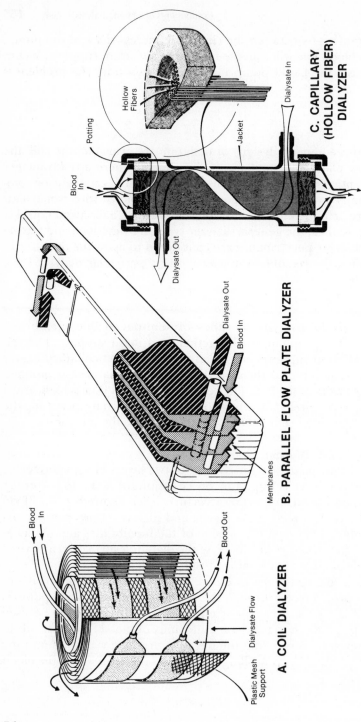

Figure 6.12. General dialyzer designs. See text for explanation.

156

Capillary (Hollow Fiber) Dialyzer

The hollow fiber dialyzer consists of fine capillaries with a semipermeable membrane (cuprophan or cellulose) enclosed in a plastic cylinder. (See Figure 6.12C.) Blood is pumped through the capillaries, and dialysate is pumped countercurrent or crosscurrent to the blood on the outside of the capillaries.

The hollow fiber dialyzer has a large dialyzing surface area, and ultrafiltration is achieved by a combination of negative dialysate pressure and positive blood channel pressure. Depending on the type of membrane used, blood may have a higher tendency to clot in the capillaries, and a larger amount of heparin may be required than with other types of dialyzers.

Dialyzer Performance

Factors that influence dialyzer performance and thus determine selection for patient use include:

1. Dialyzing membrane surface area.
2. Resistance to diffusion.
3. Membrane thickness and pore size.
4. Coefficient of ultrafiltration.
5. Ultrafiltration predictability.
6. Clearance (dialysance) of uremic toxins and electrolytes.
7. Priming volume.
8. Compliance.
9. Blood recovery.
10. Cost.
11. Availability.
12. Ease of assembly.

Dialyzing membrane surface area, membrane thickness and pore size, resistance to diffusion, coefficient of ultrafiltration, and clearance of uremic toxins and electrolytes are interrelated. The larger the dialyzing surface area and the thinner the membrane, the greater the clearance and ultrafiltration. It is important that ultrafiltration be both predictable and consistent with each treatment; that is, the coefficient of ultrafiltration for each dialyzer should be very close to that stated by the manufacturer with only small variations in any dialyzer of the same brand. The pores in the membrane should be large enough to permit uremic wastes and water to pass from blood to dialysate and for electrolytes to move in both directions, but small enough to prevent passage of blood cells and serum protein from blood to dialysate and bacteria from dialysate to blood. Resistance to diffusion is caused by a blood film layer, resistance of the membrane itself, and a dialysate fluid film layer. Resistance caused by the blood film layer is reduced by achieving a very thin blood channel; membrane resistance is reduced by using a thin membrane; and dialysate fluid film resistance is overcome by using high dialysate flow rates and by constructing the support structure to create turbulence along the dialysate pathway.

The priming volume of a dialyzer should be small and the volume should remain fairly constant with changes in the TMP throughout dialysis. If a dialyzer is compliant (as TMP increases, so does the blood volume in the dialyzer), the patient may develop problems with hypovolemia due to the increased extracorporeal blood volume. Currently most disposable dialyzers are relatively noncompliant, owing to the rigid support structure.

Since anemia is a serious problem in end stage renal disease, the dialyzer should allow total recovery of extracorporeal blood at the end of the dialysis.

Cost, availability, and ease of assembly are important to in-center and home dialysis and should be considered before selecting the dialyzer. The cost of most disposable dialyzers is comparable, and part of this cost may be offset by reuse of the dialyzer; therefore, availability and ease of assembly are the primary issues to consider.

Anticoagulation During Dialysis

When the blood comes in contact with rough or foreign surfaces, as in the blood lines and dialyzer, it tends to clot unless a method of anticoagulation is used. Anticoagulation is always necessary during dialysis to prevent clotting of blood in the tubing and dialyzer. The short-acting anticoagulant, heparin, is used in hemodialysis to prevent this clotting tendency.

The anticoagulant activity of heparin is related to its sulfuric acid content. Heparin is derived from intestinal mucosa (mucosal heparin) or from beef lung (beef lung heparin). The clinical effectiveness of the two types of heparin is the same, provided that each is prescribed in USP units rather than milligrams. If the two types are exchanged based on milligrams, mucosal heparin is more potent than beef lung heparin. Heparin is metabolized in the liver, and a weakly active form is excreted in the urine. Heparin activity is usually quite small four to six hours after administration.

Protamine sulfate is used to neutralize heparin activity. Protamine is highly alkaline and neutralizes the highly acidic heparin to form a stable salt:

$$\text{heparin} \atop \text{(acid)} \quad + \quad \text{protamine} \atop \text{(base)} \quad \rightarrow \quad \text{salt} \atop \text{(neutral)}$$

Protamine is prescribed in milligrams because it neutralizes heparin by weight, not by anticoagulant activity. Approximately 1 to 1.5 mg of protamine neutralizes 1 mg of heparin (either mucosal or beef lung). Protamine may act as an anticoagulant when given in large doses, but moderate doses do not have a significant anticoagulant effect.

During hemodialysis, heparin may be administered continuously, intermittently, or regionally. Heparin therapy must be monitored closely, because individual responses may vary. Clotting tendency may be increased by such factors as anxiety or infection and decreased by anemia (hematocrit < 14–15). The Lee-White clotting time or activated partial thromboplastin time may be used for monitoring the effect of heparin during hemodialysis.

Continuous heparinization is achieved by infusing heparin throughout dialysis via a calibrated infusion pump into the arterial blood line (inlet) of the dialyzer. Depending on the patient's response, herapin is adminstered at a rate of 1000–2000 USP units per hour.

Intermittent heparinization is done by administering a loading dose of heparin at the beginning of dialysis, and additional smaller doses are administered throughout dialysis, the doses being determined by the clotting times.

If the patient has had recent surgery, has a pericardial friction rub or pericardial effusion, or has any bleeding tendency, a regional heparinization is required. Heparin is infused continuously via an infusion pump into the arterial blood line (inlet); concomitantly, protamine sulfate is infused into the venous line (outlet), where blood is being returned to the patient. The net effect is that the heparin is neutralized before the blood inside the dialyzer reenters the body.

Occasionally, after a regional heparinization a phenomenon called "heparin rebound" may occur. It occurs most often when large doses of heparin and protamine are used, and rarely when small doses are used. The cause of heparin rebound is unclear, but is probably caused by a breakdown of the heparin-protamine complex in the reticuloendothelial system. Heparin then reenters the systemic circulation, resulting in an excess of heparin. The problems related to heparin rebound may be prevented by an awareness of its occurrence and by determining the clotting time three to four hours postdialysis and administering additional protamine if the clotting time is elevated.

Dialysate Delivery System

The purpose of a dialysate delivery system is to prepare and deliver dialysate of the required chemical composition to the dialyzer. There are two types of dialysate delivery systems: the batch system and the dialysate proportioning system. (See Figure 6.13.)

The batch system is commonly used with the coil type dialyzer. A concentrated dialysate solution or individual chemicals are added to water until the desired composition is obtained. The dialysate is pumped around the coil at a rate of 10–30 liters per minute. A new batch of dialysate must be mixed two or three times during dialysis. The recirculating single-pass (RSP) system is a modification of the batch system. The dialysate is mixed in a large container and is pumped over the coil membranes located in a second container. After passing over the coil, part of the dialysate is drained off and part recirculated over the coil. The part that is drained off is replaced by fresh dialysate. Since this is an open system, negative pressure cannot be obtained in the dialysate compartment.

Depending on individual unit preference, the dialysate proportioning system is commonly used with parallel plate dialyzers, but it may be used with all types. Dialysate concentrate is mixed with water in a ratio of 1:35 by a proportioning pump. The dialysate is pumped through the dialyzer only once before going down the drain. This closed system allows negative pressure to be obtained and controlled in the dialysate compartment. The proportioning system may supply dialysate to a single dialyzer (as in home dialysis), or a large central proportioning system may be set up to supply dialysate to several dialyzers.

Dialysate Fluid Composition

Regardless of the type of dialysate delivery system, the dialysate delivered to the dialyzer must have an electrolyte concentration corresponding to that of normal serum. The constituents and typical concentrations of each in the dialysate are listed in Table 6.3. The anions (negative ions) and cations (positive ions) are equal in number. Because of blood-dialysate concentration gradients for the various electrolytes, excess serum electrolytes move from blood to dialysate, and if there is a deficiency of any electrolyte(s) in the serum, the movement is from dialysate

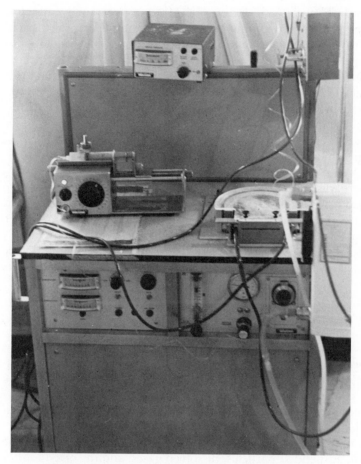

Figure 6.13. Typical hemodialysis delivery system.

Table 6.3. Typical Dialysate Composition

Ion	Dialysate Concentration Range
Sodium	135 mEq/L
Calcium	3.0 mEq/L
Magnesium	1.0 mEq/L
Potassium	0–3 mEq/L
Chloride	104 mEq/L
Sodium acetate	38 mEq/L
Glucose	0–200 mg/100 ml

161

to blood. The dialysate is relatively free of metabolic waste products (such as urea and creatinine); therefore, the movement of these is from blood to dialysate. The concentration of dialysate may be altered to treat certain electrolyte imbalances in the dialysis patient; for example, potassium is not included or is in a low concentration if the patient is hyperkalemic. The sodium acetate is converted by the body to sodium bicarbonate, which, in turn, helps maintain a normal serum pH. Glucose is usually not included in the dialysate; however, if the patient is diabetic, approximately 200 mg/100 ml of glucose may be included to prevent hypoglycemia from dialysance of glucose. Dialysate is made from clean water and chemicals, but it is not free of bacteria. Bacteria and other microorganisms are too large to cross the membrane and contaminate the blood; however, they may secrete an exogenous material and precipitate a pyrogenic reaction in the patient. Dialysate is warmed to approximately 100°F to prevent cooling of blood and to increase solute removal by diffusion. A too-high temperature is a complication of hemodialysis that is discussed in a subsequent section of this chapter.

Water Treatment

The water used to dilute the dialysate concentrate or to dissolve the chemicals must meet certain specified standards. The water supply need not be sterile, but it must contain only trace amounts of minerals and other contaminants that can cross the dialysis membrane and cause complications for the patient. Since water quality and composition vary from location to location, water treatment systems are employed to insure a uniform water supply. Three types of contaminants must be considered: suspended particles, dissolved gases, and dissolved ionized material. Suspended particles, such as mud, algae, and some bacteria, are adequately removed by filters. Dissolved gases are removed by a degasser before the dialysate enters the dialyzer. Dissolved ionized material is removed by a process of deionization or by a reverse osmosis process.

Deionization is the process of removing dissolved ionized compounds from water by ion exchangers. Dissolved positive ions (cations such as sodium, calcium, and magnesium) are removed by passing water through a cation resin. Negative ions (anions such as chlorides, sulfates, carbonates, nitrates, and phosphates) are removed by an anion resin.

Reverse osmosis is the process of forcing water under pressure through a semipermeable membrane. Water passes through the membrane; dissolved materials cannot. This process removes approximately

95% of cations and anions and is similarly efficient in the removal of microorganisms.

Monitors

A dialysate delivery system should include monitors that indicate variables in the system. Both audible and visual alarms should be present to alert the operator when preset limits are violated. Parameters that are monitored during hemodialysis include variables in the dialysate channel and variables in the blood channel. Factors monitored in the blood channel include arterial pressure, venous pressure, and air in the blood as it is returned to the patient. Factors monitored in the dialysate channel include concentration (conductivity) of dialysate, dialysate flow rate, dialysate temperature, dialysate pressure, and blood in the dialysate. Table 6.4 summarizes hemodialysis monitoring systems in terms of factor monitored, operation of monitor, and conditions causing an alarm.

Monitors must be properly used and receive periodic preventive maintenance. Shutting alarms off or improperly setting alarm limits can endanger the patient's life. Alarms can assist in providing a safe, efficient dialysis only if properly functioning and properly set before each dialysis and reset after the occurrence of an alarm.

THE DIALYSIS PROCEDURE

Although this section discusses the steps in a typical hemodialysis procedure, it is not intended to serve as a procedure manual for any specific type of dialyzer. To clarify the discussion, some of the salient aspects of dialyzing with a parallel flow plate dialyzer are illustrated and summarized in the text.

The dialysis treatment is divided into phases: predialysis, initiation of dialysis, intradialysis, and postdialysis. Predialysis activities include preparation of the dialzyer and assessment of the patient. Initiation of dialysis includes connecting the blood lines to the circulatory access site and beginning the dialysis procedure. During dialysis the patient is monitored to detect his reaction (desired and adverse) to the treatment; anticoagulation of the blood is monitored; and the dialysis system is monitored for technical problems. Dialysis is discontinued by returning the blood inside the dialyzer to the patient. Postdialysis the patient's status is evaluated and the dialyzer is either discarded or, in some centers, cleaned and sterilized for reuse on the same patient.

Table 6.4. Hemodialysis Monitoring Systems

Factor Monitored	Operation of Monitor	Conditions Causing an Alarm
SECTION I. BLOOD CHANNEL		
Arterial pressure of extracorporeal blood	Measures pressure of blood in drip chamber between patient and dialyzer inlet. Readout is in form of gauge or manometer calibrated in mmHg. Upper and lower limits set by operator. Both visual and audible alarms present.	*Low alarm:* Hypotension; occlusion of arterial side of circulatory access; disconnection of arterial line; blood pump set at rate more rapid than blood flow from patient can supply the pump; massive blood leak inside dialyzer. *High alarm:* Hypertension; clotting of dialyzer; occlusion of venous (outlet) blood line or of venous side of circulatory access.
Venous pressure of extracorporeal blood	Measures pressure of blood in drip chamber between dialyzer outlet and patient. Readout is in form of gauge or manometer calibrated in mmHg. Upper and lower limits set by operator. Both visual and audible alarms present.	*Low alarm:* Hypotension; clotting of dialyzer; disconnection of venous line; massive dialyzer leak; sudden increase in negative pressure. *High alarm:* Hypertension; occlusion of venous line or venous side of circulatory access site.
Air bubble detector	Detects air bubbles and clots in the venous blood by means of photoelectric cell or ultrasound. When alarm sounds, it stops the blood pump and clamps the venous blood line until condition is corrected.	Large amounts of air in blood line; air mixed with blood; small clots in blood line.
SECTION II. DIALYSATE CHANNEL		
Dialysate concentration (conductivity)	Continuously measures electrical conductivity (concentration) of dialysate. Upper and lower limits of safety are preset by the manufacturer for some systems and may be set by the operator for other	Alarms caused by incorrect proportion between water and chemicals (dialysate concentrate). *Low alarm:* Too much water or too little chemicals. *High alarm:* Too little water or too much chemicals.

	systems. Improper concentration of dialysate can result in blood cell and CNS damage. Alarm condition causes dialysate to by-pass dialyzer until problem is corrected.	
Dialysate flow	Measures and displays flow rate on monitor. Flow rate is preset by manufacturer for many systems and may be set by operator for others. Divergence from desired rate, unless extremely out of range, does not result in harm to the patient.	Mechanical malfunctioning of pumps. Electrical power loss. Inadequate water pressure.
Dialysate temperature	Thermostat controls electric heater or hot/cold mixing valve. Range may be preset by manufacturer for some systems and may be set by operator for others. Incorrect temperature results in blood cell damage or chilling. Alarm conditions cause dialysate to by-pass dialyzer until condition is corrected.	Mechanical malfunctioning of heater. Extremely hot water supply. Electrical power loss.
Blood in the dialysate	Photoelectric cell detects color changes in effluent dialysate line. Audible and visual alarms are activated and blood pump stops. Effluent dialysate may also be checked by Hemastix for presence of blood. Visual monitoring of effluent dialysate line for presence of blood is also important. If blood leak is severe, discontinue dialysis and set up new dialyzer.	Tear in dialyzer membrane allowing mixing of blood and dialysate. Will alarm with excessive air in dialysate.
Dialysate pressure (negative pressure)	Measures negative pressure of dialysate. Also incorporates vacuum mechanism to control amount of negative pressure. Upper and lower limits are set by the operator. Alarm condition causes audible and visual alarms and stops dialysate flow.	Mechanical malfunction of dialysate pump. Electrical power loss.

Predialysis Process

Before dialysis can be initiated, the dialyzer must be prepared, the monitoring system must be readied, and the patient must be assessed and prepared for the procedure.

Preparation of the dialyzer consists of flushing air from both blood and dialysate channels. The dialysate channel is flushed by connecting the dialyzer to the dialysate line and allowing the dialysate to flow through until all air is removed. The blood channel is primed by flushing with 400–500 ml of normal saline. Priming must be from bottom to top to insure that all air is removed from the dialyzer. The normal saline remains in the dialyzer and is displaced when the blood enters. Figures 6.14A and B illustrate the priming process for a typical parallel flow plate dialyzer.

The predialysis patient assessment includes measuring and recording vital signs and weight, observing for edema, rales, or rhonchi, and determining other problems that may be present. The blood pressure is measured in both lying and standing positions and recorded to be used as a baseline throughout dialysis. It should also be compared with the patient's previous blood pressure measurements to determine deviations from his usual reading. An apical pulse is auscultated for rate, rhythm, and the presence of a pericardial rub. The lungs are auscultated for presence of rales or rhonchi indicating excess fluid; respiratory rate, rhythm, and quality are assessed. The temperature may be subnormal if the BUN is elevated to any degree. Weight is obtained and compared to the last postdialysis weight and to the "dry" weight. Weight gain between dialyses should be 1.5–2.0 kg. The feet, ankles, hands, and eyelids are checked for edema. A determination is made of the amount of weight to be removed by dialysis. In addition, discuss with the patient any problems such as headache, nausea, vomiting, or respiratory difficulty that he has had since the last dialysis, as they may affect the process of the present treatment.

Initiation of Dialysis

To initiate dialysis the circulatory access site is prepared (see Chapter 7 for details) and the arterial and venous blood lines of the dialyzer are connected to the appropriate sides of the shunt or to the appropriate fistula needle. (See Figure 6.14C.)

A few milliliters of blood may be removed at this time for BUN, creatinine, electrolyte, hematocrit, and baseline clotting time determinations.

The administration of heparin (and protamine, if required) is started shortly after the blood lines are connected.

The blood flow is started slowly (50–75 ml/min) and increased gradually to avoid a fall in blood pressure. An optimum blood flow is reached within 30 minutes after starting dialysis. (See the section on dialysance for discussion of blood flow rate and solute removal.) The blood pressure is checked frequently as the blood fills the dialyzer, and the patient is observed for signs and symptoms of hypotension—yawning, restlessness, nausea, vomiting, confusion, dizziness, feeling of warmth, chest or back pain, and/or diaphoresis.

Monitoring During Dialysis

After the initiation of dialysis the following parameters are monitored until completion of the procedure: vital signs, weight, clotting time of the blood, desired and adverse reactions to the treatment, comfort and diversion for the patient, and technical problems in the delivery system and/or dialyzer.

Depending on the patient's status, blood pressure is measured every 15 minutes to an hour. The patient should be taught to recognize and report early signs of hypotension so measures may be taken before there is a significant decrease. An increase in the diastolic pressure as a compensatory mechanism to decreasing vascular volume is a sign of impending hypotension. If the blood pressure drops significantly and/or the patient is symptomatic (nausea, vomiting, diarrhea, perspiration, restlessness, confusion), one or more of the following measures is implemented:

1. Decrease the blood flow rate from the patient to the dialyzer.
2. Lower the TMP to decrease ultrafiltration and thus the amount of fluid removed from the vascular volume.
3. Elevate the patient's feet and legs above the level of the heart. This returns approximately 500 ml per minute to the cardiac output.
4. Increase the circulating fluid volume by administering normal saline boluses of 100 to 500 ml into the blood lines. Frequent blood pressure determinations must be made during administration. In children 50–100 ml may be sufficient.
5. Increase the circulating fluid volume by administering a colloid osmotic agent such as albumin. Albumin draws fluid from the extravascular into the vascular space, thus increasing the vascular volume and blood pressure. Albumin is especially helpful to increase the blood pressure if the patient has a low serum albumin level. If the patient

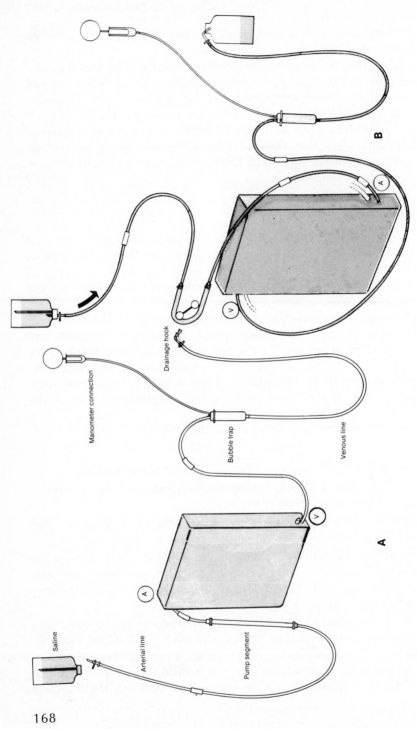

Saline

Arterial line

Pump segment

A

Manometer connection

Drainage hook

Bubble trap

Venous line

V

A

B

168

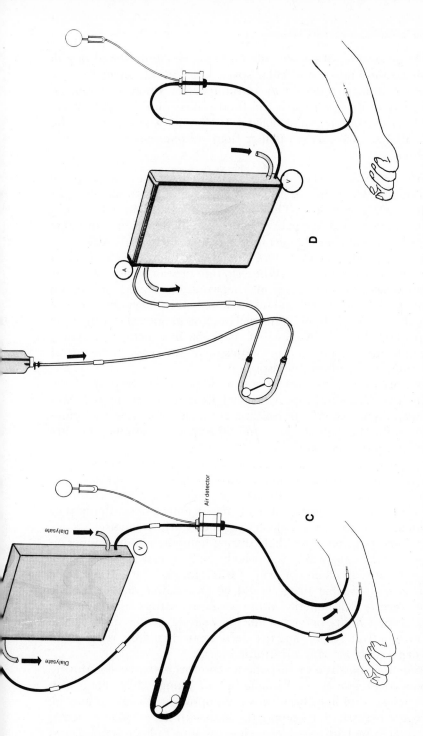

Figure 6.14. A. Preparation for priming dialyzer with normal saline. B. Flushing dialyzer with normal saline to expel air from the blood compartment and to prepare for connection to the patient. C. Dialyzer connected to the patient and dialysis procedure in progress. D. Termination of dialysis and rinsing of dialyzer blood compartment with normal saline to return as much blood as possible to the patient.

has a large amount of edema, albumin may be administered to pull the edema fluid into the vascular space. Once in the vascular space, the excess fluid is removed by ultrafiltration. Albumin should be given early in dialysis so that the fluid pulled into the space is removed before completion of dialysis. If albumin is given toward the end of dialysis, the excess vascular fluid volume may cause pulmonary edema.

The weight may be checked during dialysis to determine the adequacy of ultrafiltration. Many dialysis units have bed scales for constant weight monitoring during treatment. If bed scales are not available and a weight determination is needed, the patient may carefully stand (don't dislodge fistula needles or kink blood lines) with assistance on bedside scales.

The adequacy of heparinization of blood in the dialyzer is determined frequently by performing a Lee-White clotting time or an activated partial thromboplastin time. If a regional heparinization is used, a clotting time must be performed on blood taken directly from the patient as well as on blood from the dialyzer. A normal or close to normal clotting time for the patient's blood indicates that the heparin is being adequately neutralized by the protamine; if not, adjustments are made in the rate of heparin and/or protamine administration.

All monitors and alarms must be functioning and must be properly set during dialysis. Technical aspects of dialysis that are monitored have already been discussed. Any technical malfunction may cause a serious complication for the patient; these and other patient complications are discussed later in this chapter.

If the patient desires, meals are served during the dialysis procedure; however, large or heavy meals should be avoided, because they can cause a hypotensive episode. Some dialysis centers allow a less restricted dietary and fluid intake during treatment; most centers stress the importance of maintaining the usual dietary regimen during dialysis.

Medications are given or withheld during hemodialysis depending on whether or not the drug will be removed by dialysis. (See Chapter 9 for a discussion of the dialyzability of drugs.) If it is known that a drug will be removed by dialysis, that drug should be given after dialysis for the patient to receive full benefit. Antihypertensive drugs should not be given for several hours before or during dialysis, as they prevent the vascular system from responding to a decrease in circulating volume due to extracorporeal blood and ultrafiltration.

Attention must be given to the patient's comfort and diversion during the dialysis treatment. A comfortable bed or lounge chair along with position changes and light back rubs are important. Diversion may be limited by the necessity for keeping the limb with the circulatory access site somewhat immobile. Activities such as reading, radio, television, and some crafts may be arranged for the patient. Conversation among in-center dialysis patients is encouraged. If chairs or beds can be moved closer together, chess, checkers, and card games are also diverting.

Discontinuing Dialysis

To terminate dialysis the arterial line is clamped and disconnected from the circulatory access. The heparin infusion is discontinued 15 minutes to an hour before termination of dialysis. The arterial line of the dialyzer is connected to a bottle of normal saline. (See Figure 6.14D.) Approximately 100 to 200 ml of normal saline is infused into the dialyzer to rinse the blood compartment and return as much blood as possible to the patient. The saline rinse may be followed by an air rinse. If an air rinse is used, the operator must be particularly cautious to prevent an air embolism.

After all of the blood in the dialyzer has been returned to the patient, the external shunt is reconnected and dressed or the needles are removed from the arteriovenous fistula, and pressure is applied over the needle insertion sites until bleeding stops. A pressure dressing may be applied over the insertion sites and removed within four to six hours after dialysis.

According to unit policy, the dialyzer is either discarded or cleaned and sterilized for reuse on the same patient. The delivery system is cleaned and prepared for reuse.

Postdialysis Observations

After dialysis the patient's status and response to the procedure are evaluated. Vital signs and weight are obtained and compared with pre-dialysis measurements. It is expected that the blood pressure and weight will be lower, owing to fluid removal. The temperature may be higher, because the BUN has been decreased (urea is a hypothermic agent). If the temperature is above 99.6°F, sepsis is suspected and blood cultures should be obtained.

If regional heparinization has been used, the patient should be monitored for heparin rebound for several hours postdialysis. (See the section on anticoagulation.)

Complications of Hemodialysis

In this section dialysis disequilibrium syndrome and hemodialysis-associated hepatitis are discussed. Table 6.5 places the other principal complications of hemodialysis in three categories: immediately lethal;

Table 6.5. Complications of Hemodialysis

SECTION I. IMMEDIATELY LETHAL

A. *Air Embolism*

Causes	Prevention
1. Retained air in the dialyzer.	1. Prime dialyzer thoroughly with venous (outlet) end up.
2. Loose connections or leaks in the blood lines.	2. Bridge all connections tightly.
3. Blood pump set too fast during reinfusion.	3. Turn blood pump "On" slowly.
4. Empty saline bottle or bag:	4. Air detector should be used, but is not foolproof.
a. failure to clamp infusion line	5. Reinfuse slowly, and have double clamps in position at all times.
b. constant saline drip	6. During dialysis, administer saline as a bolus, never as a constant saline drip.
	7. Discard clamps with weak jaws.

Signs and Symptoms	Treatment
1. Chest pain, dyspnea, coughing, cyanosis.	1. Stop infusion of air.
2. Visual problems—"seeing stars," diplopia, blindness.	2. Position patient on left side with feet elevated for at least 30 minutes.
3. Neurological deficits—confusion, coma, hemiparesis.	3. Administer oxygen.
4. Evidence of air in blood lines.	4. Call physician.

B. *Hemolysis (hypotonic dialysate)*

Causes	Prevention
Usually requires two simultaneous errors:	1. *Always* check dialysate with hand conductivity meter before dialysis.
1. Failure to fill delivery system with dialysate concentrate.	2. Clean concentrate tank, lines, and filter frequently.
2. Obstruction of dialysate concentrate line.	3. All delivery systems should include a conductivity alarm with preset limits.
3. Incorrect setting of conductivity alarm limits.	4. Regular preventive maintenance of alarm system.
4. Absence of conductivity alarm (on older systems).	
5. Malfunction of conductivity monitors.	

Signs and Symptoms	Treatment
1. Burning in circulatory return site.	1. *Immediately* clamp return (venous) line. Do not reinfuse hemolyzed blood.
2. Warmth in throat.	2. Monitor vital signs and observe for arrhythmias.
3. Chest pain and dyspnea.	3. Check postdialysis hematocrit and electrolytes. Acute anemia is most often the critical problem.
4. Arrhythmias.	4. Consider blood transfusion if symptoms are severe.
5. Clear blood in return lines.	5. Repeat dialysis if electrolyte abnormalities are severe.
6. Sodium concentration low in hemolyzed blood.	

C. Hyperthemia (overheated dialysate)

Causes	Prevention
1. Malfunction of heater and/or temperature monitor.	1. All electrical components should be shielded from corrosive effects of dialysate.
2. Absence of separate temperature monitor on delivery system.	2. Two temperature monitors should be present: one to control the heater and one to monitor the final temperature.
3. Absence of high-temperature alarm and by-pass mechanism.	3. Regular preventive maintenance of monitors.
	4. Check dialysate temperature when patient complains of feeling hot.

Signs and Symptoms	Treatment
1. Patient will complain of feeling hot.	1. *Immediately* discontinue dialysis.
2. Blood may be very dark.	2. Do not return heat-damaged blood.
3. Eventual coma and death.	3. Obtain serial measurement of patient's temperature.
	4. Record temperature of dialysate.
	5. Determine hematocrit and electrolytes.
	6. Observe for signs and symptoms of hemolysis.
	7. Provide external cooling for temperatures over 106°F.

Table 6.5. (*continued*)

D. Exsanguination

Causes	Prevention
1. Accidental separation of blood lines.	1. Tightly secure and bridge *all* connections.
2. Needles accidently dislodged from circulatory access site.	2. Tape needles at two points.
3. Ruptured blood lines.	3. Do not allow patient to dialyze alone.
4. Ruptured dialyzer membrane.	4. Check blood pump for proper occlusion monthly.
5. Separation of external cannula from itself or from vessel.	5. Place blood lines in pump properly.
6. Internal bleeding.	6. All delivery systems must have functioning blood leak detector.
	7. Visually monitor dialysate outflow line for evidence of blood.
	8. Proper shunt care and observation.
	9. Use regional heparinization if patient has bleeding tendency.

Signs and Symptoms	Treatment
1. Source of bleeding is usually obvious.	1. Immediately clamp on both sides of separated line.
2. Shock, often with convulsions and/or vomiting.	2. Turn blood pump "Off."
3. Melena and/or hematemesis in GI bleeding.	3. Apply local pressure to bleeding point.
	4. Do not return blood from a badly ruptured dialyzer.
	5. Give protamine for bleeding developing during dialysis.
	6. Administer oxygen.
	7. Administer volume expander if hypotensive.

E. Cardiac Tamponade

Causes	Prevention
1. Acute pericarditis.	1. Auscultate for a rub and for a paradox when a patient has chest pain or unexpectedly low blood pressure.
2. Chronic pericarditis.	2. Dialyze using a regional heparinization when pericarditis is known.
3. Constrictive pericarditis.	3. Replace volume liberally and rapidly for hypotension in a patient with known pericarditis.
4. Precipitated by a reduction in blood volume in any of the above conditions.	

Signs and Symptoms	Treatment
1. Central chest pain, often worse when supine, improves when upright. 2. Pericardial friction rub. 3. Hypotension, especially during dialysis, often apparently inappropriate. 4. Paradoxical pulse greater than 10 mmHg. 5. Distended neck veins. 6. Muffled heart sounds. 7. Absent apical impulse. 8. Low EKG voltage.	1. Intensive dialysis for pericarditis. 2. Subtotal pericardiectomy for pericardial effusion. 3. Pericardiocentesis in an extreme emergency while preparing the patient for surgery. 4. Keep a pericardiocentesis tray at the bedside of all patients with known pericarditis.

SECTION II. OFTEN SERIOUS, POSSIBLY LETHAL

Problem	Causes	Prevention	Treatment
A. Fever	1. Pyrogens 2. Infection	1. Proper water treatment.	1. Blood culture for all fever during dialysis. 2. ASA or Tylenol for fever. 3. Antibiotics. 4. Culture dialysate and water.
B. Seizures	1. Dialysis dis-equilibrium syndrome	1. Avoid excessively rapid BUN drop during dialysis. 2. Avoid severe uremia. 3. Anticonvulsant medication. 4. Blood pressure monitoring and support during dialysis.	1. Slow blood flow and short dialysis to decrease BUN slowly. 2. Begin dialysis early in course of uremia. 3. Measure blood pressure frequently during dialysis and administer volume expander as necessary.
C. Major arrhythmias	1. Electrolyte and pH changes 2. Underlying heart disease 3. Removal of anti-arrhythmic drugs by dialysis	1. Use 3 mEq potassium dialysate if patient has known heart disease or is on a digitalis preparation. 2. Give additional antiarrhythmic drugs during dialysis	1. Antiarrhythmic drugs as required. 2. Potassium as required. 3. Discontinue dialysis for severe, persistent arrhythmias. 4. Monitor EKG.
D. Hyperosmolarity	1. Hyperglycemia 2. Hypernatremia	1. Glucose in dialysate for diabetics. 2. Proper dialysate mixture.	1. Monitor blood glucose. 2. Constant monitoring of dialysate conductivity.

Table 6.5. (continued)

SECTION III. LESS SERIOUS BUT SIGNIFICANT

Problem	Causes	Prevention	Treatment
A. Headache, cramps, back pain	Early dialysis disequilibrium syndrome	1. Proper dietary control 2. Avoid rapid dialysis.	1. Administer saline intravenously. 2. Slow blood flow.
B. Angina	1. Anemia 2. HASCVD	1. Blood transfusion if necessary. 2. Administer nitroglycerin and related drugs. 3. Increase blood pump speed slowly.	1. Discontinue dialysis if severe. 2. Administer oxygen. 3. Administer nitroglycerin. 4. Mild sedation. 5. Decrease blood flow. 6. Decrease ultrafiltration rate.
C. Hypotension	1. Hypovolemia from excessive fluid removal	1. Proper fluid intake. 2. Remove fluid as slowly as possible. 3. Monitor hematocrit.	1. Administer volume expanders: saline and/or colloid osmotic agents. 2. Blood transfusion for anemia.

often serious, possibly lethal; and less serious but significant. In each category the causes, prevention, signs and symptoms, and treatment for the various complications are listed.

Dialysis Disequilibrium Syndrome

The patient should be observed for signs and symptoms of the dialysis disequilibrium syndrome toward the end of dialysis and for several hours postdialysis. The signs and symptoms of the syndrome range from mild confusion and headache to convulsions, cardiopulmonary arrest, and death. The etiology of this problem is unclear but is thought to be due to a rapid change in the BUN during dialysis. During dialysis the concentration of the serum urea nitrogen is reduced more rapidly than the urea nitrogen in the cerebrospinal fluid and brain tissue because of the slow transport of urea across the blood-brain barrier. Urea acts as an osmotic agent and draws water from the serum and extracellular fluid into the central nervous system, causing edema of the brain. Other factors that may be involved include rapid pH changes and electrolyte shifts. The signs and symptoms are those of any patient suffering increased intracranial pressure: headache, nausea, vomiting, restlessness, rising pulse pressure, decrease in sensorium, convulsions, coma, and death.

Guidelines for the prevention and treatment of dialysis disequilibrium syndrome include (7,8):

1. Addition of an osmotic solute, such as glucose, mannitol, urea, or sodium chloride, to the dialysate to prevent a rapid fall in serum osmolality.

2. Short, frequent dialyses with an inefficient dialyzer and a slow blood flow rate to prevent rapid removal of solute.

3. Prophylactic or therapeutic use of anticonvulsant medications such as short-acting barbiturates (amytal), long-acting barbiturates (phenobarbital), diazepam (Valium), or diphenylhydantoin (Dilantin).

In addition, early recognition of signs and symptoms of dialysis disequilibrium syndrome and termination of the procedure may prevent a life-threatening situation. Resuscitation equipment should be readily available in all dialysis units.

Hemodialysis-Associated Hepatitis

Hemodialysis-associated hepatitis is a significant problem for patients receiving hemodialysis and for staff in hemodialysis units. Since the first epidemics of hepatitis in dialysis units in 1966, the number of cases has been steadily rising (9).

The hepatitis B surface antigen (HBsAg) was discovered in 1965. HGsAg was formerly called Australia (Au) antigen, hepatitis-associated antigen (HAA), or serum hepatitis (SH) antigen.

The hepatitis B virus is composed of a core structure (HBcAg) and a surface structure (HBsAg). The surface structure may be present by itself. The core structure probably represents the true hepatitis B virus and is required for actual infection of liver cells. Apparently the core structure reproduces in liver cell nuclei and migrates to the cytoplasm, where it is enveloped with the surface structure. The surface antigen is reproduced in excess of the core antigen and may appear in the serum weeks to months before the development of abnormal liver function tests and may be present in the serum after the whole virus has disappeared (10).

Following infection, the surface antigen appears first, DNA polymerase next, followed by antibody to the core antigen; elevation of liver enzymes appears last. Antibody to surface antigen appears late in the course of infection—weeks to months after HBsAg and abnormal SGOT levels (10).

Laboratory tests for HBsAg include agar gel diffusion, complement fixation, counter-immunoelectrophoresis, and radioimmunoassay. There is no currently available test for HBcAg. Antibodies to surface and core antigens may be determined by radioimmunoassay and complement fixation tests.

Carriers of HBsAg may have no clinical signs of liver disease and may not develop detectable levels of antibodies to HBsAg. A positive HBsAg indicates acute or chronic hepatitis B or may indicate an asymptomatic carrier (10).

Transmission of the hepatitis B virus in hemodialysis units may be from percutaneous inoculation with contaminated instruments, needles, or other objects; entry of contaminated blood through wounds or breaks in the skin or mucous membrane; or ingestion of contaminated blood or other material. Blood that is HBsAg-positive is the most common vehicle for transmission; however, other substances, such as saliva, feces, urine, semen, breast milk, tears, sweat, synovial fluid, and bile, may also be suitable vehicles for transmission of infection (9).

The incubation period for acute icteric hepatitis is six weeks to six months (average two to three months). Prodromal symptoms include malaise, anorexia, vomiting, fatigue, mental depression, and elevated serum glutamic oxalacetic transaminase (SGOT) and serum glutamic pyruvic transaminase (SGPT); urticaria and arthralgia may occur. Icterus if present appears two or more weeks after the beginning of prodromal symptoms and usually lasts one to two weeks. Full recovery may take months. The death rate from hepatitis B is approximately 1%. Anicteric hepatitis B occurs two to three times more frequently than the icteric type and often goes undiagnosed (11).

Detection, Prevention, and Control in Hemodialysis Units. Surveillance of patients and staff in hemodialysis units for hepatitis B infection is imperative. The Center for Disease Control recommends the following measures for detection, control, and prevention of hepatitis B infection in hemodialysis units (9).

1. Patients and staff should have the following blood tests performed monthly: HBsAg, antibody to HBsAg (anti-HBs), SGOT and SGPT.
2. After thorough cleaning of articles, one of the following sterilization or disinfection procedures is used:
   a. Heating is the method of choice (autoclaving at 121°C (250°F) for 15 minutes, boiling for 20 minutes, or exposing to dry heat at 170°C (340°F) for 60 minutes).
   b. Chemical germicidal solutions that kill the hepatitis B virus are hypochlorite (Clorox), formaldehyde, and activated glutaraldehyde (Cidex). Sodium hypochlorite solution containing 5000 to 10,000 ppm available chlorine is strongly recommended to disinfect equipment soiled with blood. These solutions should be prepared fresh daily. Hypochlorite corrodes metal; therefore, metal should be autoclaved or disinfected with formaldehyde or glutaraldehyde.
3. Standard immune serum globulin is not routinely recommended for hepatitis B prophylaxis, since it has little or no effect in preventing or modifying the clinical course of the disease. Immune serum globulin with large amounts of anti-HBs are being studied and may prove beneficial in preventing or lessening the severity of hepatitis B infection.
4. Patients should receive as few blood transfusions as possible. Studies show that frozen packed red blood cells have less chance of transmitting hepatitis (12).
5. Eating, smoking, and drinking in hemodialysis units must be prohibited by staff and kept to an absolute minimum for patients.
6. All hemodialysis equipment should be cleaned and sterilized before reuse.
7. Acute and chronic renal failure patients should be treated in completely separate areas.
8. Patients who are known to be HBsAg-positive should be isolated in a separate area of the unit and should receive care by staff who are not assigned to HBsAg-negative patients.

9. Disposable gloves should be worn to perform any activity that could contaminate the hands, such as cleaning shunts, inserting fistula needles, drawing blood, offering bedpans, disassembling dialysis machinery, or changing dressings.

10. Hemodialysis staff should wear a gown while working in the unit and should cover the gown by a laboratory coat when going outside the unit.

11. Blood or other laboratory specimens should be clearly labeled as having come from hemodialysis patients. Specimens from known HBsAg-positive patients should be so labeled.

12. An ongoing educational program for dialysis unit staff and for patients and families is essential to prevention and control of hepatitis B infection.

REFERENCES

1. C L Hampers, E Schupak, E G Lowrie, et al.: *Long-Term Hemodialysis*. New York, Grune & Stratton, 1973.

2. D J Brundage: *Nursing Management of Renal Problems*. St Louis, Mosby, 1976.

3. E G Lowrie, C L Hampers, J P Merrill: Physical principles in hemodialysis, in Bailey G (ed): *Hemodialysis Principles and Practice*. New York, Academic, 1972, pp 195–210.

4. Y Nosé: *Manual on Artificial Organs, Vol I: The Artificial Kidney*. St Louis, Mosby, 1969.

5. _____: *Hemodialysis Manual*. Washington, DC, US Dept of HEW, 1971.

6. _____: *Fluid Removal Management*. Lakewood, Colorado, Cobe Laboratories, Inc, 1976.

7. A I Arieff, S G Massry: Dialysis disequilibrium syndrome, in Massry S and Sellers A (eds): *Clinical Aspects of Uremia and Dialysis*. Springfield, Ill, Charles C Thomas 1976, pp 34–48.

8. A J Mocelin: Complications of treatment with hemodialysis, in Bailey G (ed): *Hemodialysis Principles and Practice*. New York, Academic 1972, pp. 397–408.

9. D Snydman, J A Bryan, R E Dixon: Prevention of nosocomial viral hepatitis, type B (hepatitis B). *Ann Int Med* 83: 838–845, 1975.

10. M R Robinson: Viral hepatitis, parts I and II. *Assn for Prac in Infection Control Newsletter*. 3: 1–9, 1975.

11. Center for Disease Control: Perspectives on the control of viral hepatitis, type B. *Morbidity and Mortality Weekly Report* 25(17): 3–8, May 7, 1976.

12. J L Tullis, J Hinman, M Sproul, et al.: The incidence of posttransfusion hepatitis in previously frozen blood. *JAMA* 214: 719–723, 1970.

BIBLIOGRAPHY

Bailey G (ed): *Hemodialysis Principles and Practice.* New York, Academic 1972.

Barbour B H: Hemodialysis equipment, in Massry S and Sellers A (eds): *Clinical Aspects of Uremia and Dialysis.* Springfield, Ill, Charles C Thomas 1976, pp 659–670.

_____: *Basic Information: Anticoagulation.* Chicago, Abbott Labs, 1976.

Brundage D J: *Nursing Management of Renal Problems.* St Louis, Mosby, 1976.

Bond W W, Peterson N J, Favero M S: Viral hepatitis B: aspects of environmental control. *Health Laboratory Science* (in press).

_____: *Dialysis Manual.* Northbrook, Ill, Gambro Inc, 1972.

Ederer G M, Van Drunen N, Matsen J M: Guidelines for the prevention of hepatitis B infections among hospital personnel. *APIC Newsletter* 2: 5–8, 1974.

Favero M S: Microbiological hazards associated with artificial kidney machines. *APIC Newsletter* 2: 9–16, 1974.

_____: *Fluid Removal Management.* Lakewood, Col, Cobe Laboratories, Inc, 1976.

Gotch F A: Solute transport and ultrafiltration in hemodialysis, in Massry S and Sellers A (eds): *Clinical Aspects of Uremia and Dialysis.* Springfield, Ill, Charles C Thomas, 1976, pp 639–658.

Gutch C F, Stoner M H: *Review of Hemodialysis for Nurses and Dialysis Personnel,* ed 2. St Louis, Mobsy, 1975.

Hampers C L, Schupak E, Lowrie E G, et al.: *Long-Term Hemodialysis.* New York, Grune & Stratton, 1973.

Malchesky P S, Kiraby R J, Surovy, et al.: Evaluation of hemodialyzers. *Dialysis and Transplantation* 4 (5), 1975.

Muehreke R C: *The Use of Heparin in Hemodialysis.* Chicago, Abbott Labs, 1976.

Sellers A L, Gral T: Morbidity and mortality in patients undergoing maintenance hemodialysis, in Massry S and Sellers A (eds): *Clinical Aspects of Uremia and Dialysis.* Springfield, Ill, Charles C Thomas Pub, 1976, pp 616–638.

Shinaberger J: Indications for dialysis, in Massry S and Sellers A (eds): *Clinical Aspects of Uremia and Dialysis.* Springfield, Ill, Charles C Thomas, 1976, pp 490–503.

Weseley S: Air embolism during hemodialysis. *Dialysis and Transplantation* 1 (3), 1972.

7
Access to the Circulation for Hemodialysis

Sharon R. Parker, R.N.

Larry E. Lancaster, R.N., M.S.N.

Access to the circulatory system has been the singularly most important factor in the development of hemodialysis as a successful treatment modality for the patient with end stage renal disease. The history and development of vascular access has paralleled the increased use of hemodialysis for treatment of both more and different types of acute and chronic renal failure.

This chapter offers the nurse caring for the patient with end stage renal disease receiving dialysis an understanding of:

1. The advantages and disadvantages of various types of circulatory access methods.
2. The basic procedure for surgical construction of various types of circulatory access.
3. The complications related to circulatory access and the management of each.
4. The points that should be stressed while teaching the patient and family about circulatory access.

The initial landmark in circulatory access for chronic dialysis was achieved by Quinton, Scribner, and Dillard in 1960 with the successful semipermanent cannulation of vessels forming an arteriovenous shunt. The use of Teflon (initially for the entire shunt, then later for only the vessel tip) made this shunt remarkable, as it had amazingly low thrombogenicity (1).

Before the introduction of the Quinton-Scribner shunt dialysis had been practical only for those patients with acute renal failure. A wide range of vascular access methods had been used with these people, beginning with Kolff's early trials of dialysis in man using 50-ml aliquots of blood taken by venipuncture and dialyzed before being returned to the patient. This method was time-consuming and impractical and pointed up the need for continuous-flow access (2). The next forward move was the use of arterial puncture for access and venous puncture for blood return. Again this method was rendered impractical by the problems encountered with repeated arterial punctures. At about the same time surgical exposure and cannulation of an artery and a vein was being employed for each dialysis treatment. However, with all of these methods there was a "life-and-death race" between the decreasing availabilty of access sites and the return of renal function (3).

In recent years, progress has been achieved with circulatory access; however, providing long-term access has alternately stimulated, frustrated, and taxed the skills of vascular surgeons. The search for the "ideal" access continues. A perfect vascular access would meet four criteria:

1. A high blood flow rate.
2. Ease of use either by puncture or the ability to quickly disconnect externally.
3. Negligible infection rates.
4. Absence of clotting (4).

Many attempts have been made to provide this type of "perfect" access, but none has been universally ideal.

Today, the long-term nature of chronic hemodialysis has insured that the major goal in vascular access be conservation of the utilization of access sites. Pre-end stage planning for vascular access seems to be the ideal way of conserving these sites.

Since success of vascular access is highly dependent on healthy, undamaged blood vessels, an attempt is made, starting as early as possible, to prevent further damage to the chosen vessels. If the patient is hospitalized, the staff and patient are instructed no venipunctures in the chosen limb, and signs are placed on the patient's bed to that effect. Highly visible signs are of great assistance in large institutions where there are many different people starting intravenous infusions and taking blood specimens.

Vascular assessment important to long-term planning includes the examination of all peripheral vessels to select the location and type of access best suited to the needs of the individual patient. The patient's underlying disease state and other health-related problems and social situation are considered. An adequate assessment is made under good lighting by direct and manual examination. A tourniquet and blood pressure cuff are used to dilate veins so they may be adequately examined for filling and patency. For the experienced observer palpation and estimation of peripheral pulse amplitude will give sufficient information about the health of arterial vessels (4). Angiography is not necessary in preoperative evaluations unless veins are not visible or pulses are absent (4).

Size and superficiality of vessels in the forearm are noted. Patency of radial and ulnar arteries are verified using the Allen test, especially if the chosen method of circulatory access requires ligating the distal artery. A modified Allen test may be done using the following procedure:

1. The patient induces blanching of the chosen hand by tightly clenching his fist.

2. The examiner occludes both the radial and ulnar arteries while the patient's fist is clenched.

3. The patient is instructed to open his fist. The palm will be blanched.

4. The examiner releases pressure on either the radial or the ulnar artery and carefully observes for return of color to the palm. This color return should occur within about five seconds.

5. The procedure is repeated, beginning with step one and releasing the artery that remained compressed in step four.

If there is rapid color return to the palm on release of both arteries, the implication is that there is adequate flow through both ulnar and radial arteries; therefore, if one vessel is used in creating vascular access, there will be adequate circulation to the extremity through the remaining artery (5).

EXTERNAL SHUNTS

External shunts basically consist of two rigid Teflon tips implanted in an artery and a vein. Silastic tubing is attached to the Teflon vessel tips and brought to the outside through puncture wounds in the skin. The Silastic tubes are connected together to allow for uninterrupted blood flow.

External shunts are now less widely used as a means of vascular access for chronic dialysis, although historically and practically they are still important to hemodialysis. The external types of vascular access are now used for patients with reversible renal failure, patients awaiting immediate transplantation, and initial management of rapid-onset chronic renal failure. Also, alternative types of external shunts may be used in those patients who have inadequate vessels to develop an arteriovenous fistula (4).

The major advantage of an external shunt is that it may be used immediately after placement without a maturation period. Consideration can also be given to the use of external devices in small children and in adults who have real fears of venipuncture.

The problems encountered with external shunts, particularly in long-term situations, far outnumber the advantages. The disadvantages include high incidence of infections, mechanical complications requiring revision, repeated clotting episodes necessitating anticoagulation, failure due to intimal proliferation or stricture, and the day-to-day disability associated with an external device.

Choice of Placement Sites

The choice of placement sites for external shunts depends on two criteria: the type of renal failure (acute or chronic) and the availability of undamaged vessels of the proper size. The nondominant upper extremity is the site preferred for external placement in those patients with reversible or acute renal failure. Generally at this site the radial artery and cephalic vein are the chosen vessels, as they are the most conveniently located for creating an external shunt in the wrist. (See Figure 7.1.) If the cephalic vein is thrombosed, as frequently occurs in patients who have prolonged illnesses, the vena comitantes of the radial artery

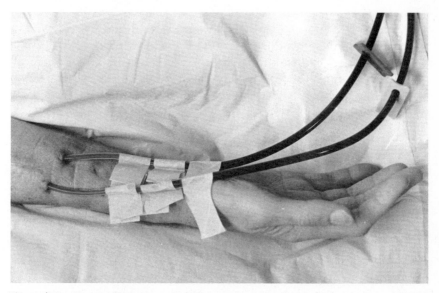

Figure 7.1. External arteriovenous shunt placement in the wrist. External shunt is connected to blood lines for hemodialysis.

may be used despite their ultrathin walls. The basilic vein in the mid-forearm or close to the elbow may be used, although it is frequently overlooked. A combination of artery at the wrist and vein above the elbow should be avoided because of the long extracorporeal connection required.

Ankle shunts are usually used for patients when dialysis will be long-term, thus "saving" the vessels in the arm for an arteriovenous fistula. The vessels commonly used in the leg are the saphenous vein and either the anterior tibial artery or the tibial artery.

Types of External Shunts

Scribner Shunt

The classic Quinton-Scribner shunt consists of Teflon tips inserted into the vessels. The remainder of the shunt is constructed of Silastic, which has a reverse curve so that the external portion of the shunt is directed away from the joint of the extremity.

The primary advantages of the Scribner shunt are its availability for immediate use and the additional freedom of movement it provides in the joint of the extremity.

Its disadvantages are that, because of the curve, it is difficult if not impossible to declot, and possibly it has a higher incidence of thrombosis than other types of external prostheses.

Ramirez Shunt

The Ramirez is an example of a straight cannula shunt with Silastic wings added to the embedded portion to provide for more stability and to help prevent accidental dislodgement. (See Figure 7.2A.) Besides offering the same advantages as other shunts, it has more stability and is easier to restore to patency when thrombosis does occur (6). This shunt must be placed high enough above the joint so that motion of the extremity is not impaired (7).

Buselmeier Shunt

This shunt has Teflon tips inserted into vessels in the same manner as the standard external shunts. The outer portion of the cannula is U-shaped with two short branches coming off each side of the curve. Most of the device is subcutaneous; only a small portion is exteriorized. When the patient is started on dialysis, obturators that are kept in the branches are removed and connection to blood lines is made (8).

The following advantages are attributed to the Buselmeier shunt: comparatively higher blood flow rates because the shorter tubing lessens blood flow resistance; less chance of accidental dislodgement and intimal

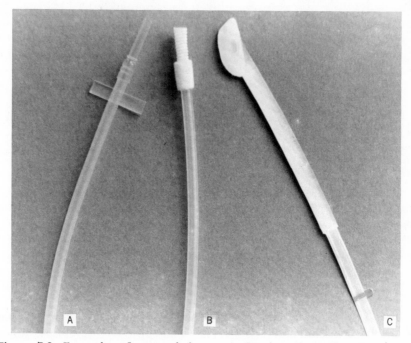

Figure 7.2. Examples of external shunts: A. Ramirez shunt. B. Allen-Brown shunt. C. Thomas femoral shunt.

injury, owing to the smaller length of tubing external; and, because of the built-in capacity for recirculation, an avoidance of excessive suction on the arterial wall (7).

The major disadvantage is the possibility of septic episodes during dialysis, which have been traced to the plugged portions of the shunt (7).

Thomas Shunt

A device for using large thigh vessels in constructing external arteriovenous shunts was described in 1969 (9). It consists of a face plate made of Dacron fabric attached to Silastic tubing via a sleeve of Dacron. (See Figures 7.2C and 7.3.) The plate is sutured onto the side of the superficial femoral artery using a vascular suturing technique. The venous return may be of the regular type or of the Thomas applique type (7).

Advantages of the Thomas shunt include unimpeded flow to the distal extremities, as there is no interruption of the vessel; small incidence

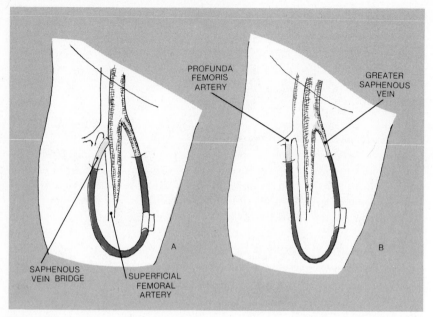

Figure 7.3. Schematic drawing of external arteriovenous shunt placement in the thigh using: A. Bridged (saphenous vein) technique. B. Direct technique.

of thrombosis because of high blood flow rates; and lack of vessel stenosis because of the technique for insertion (7).

Disadvantages include greater possibility of inducing congestive heart failure; infection of the shunt (in the femoral triangle), which may cause sepsis; and formation of pseudoaneurysms, which may be complicated by hemorrhage. If, because of the complications, the superficial femoral artery is destroyed, there will be compromise of the distal circulation; therefore, at most institutions this type of shunt is used only in patients who have no other available circulatory access site (4,7,10,11).

Allen-Brown Shunt

The Allen-Brown shunt is a composite device made of an accordion-pleated sleeve of knitted Dacron to which a Silastic tube is glued. (See Figure 7.2B.) An end-to-end anastomosis is made between the vessel and the Dacron sleeve instead of inserting a Teflon tip into the lumen of the vessel (7).

The advantage of the shunt is that it can be anastomosed onto short segments of vessels, allowing use of an expended vessel (10).

The disadvantages are similar to those of the standard external shunts or the Thomas device.

Complications of External Circulatory Access

The major complications causing failure of external circulatory access devices are thrombosis and infection. Less frequently shunts fail because of dislodgement (accidental or suicidal) and hemorrhage. Limitation of activity must also be considered a severe disadvantage if not a complication.

Thrombosis

Clotting is the most common complication of external shunts. Hallmarks of impending thrombosis are increased venous resistance and decreased arterial flow (11). If such a situation (decreased flow or increased resistance) is noted, angiography has proven valuable in determining the cause of the suspected thrombosis (12). During the angiographic procedure a bolus of dye is injected into the artery and vein, and a series of films follow the injection of dye as it progresses up the vessel. The patient usually experiences a burning sensation, which can be painful especially if a declotting procedure has been performed.

Early clotting is usually caused by malalignment of vessel tips. This can be determined by angiography and can be corrected by surgical revision. Early thrombosis can also be caused by intimal stripping during insertion of the shunt. This problem also requires surgical correction. Late arterial thrombosis is usually due to intimal proliferation and fibrosis from repeated trauma (7). Early thrombosis on the venous side may be the result of malalignment; later thrombosis can be caused by a phlebotic process, recent thrombi, or fibrosis at the vessel tip. Clotting is also caused by excessive external pressure or prolonged bending of the joint proximal to the shunt (7). Exposure to extremes of heat or cold also seems to have some effect on thrombosis, especially if the extracorporeal circuit is excessively long or exposed to the temperature extremes for prolonged periods.

Declotting

Declotting is most effectively accomplished using a small embolectomy catheter (3–4F). The person performing the proceudre should have considerable experience in declotting. Our experience shows that dialysis nurses have been a stable and knowledgeable group to perform this procedure.

Aspiration of the clot is attempted initially and is occasionally successful. If aspiration is unsuccessful, then an embolectomy is attempted. The equipment needed for declotting includes: an embolectomy catheter (3–4F); a basin of povidone-iodine solution; a basin of heparinized saline for flushing (2000–4000 U of heparin per 1000 ml saline); sterile gloves, gown, mask, and drapes; and two sterile bulldog clamps. (See Figure 7.4.)

The procedure for declotting is:

1. Remove the dressing from the shunt.
2. Put on mask, sterile gown, and gloves.
3. Carefully and aseptically scrub the area of the shunt with povidone-iodine solution.
4. Change gloves after skin preparation.
5. Place sterile drapes around the extremity. Leave the limbs of the shunt exposed and make a rather large sterile field, which is needed to accommodate the length of the embolectomy catheter.
6. Place the bulldog clamps and sterile gauze sponges on the sterile field. Have an assistant hand the following to the person declotting: two 20- to 35-cc syringes without needles, one tuberculin size syringe without needle, and one 3 to 4 French embolectomy catheter. Have the assistant pour heparinized saline into a sterile basin.
7. Disconnect the shunt and clamp the Silastic tubing with bulldog clamps if there is an unexpected blood flow.
8. If only one side of the shunt is clotted, clamp the limb of the shunt that is not clotted before disconnecting. If clamps are used on a clotted shunt, the clot may break apart, making it potentially more difficult to retrieve.
9. Test the embolectomy catheter for balloon patency and volume by attaching the tuberculin syringe and inflating the balloon with air or normal saline solution. The balloon should be firm but not taut. Leave the syringe filled with the proper amount of normal saline to inflate the balloon connected to the catheter.
10. Using one hand to stabilize the limb of the shunt being declotted, gently insert the embolectomy catheter until resistance is met; if no resistance is felt, insert the catheter full length.
11. Inflate the balloon, using the attached syringe.
12. Slowly withdraw the catheter with the balloon inflated. If tightness or resistance is met during withdrawal, deflate the balloon very slightly. Continue to maintain traction on the catheter while withdrawing the balloon from the vessel without damaging the vessel lining or the vessel tip. The most difficult area through which to manipulate the balloon is the vessel tip, and the problem (clot) is often in this area.
13. If a clot is removed or blood flow is obtained, fill a 35-ml syringe with heparinized saline and aspirate; then flush the shunt. When flushing, never use more than 5 ml at a time to prevent pushing

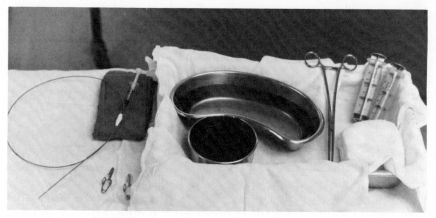

Figure 7.4. Equipment used for declotting an external shunt. See text for explanation.

emboli into the systemic circulation, and never push against large amounts of resistance.

14. If sufficient flow is obtained on the arterial side or no resistance is felt on the venous side when flushing, and the person performing the procedure thinks that all clots are retrieved, the procedure is completed. The maneuver, however, may need to be repeated several times to accomplsih complete clot removal.

When the declotting procedure is completed, the shunt may be reconnected. However, often the complications that were responsible for the thrombosis preclude reconnection, and the patient may need further assessment. If the person who has performed the declotting procedure believes that the shunt will not remain patent, the shunt should be placed on unilateral or bilateral heparin infusion pumps until angiography and/or revision can be done.

Few complications have been reported in the use of this declotting procedure, especially when the person performing it has been well trained in its theory and technique. The complications during and following a shunt embolectomy include systemic emboli, rupture of the vessel by the catheter tip, and dislodgement of the shunt tip from the vessel.

Infection

Infection is an almost inevitable complication of external shunts. Many of the infective episodes consist of only localized cellulitis, although they can result in septicemia and death. Most shunts are infected with *staphylococci* (approximately 90%) with the remainder attributed to *pseudomonas* and *enterobacteriaceae*. Because of the high rate of infections largely due to *staphylococci* some centers routinely place the patients with shunts on prophylactic antibiotic therapy. The best prophylaxis for infection appears to be meticulous daily shunt care (7) and prevention of trauma when handling the shunt (11).

Dislodgement

Accidental or purposeful dislodgement can be a life-threatening complication of external shunts. In our experience over the last five years there has been one documented and one suspected suicide caused by hemorrhage from a disconnected shunt.

Prevention of accidental dislodgement or disconnection is imperative. The dressing should cover the entire external portion, especially if there is a large amount of activity involving the limb with the external shunt.

Spontaneous dislodgement of the tip from the vessel occurs frequently when there is a smoldering infection at the vessel tip. This condition may be heralded by a leak around the vessel tip, which may form a pseudoaneurysm. If a pseudoaneurysm (which appears as a pulsatile mass at the area of leakage) is noted, the vessel should be ligated and the shunt revised proximally if possible. Appropriate antibiotic therapy should also be started.

Skin Erosion

It is reported in the literature (7) that erosion of the wings and tip through the skin is being decreased by the use of straight instead of recurved cannulae and by deeper subcutaneous placement. We are, however, seeing this problem fairly frequently with the Ramirez cannula, especially when the patient is very thin and there is a clinical or subclinical infective process.

Patient Education

Patient-family education is vital for prevention of complications related to the external shunt. The more knowledgeable and competent the patient is in handling his shunt, the less likely he is to develop serious complications.

Cleaning and dressing the external shunt is usually the first technical skill the nurse teaches the patient. The procedure can be mastered by everyone including small children. We try to impress upon the patient that shunt care is primarily his responsibility and that a family member learns how to do the procedure only in case the patient is unable to manage this for a period due to illness.

External Shunt Care Procedure
Equipment used for shunt care includes peroxide, povidone-iodine solution, sterile cotton-tipped swabs, sterile gauze sponges, gauze bandage, scissors, tape, and povidone-iodine ointment.

1. Carefully remove the dressing from the shunt. If dried blood has caused the dressing to adhere to the skin, pour peroxide over the dressing until easy removal is possible.
2. Place a sterile towel (clean towel when at home) under the shunt extremity.
3. Pour peroxide over the cannula insertion sites and around the shunt area. Clean the area around the shunt insertion sites with a gauze sponge to remove dried blood. Gently cleanse each cannula insertion site, using a sterile cotton-tipped applicator. Carefully clean underneath the cannula. Use a separate applicator for each side, and clean from insertion site outward.
4. Repeat step 3, using povidone-iodine solution.
5. A small amount of povidone-iodine ointment may be applied around each cannula insertion site if signs of infection are noted.
6. Place one sterile gauze sponge under the shunt and one sterile gauze sponge over the shunt. (In the hospital and at home when no strenous activity is expected, a small portion of the shunt may be left visible so the shunt may be easily checked for patency.)
7. Apply a gauze bandage securely around the shunt. The dressing should not be constrictive. Tape the dressing in place.
8. Place bulldog clamps on the edge of the gauze bandage so they are readily available. (See Figure 7.5.)

Patient education must also include methods to manage emergencies involving external shunts. Clotting is not seen as an emergency; however, it is a stressful event for the patient. The patient is instructed to call his physician when signs of shunt clotting are noted. The physician will instruct the patient in the proper procedure to follow. Other more emergent situations include hemorrhage from a disconnected shunt or from dislodged vessel tips. If the shunt has been disconnected at the connection site, the patient is instructed to clamp both sides of the shunt with the fingers and/or bulldog clamps. The shunt is reconnected with a sterile connector. If blood loss has been considerable, the physician should be notified. If the vessel tip comes out of the vessel, the patient is instructed to hold pressure on the bleeding site and clamp the remaining limb of the shunt. He should call the physician and proceed as directed. If the patient lives a great distance from his primary treatment center,

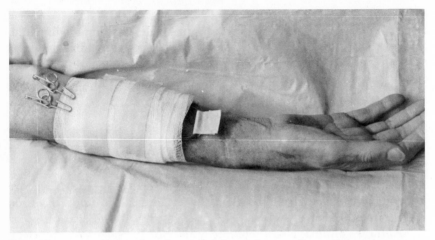

Figure 7.5. Properly bandaged external shunt. See text for explanation.

consideration may be given to having him go to a local emergency room for initial treatment.

The nurse must be sure the patient is totally familiar with the actions to take in event of emergencies; however, care should be taken to avoid unduly frightening the patient with a new external shunt. It is sometimes difficult to offer support without being overly cautious and thus alarming the patient. The patient needs to know that emergencies may occur and the steps to take if they do occur; at the same time he needs to be reassured that the true emergencies do not happen frequently and that when they do, by using common sense and by following instructions he can manage the problem.

INTERNAL ARTERIOVENOUS FISTULA

Venipuncture for repeated hemodialysis was first reported in 1962 by Cimino and Brescia. Large-bore needles could be inserted into the patient's vessels and then connected to the dialyzer. The venipuncture method of vascular access circumvented many of the problems inherent with the external arteriovenous shunt. It could be performed repeatedly with only slight discomfort to the patient and without permanently injuring the vessels. The primary drawback to this method was the necessity of having sufficiently large vessels to supply the needed blood flow for dialysis; normal sized veins could not always provide the blood flow rates of 250 to 400 ml per minute that were needed for dialysis (13).

Encouraged by their success in using venipuncture, Cimino and Brescia began refinement of the procedure to produce consistently adequate blood flow rates for dialysis. In 1966, they reported a method of creating a relatively small superficial arteriovenous fistula that caused progressive enlargement and arterialization of the anastomosed vein. The vein could then be used as a venipuncture access site for hemodialysis (14). This development overcame many of the problems that had been encountered in using external shunts. After a decade of use the arteriovenous fistula remains far superior to the external AV shunt in terms of longevity and complication rates.

Advantages of the AV fistula in comparison to the AV shunt include less propensity for clotting; decreased infection rates; no problems of accidental dislodgement; and no restriction in activity. Disadvantages include the length of time required for maturation before the fistula may be used and the reluctance of some patients to undergo repeated venipunctures.

Hemodynamic Considerations

Surgeons have traditionally attempted to correct or eliminate arteriovenous fistulae that were traumatic in origin and caused cardiac enlargement and decompensation (4). However, surgically created AV fistulae seldom cause cardiac decompensation because of the small diameter of the artery and the purposefully limited size of the fistula orifice.

In 1923, Emile Holman documented the natural history of traumatic AV fistulae and their progressive increase in size, which caused increased cardiac output and eventual cardiac failure. Holman also described two early experiments in creating AV fistulae of 6-mm size. These fistulae failed to enlarge and produced no cardiac problems. He believed that his inexperience in vessel anastomosis caused scarring, thus preventing fistula enlargement. Later Holman described techniques that would insure fistula growth. These included using interrupted sutures to avoid "purse stringing." Unknowingly Holman provided the precedent for creation of small, confined AV fistulae that would not cause cardiac decompensation (4).

Brescia, Cimino, and others, in rediscovering the method for creating confined AV fistulae, used a technique consisting of a 3- to 5-mm side-to-side anastomosis between the radial artery and the cephalic vein, although other large adjacent veins may be used (14).

It is essential that growth of the fistula orifice be restricted as much as possible to prevent cardiac complications. A continuous rather than intermittent technique should be used along with synthetic nonabsorbable materials when suturing the anastomosis (4).

Placement Sites and Time of Placement

Placement sites for AV fistulae are generally in either forearm, with the nondominant arm being preferred to allow the patient more freedom while on dialysis. AV fistulae are also commonly placed in the upper arm, using the brachial artery and cephalic vein. If the commonly used vessels (radial artery, brachial artery, and cephalic vein) are not available, the surgeon can usually find other sufficiently large superficial vessels. However, if there are absolutely no vessels available, a graft fistula can usually be formed (these are discussed in more detail in another section of this chapter).

Time of placement can be as critical as the placement site. Creation of an AV fistula that will develop well and have a long life span requires careful timing, proper site selection, and exacting surgical technique. In a patient being followed for progressive renal failure, an AV fistula should be created when the endogenous creatinine clearance falls to 15 ml per minute. This allows a three-to-six month maturation time before maintenance dialysis is initiated. When the course of renal failure is expected to be rapidly progressive, as in rapidly progressive glomerulonephritis or diabetic nephropathy, the AV fistula should be created when the creatinine clearance is 25 ml per minute (7).

Types of Arteriovenous Fistulae

AV fistulae of any type are constructed in the same manner. The alternative methods that have been derived from the basic Brescia-Cimino procedure are an attempt to solve some of the problems encountered (these problems are discussed later). Types of AV fistula anastomoses include:

1. Side-artery to side-vein with the distal vessels left open.
2. Side-to-side converted to end-artery to side-vein by ligating the distal portion of the vein.
3. Side-to-side converted to end-artery to side-vein by ligating the distal artery.
4. Side-to-side converted to end-to-end by ligating both the distal artery and vein.
5. Side-artery to end-vein in a smooth loop fashion.
6. End-artery to side-vein in a smooth loop fashion.
7. end-to-end in a smooth loop fashion.

The illustrations in Figure 7.6 show only the radial artery and cephalic vein; however, all types of anastomoses are applicable to other artery-vein parts.

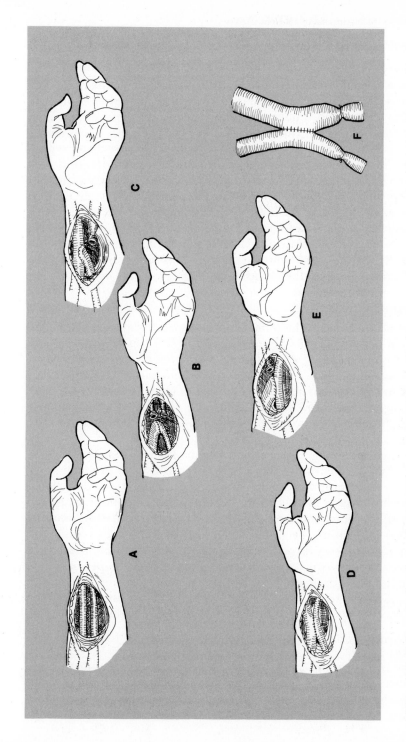

Figure 7.6. Schematic drawings of various internal arteriovenous fistulae anastomoses: A. Normal artery-vein relationship. B. End-to-end anastomosis. C. End-vein to side-artery anastomosis. D. Side-to-side anastomosis as described by Brescia and Cimino. E. Side-vein to end-artery anastomosis. F. Side-to-side anastomosis converted to end-to-end anastomosis.

Complications

Thrombosis

Thrombosis should not commonly occur in AV fistulae in the first weeks or months if the basic prerequisites for a good fistula are met—that is, good arterial flow and venous runoff as well as meticulous technique in making the anastomosis. However, assuming the above prerequisites are met, early clotting may occur because of extrinsic pressure either from a tight bandage or from positioning of the patient that might cause such pressure (7). Clotting, early or late, may be caused by hypovolemia or marked prolonged hypotension (as during a cardiac arrest or possibly during a long surgical procedure).

Turbulence at the anastomosis has been theorized as one factor in causing thrombosis of AV fistulae. Although no data support this theory conclusively, several techniques designed to reduce turbulence have been described, such as the smooth loop anastomoses (15).

Venous Hypertension

Swelling of the hand in the immediate postoperative period after creation of an AV fistula may be normal and of little consequence. Distal venous hypertension as a continuing phenomenon can be extremely debilitating. The entire hand may become edematous with resulting varicosities and ulceration; however, the usual disabling symptom is a "sore thumb" syndrome. Sore thumb syndrome consists of an edematous cyanotic thumb with eczematous skin changes and oozing of serosanguinous fluid around the nail bed (7).

The cause of venous hypertension may be high resistance to flow in the proximal portion of the vein or any effect causing a predominantly distal flow. Angiographic studies in these cases are helpful in delineating the problem. If the proximal vessel is open with no stenotic areas, then it is assumed that the hypertension is due to a Venturi effect and may be eliminated by ligating the distal portion of the vein, thus creating an end-vein to side-artery fistula. If angiography shows stenosis or increased resistance in the proximal vessel, then angioplasty may be performed to alleviate the areas of stenosis; or if there are multiple stenotic areas, it may be necessary to use another open vein. In either case the surgeon usually chooses to convert the fistula to an end-vein to side-artery access.

Ischemia

Ischemic complications caused by an AV fistula are commonly referred to as "steal syndrome." Steal syndrome occurs when the limb usually supplied by antegrade flow is deprived by retrograde flow or short-circuiting in that artery to an area of lower resistance (4). Symptoms of steal syndrome may vary from cold, possibly painful fingers to gangrene. Steal syndrome develops in less than 2% of the population with AV fistulae. Steal syndrome can be corrected by ligating the distal portion of the artery utilized in forming the fistula, thus redirecting the retrograde flow. However, if collateral circulation is inadequate, the fistula may have to be sacrificed by ligating both the proximal and distal portions of the vein used in creating the fistula. Proximal fistulae, such as a brachial-cephalic or brachial-basilic, tend to cause a higher incidence of ischemic problems because of the larger size of the fistula opening and the larger diameter of the vessels involved (7).

Aneurysms

Aneurysms of the fistula usually form as a result of repeated needle punctures at the same site. Formation of aneurysms may pose problems such as pain, decreased blood flow, formation of thrombi, and risk of rupture due to the sacular nature of the aneurysm or the thin skin over it. If necessary, the aneurysm may be surgically repaired.

Pseudoaneurysms result from hematoma formation at a puncture site. These are rare and may be easily corrected by surgical removal of the clot and direct suturing of the puncture in the vessel.

High-Output or Congestive Heart Failure

The problem of high-output cardiac failure is frequently raised and has been described; however, in most cases it is difficult to pinpoint the fistula as the cause of heart failure in dialysis patients (10). When congestive heart failure occurs because of AV fistulae, it is usually in the patient with a limited cardiac reserve, a high-flow fistula, or a fistula orifice of more than 8 mm. Using methods where cardiac output could be measured with an AV fistula opened and closed, it was shown that opening the fistula increased the cardiac output an average of 10% (16). Occluding the AV fistula by digital compression, thus increasing peripheral resistance, will in some patients lower the heart rate and correspondingly decrease cardiac output (Branham's sign).

Infection

The incidence of infection in AV fistulae has been reported as 1 per 100 patient years compared with 50 per 100 patient years in external shunts (7, 11). When infection occurs in the AV fistula, it may be seen at the suture line or puncture site. There have been reports of septic pulmonary embolism and septicemia traced to AV fistulae with aneurysm formation (17).

Patient Education

The patient with an AV fistula has fewer techniques to learn than the patient with an external shunt. The nurse will initially instruct the patient how to elevate the extremity in the immediate postoperative period to prevent and/or relieve edema. The patient should also be reassured that elevation will aid in relief of discomfort. Also, any initial discomfort should be mild and will last only a few days.

The next task to be confronted will be exercising the extremity to promote rapid maturation of the vessel. Exercises should be started a week after formation of the fistula. These exercises are essential if the fistula will be used soon. The exercises are necessary but not as important if the fistula has been formed well in advance of initiation of dialysis.

The patient is instructed to apply a tourniquet to the fistula extremity (apply snugly but not so tight as to occlude arterial flow) and at the same time to squeeze a small rubber ball in the hand. This should be done for three to five minutes each time. The frequency of exercise is determined by how soon after construction the fistula will be used. The exercise may be done three to five minutes every hour during waking hours or as infrequently as once a day. Another method of exercise consists of applying a tourniquet and immersing the fistula extremity in warm water for five to ten minutes at a time.

Good technique for insertion of needles into the fistula is important to maintaining the life of the fistula. If the patient will be dialyzing at home or performing self-venipunctures, several points should be stressed:

1. The most important point should be rotation of puncture sites. Rotation serves to prevent excessive scar tissue formation, to prevent aneurysm formation, and to promote better healing of old puncture sites, thus giving the fistula a longer life.

2. The patient should be taught that to prevent recirculation of blood, the arterial and venous needles must be placed a minimum of 1½ inches apart, with the arterial needle pointing toward the anastomosis of the fistula and the venous or return needle pointing away from the anastomosis. (See Figure 7.7)

3. Patients should be cautioned to watch the fistula for signs of infection, to observe for aneurysm formation, to check for loss of a palpable thrill (loss of thrill would indicate clotting), and to avoid constriction of the fistula vessel by sleeves or heavy purses carried on that arm.

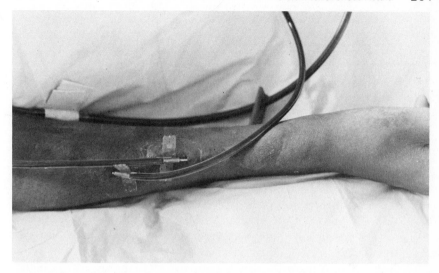

Figure 7.7. Proper placement of needles in internal arteriovenous fistula for hemodialysis. See text for explanation.

GRAFT ARTERIOVENOUS FISTULA

Most circulatory access needs are met by use of an arteriovenous fistula; however, for some patients with inadequate vessels the best alternative may be interposing a graft between an artery and a vein. Graft AV fistulae tend to be used as a secondary or alternative access method, although in the following groups of patients grafts may be the access of choice: patients with nutritional problems, iatrogenic vein loss, severe obesity, marked cachexia, or self-inflicted vein loss (7).

Many materials are available for constructing graft AV fistulae. The major classifications of grafts are biologic, semibiologic, and prosthetic. Biologic graft materials include autogenous and homologous saphenous veins, umbilical veins, and bovine artery or xenografts (18). Semibiologic grafts are primarily Mandril grown grafts. Prosthetic grafts include Dacron velour grafts, expanded polytetrafluoroethylene (PTFE or Teflon) grafts, Impra grafts, and Gore-Tex grafts (19).

Sites frequently used for graft placement are straight or looped grafts in the upper arm, forearm, or thigh. The graft may be interposed between any patent artery and vein of adequate size. (See Figure 7.8.) Ischemia may become a problem more frequently when larger vessels are used.

There are several advantages peculiar to graft AV fistulae. Most grafts can be used sooner than regular AV fistulae. The subcutaneous place-

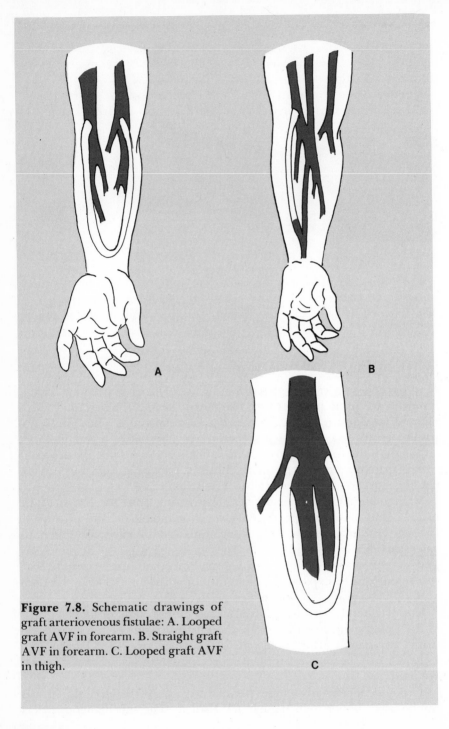

Figure 7.8. Schematic drawings of graft arteriovenous fistulae: A. Looped graft AVF in forearm. B. Straight graft AVF in forearm. C. Looped graft AVF in thigh.

ment and size of the graft generally make graft puncture easier to accomplish. Vessel size and blood flow are not dependent on vein maturation, as the graft itself is already of an adequate size.

Complications of graft AV fistulae are similar to those of regular AV fistulae but may occur more frequently and be more difficult to manage.

Thrombosis

Clotting in graft AV fistulae may be caused by:

1. Poor venous runoff.
2. Inadequate arterial flow.
3. Extrinsic compression.
4. Hemodynamic changes (7).

Poor venous runoff may be caused by stenosis at the venous anastomosis and is frequently evidenced by enlargement of the graft itself (graft hypertension). Venous stenosis may be surgically corrected by angioplasty or bypass.

Excessive extrinsic pressure is a frequent, but preventable, cause of graft clotting. Great care should be taken to avoid tight bandages and clothing. When applying pressure on a graft after needle removal, one should apply only light digital pressure, thus allowing continuous flow through the graft. One can feel the flow in the graft while holding pressure, and we believe that bleeding from puncture sites is stopped more easily by light pressure than by heavier and potentially damaging pressure.

Decreased arterial flow through the graft due to hypotension or hypovolemia may cause clotting. Grafts frequently clot while patients undergo prolonged operative procedures.

Infection

Infection is a major problem with graft AV fistulae. Infection must be treated vigorously and quickly, especially in the early postoperative period. Some centers suggest sacrifice of the graft if a primary early postoperative infection develops (7). These early infections tend to involve the entire graft and are difficult to eradicate.

Hematoma formation can be a source of infection at graft sites. It is important to achieve absolute hemostasis on needle removal, particularly if the graft is used in the first week after placement. Hematoma formation during this period tends to dissect the entire length of the graft.

Later, hematoma formation tends to be more localized, as fibrous tissue grows into the space around the graft itself.

Pseudoaneurysms and Aneurysms

Pseudoaneurysms can be avoided totally by achieving good hemostasis on needle removal, thus avoiding hematoma formation. Also, rotating puncture sites to prevent excessively weakening any one area of the graft controls the formation of both aneurysms and pseudoaneurysms. Pseudoaneurysms that are enlarging require immediate surgical intervention; however, aneurysms require repair only if there is thinning of overlying tissue.

Ischemia

Ischemia tends to be more of a problem with graft AV fistulae, as larger vessels are generally employed in making the anastomosis. Symptoms of ischemia with graft AV fistulae are the same as with regular AV fistulae. Prevention of ischemia depends on limiting the size of the orifice between the arterial vessel and the graft. Orifice size in large vessels may be limited by banding the arterial end of the graft with Teflon tape until the flow through the graft is reduced to 250 or 300 ml per minute. This blood flow is adequate to maintain patency of the graft and for dialysis. Cardiac failure caused by a high-flow graft may be managed by the same technique (7).

Patient Education

Education of the patient and the family concerning graft AV fistulae follows the same principles as outlined for regular AV fistulae. Added emphasis should be placed on observing for infection and seeking prompt treatment. Techniques of achieving good hemostasis without occlusive pressure should be emphasized and practiced by those patients who are on self-care or home dialysis.

FEMORAL VEIN CANNULATION

Percutaneous cannulation of the femoral vein provides an excellent circulatory access site for emergency hemodialysis as well as one that can be easily used when permanent access sites fail.

Shaldon type catheters are introduced into the femoral vein with a

Seldinger or Potts Cournand type needle and a guide wire. The femoral artery is palpated, and a small stab incision is made with a scalpel. The incision is made medially to the artery and should be just large enough to allow introduction of the needle. The femoral needle is used with the sharp stylet in place to puncture the vessel. The stylet is withdrawn and a flexible guide wire is inserted into the vein, leaving approximately the length of the femoral catheter plus one inch outside the skin. The needle is then withdrawn and the catheter is threaded into the vessel over the guide wire. When the catheter is in the vein, simultaneously the catheter is threaded further into the vessel and the guide wire is withdrawn. If a Seldinger or Potts Cournand needle is not available, a large-gauge angiocath may be substituted.

Single femoral vein cannulation may be used for access with a blood return placed in a peripheral vein. If no peripheral return sites are available, several options may be taken:

1. One femoral catheter may be inserted and used with a single needle or alternating device.
2. A catheter may be inserted into the femoral vein in both groins.
3. Two femoral catheters may be inserted into the same femoral vein; one catheter is threaded high into the vessel and is used to return the blood, while the other catheter is inserted only far enough into the vessel so that the holes at the tip are well inside the vessel and is used to withdraw blood. The distance between the tips of the two catheters prevents recirculation; therefore, it is essential that they are spaced and attached to the dialyzer in the manner described. (See Figure 7.9.)

Femoral vein cannulation can be used with any patient, excepting those suspected of having iliofemoral thrombosis because of the possibility of embolism. The procedure is easily accomplished and causes few complications. Disadvantages include the amount of equipment and staff time the procedure requires. It also requires 10 to 15 minutes of extra time at the end of dialysis to apply pressure to the puncture site(s).

Complications of femoral cannulation are few. The major complications are local hematoma and retroperitoneal bleeding; the latter is difficult to recognize and is potentially serious. Indications of this complication are reduced flow from the catheter due to pressure from the hematoma and an unexplained drop in blood pressure. Hematoma formation is best managed by applying pressure on the puncture site. Retroperitoneal bleeding can be avoided by not forcing the guide wire when resistance is met; however, if it is suspected, pressure should be held at the puncture site for at least 10 to 15 minutes, preferably after

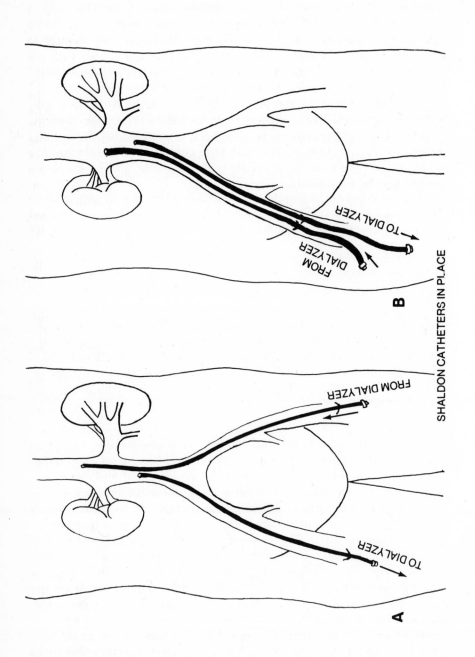

FROM DIALYZER

TO DIALYZER

B

SHALDON CATHETERS IN PLACE

FROM DIALYZER

TO DIALYZER

A

206

removing the catheter. Bleeding around the catheter may occur if the stab incision is too large. This is managed by prevention; however, if it does occur, light pressure may be applied over the site until bleeding stops or subsides.

Recognition of complications from femoral vein cannulation is primarily a nursing responsibility. Constant nursing observation provides the opportunity to be aware of moment-to-moment changes in the condition of the patient during dialysis. Nursing observations include:

1. Checking peripheral pulses in the involved extremity before, during, and after cannulation.
2. Observing the puncture site(s) for hematoma formation.
3. Observing for decreased outflow of blood and increased venous resistance.
4. Carefully assessing blood pressure.
5. Assuring that adequate pressure is applied to the puncture site for a sufficient length of time postdialysis.
6. Applying a pressure dressing postdialysis that is sufficiently tight but does not occlude peripheral pulses.
7. Assuring that an ice pack is applied if needed for hematoma formation postdialysis.

REFERENCES

1. W Quinton, D Dillard, B H Scribner: Cannulation of blood vessels for prolonged hemodialysis. *Trans Am Soc Art Int Organs* 6: 104, 1960.
2. W J Kolff, H I J Berk: Artificial kidney: dialyzer with great area. *Acta Med Scand* 117: 121, 1944.
3. G L Bailey, A P Morgan: Circulatory access for hemodialysis, in G Bailey (ed): *Hemodialysis Principles and Practice.* New York, Academic, 1972, pp 210–231.
4. R F Foran, E Shore, P M Levin, et al.: Vascular access for hemodialysis, in S G Massry, A L Sellers (eds): *Clinical Aspects of Uremia and Dialysis.* Springfield, Ill, Charles C. Thomas, 1976, pp. 504–529.
5. B Bates: *A Guide To Physical Examination.* Philadelphia, Lippincott, 1974, p 219.

Figure 7.9. Alternative placement of catheters for femoral vein cannulation: A. One catheter placed in right and one in left femoral veins. B. Two catheters placed in same femoral vein. See text for explanation.

6. O Ramirez, C Swartz, G Onestiz, et al.: The winged in-line shunt. *Trans Am Soc Artif Int Organs* 12: 220, 1966.

7. K M H Butt, E A Friedman, S Kountz: Angioaccess. *Current Problems in Surgery* XIII (9), Chicago, Medical Yearbook Pub, Sept 1976.

8. T J Buselmeier, C M Kjellstrand, L C Rattazzi, et al.: A new subcutaneous prosthetic A-V shunt: advantages over the Quinton-Scribner Shunt and A-V fistula. *Proc Dial Transp Forum,* 1972, p 67.

9. G I Thomas: A large vessel applique arteriovenous shunt for hemodialysis. *Trans Am Soc Artif Int Organs* 15: 288, 1969.

10. A P Morgan: Access to the circulation, in C Hampers, E Schupak, E Lowrie, et al.: *Long-term Hemodialysis.* New York, Grune & Stratton, 1973, pp 40–63.

11. K M H Butt: Vascular concerns in preparing for end stage care, in E Friedman (ed): *Strategy in Renal Failure.* New York, Wiley, 1978, p. 187.

12. T V Berne, A F Turner, B H Barbour: Angiographic evaluation of Quinton-Scribner shunt malfunction. *Surgery* 69: 588, 1971.

13. J E Cimino, M J Brescia: Simple venipuncture for hemodialysis. *N Eng J Med* 267: 608, 1962.

14. M J Brescia, J E Cimino, K Appel, et al.: Chronic hemodialysis using venipuncture and surgically created arteriovenous fistulae. *N Eng J Med* 275: 1089, 1966.

15. A M Karmody, N Lempert: "Smooth loop" arteriovenous fistulae for hemodialysis. *Surgery* 75: 238, 1974.

16. G J Johnson, W B Blythe: Hemodynamic effects of arteriovenous shunts for hemodialysis. *Ann Surg* 171: 715, 1970.

17. J Levi, M Robson, J B Rosenfeld: Septicemia and pulmonary embolism complicating use of arteriovenous fistula maintenance. *Lancet* 2: 228, 1970.

18. B P Mindich, B S Levowitz: Human umbilical cord vein fistula: a novel approach for hemodialysis. *Dialysis and Transplantion* 5: 4, 1976.

19. J J Bahuth: Expanded polytetrafluoroethylene as an arteriovenous conduit for hemodialysis. *Dialysis and Transplantation* 6: 11, 1977.

8
Maintenance Peritoneal Dialysis

Lowanna S. Binkley, R.N., M.A.

Peritoneal dialysis is an old technique of peritoneal lavage that was first used in man by Ganter in 1923. But it was Maxwell who, in 1959, first described his technique of inserting a catheter into the peritoneum by using a large trocar (1). This permitted the infusion of dialyzing fluid by gravity and the outflow of the fluid by gravity through the same tubing (see Figure 8.1) and made repetitive punctures for multiple dialyses a reality. The catheter was removed at the end of the dialysis procedure.

Acute dialysis, or peritoneal dialysis for patients in acute renal failure or in hyperkalemia, can be performed in this manner. The one- or two-liter bottles of dialysate are hung so that the fluid flows by gravity into the peritoneal cavity, where diffusion and osmosis take place. Those substances thus removed flow by gravity into the drainage bottle or bag. This is called an *exchange*, and 40 liters of exchange is usually considered one dialysis. Because this method, sometimes called the *manual method*, uses an open system, the patient is quite susceptible to infection. However, this technique is extremely simple, requires little or no equipment, and can be performed in even the most remote or tiny hospitals on an emergency basis.

Peritoneal dialysis, while popular as the first choice of treatment for patients with acute renal failure who require dialysis, has not reached the degree of popularity for chronic renal failure that has been attained by hemodialysis. However, peritoneal dialysis is increasingly being chosen as the primary method for long dialytic therapy for a larger expanse of the patient population with end stage renal disease.

In review, peritoneal dialysis takes place within the abdominal cavity. Although the exact physiologic phenomena are not completely understood, it is thought that the mass transfer of solutes from the blood

209

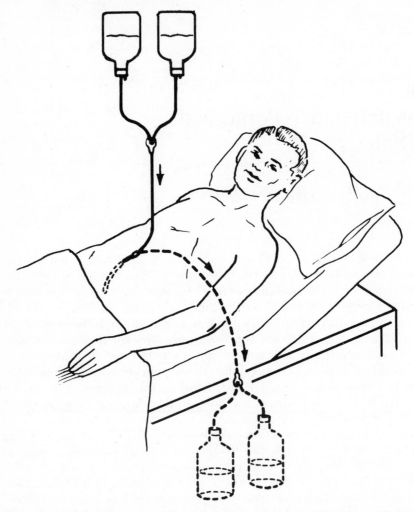

Figure 8.1. Illustration of peritoneal dialysis using the "bottle" or "hand" method. Fluid flows by gravity into the peritoneal cavity, where diffusion and osmosis take place. The waste-laden dialysate then flows by gravity into the drainage bottles.

stream occurs through the single-cell walled capillaries of the peritoneum. These plentiful capillaries are also imbedded in supportive tissues within the peritoneal cavity. Thus, any substance being dialyzed out of the patient may have several diffusion barriers to traverse, especially blood vessel walls, the supportive interstitial tissues, and ultimately the peritoneal membrane and its lining cells (2).

The peritoneal membrane itself is quite porous, which contributes to the loss of large-molecular substances, notably proteins. However, this permeability can be influenced by irritation, infection, or even blood flow changes within the peritoneum itself. Thus, capillary vasoconstriction or other vascular disease will severely reduce the effectiveness of peritoneal dialysis (3).

This may help one understand why peritoneal dialysis is so much less efficient than hemodialysis, despite the large peritoneal surface area. It takes four to five times as many hours of peritoneal dialysis to achieve the same status clinically as one can with hemodialysis.

The principles governing peritoneal dialysis are the same as those for hemodialysis. Substances contained in the dialyzing fluid and in the blood stream will equilibrate across the membrane toward the area of lesser concentration. Those substances that can cross the membrane but are not contained in the dialysate will move from the blood and interstitial fluids into the dialysate contained within the peritoneal cavity. Because the dialysate within the abdominal cavity is constantly being replenished with fresh dialysate, a high mean diffusion gradient between body fluids and dialysate can be maintained, thus enhancing solute removal.

The rapidity with which substances can be removed is determined by molecular weight or molecular configuration. A characteristic pattern is followed, with water moving faster than all other substances. Water is followed in sequence by urea, potassium, chloride, sodium, phosphate, creatinine, and uric acid. Dialysis is concerned with the removal of the by-products of protein breakdown; since these can be relatively easily measured, the efficiency of dialysis can be determined.

Water removal, or ultrafiltration, is achieved in peritoneal dialysis through an osmotic effect created with the addition of dextrose to the dialysate. Generally speaking, particularly in patients with adequate serum protein levels and moderately elevated blood urea levels, a dialysis solution containing dextrose 1.5 gm% will about equal the combined osmotic, colloid osmotic, and hydrostatic pressures on the blood side, and little or no fluid removal will occur. (See Table 8.1.) However, because of individual variations in vascular or membrane permeability, because of disease, or because of reduction in individual serum osmolality, some patients will still lose water across the membrane when dialyzing against a dialysate containing only 1.5 gm% of dextrose.

By increasing dialysate dextrose concentration and thereby increasing the osmotic gradient, fluid removal can be enhanced. Care must be taken to not use dialysate containing more than 4.5 gm% dextrose, except in extremely unusual cases, because of the side effects created by the "solvent drag effect" (2). With very high gradients, water movement

Table 8.1. Composition of McGaw Peritoneal Dialysate per Two-Liter Bottle

Hydrous dextrose	1.5 gm
Sodium acetate	0.61 gm
Sodium chloride	0.56 gm
Calcium chloride	0.029 gm
Magnesium chloride hexahydrate	0.015 gm
Sodium bisulfite	<0.010 gm
Water for ingestion	

may be so rapid as to cause hypernatremia, and hypovolemia with shock, because the water moving across the membrane also pulls a certain amount of solute with it. The consequences of this rapid movement can be fatal; thus patients dialyzing with this solution should be followed closely, with frequent determination of serum sodium, blood sugar, and volume status.

Dextrose in the dialysate will be absorbed and result in increased blood sugar levels. Blood sugar levels between 200 and 400 mg% are somewhat common and require no special intervention. However, patients with diabetes may need insulin, and they certainly will require close monitoring, to prevent them from becoming hyperosmolar or going into hyperglycemia, coma, and death. Nursing assessment for increased thirst, mental sluggishness, or lethargy should be part of the routine of patient monitoring.

Interestingly, in an attempt to ultrafiltrate or remove excess fluid from a patient, a reverse effect may be achieved by using higher concentrations of dextrose in the dialysate. The hypertonic fluid may make the patient hyperosmolar or hypovolemic, thus causing him to become excessively thirsty. The patient may respond in the first case by drinking more fluids and in the second case by drinking more fluids with excessive salt ingestion. Both situations will cause the patient to gain more fluid weight, necessitating ultrafiltration during the next dialysis to remove the excess fluid, and the whole cycle starts again.

Good teaching helps the patient understand what is happening to his body physiologically, so that he may be able to interrupt the hyperosmolar thirst–ultrafiltration–hyperosmolar thirst cycle, thus maintaining better control over interdialytic weight gains.

PATIENT SELECTION

Patients may be selected for either hemodialysis or peritoneal dialysis for the long-term dialytic treatment of chronic renal failure. For some patients peritoneal dialysis may be the preferred mode of therapy. This is especially true in small children because of the problems in developing adequate blood access; in the older patients with cardiovascular problems; in patients whose loss of shunt sites makes peritoneal dialysis a "last resort"; in patients living alone who still want to go on home dialysis; and in patients whose religious beliefs prevent the use of blood transfusions. Tenckhoff, in Seattle, believes that 25% of all patients presenting with end stage renal disease would be better with peritoneal dialysis as the primary mode of treatment (2,4).

Other patients considered prime candidates for peritoneal dialysis rather than hemodialysis include those who desire home dialysis but cannot learn its technically more demanding aspects. Some patients, for unknown reasons, just do not do well with hemodialysis; they may fare better on peritoneal dialysis. Some patients on hemodialysis may be temporarily diverted to peritoneal dialysis if their condition is such that anticoagulation would be too hazardous. This is especially true in patients with pericarditis or subdural hematoma. In some institutions a patient with a new arteriovenous fistula is placed on peritoneal dialysis as a holding procedure to await maturation of the blood access for hemodialysis. Many people believe that peritoneal dialysis is the treatment of choice for the older patient and for the young patient.

Peritoneal dialysis has been used quite successfully as a holding pattern for those patients who are awaiting a renal transplant in the near future. Since home training for peritoneal dialysis can be accomplished within three weeks, a considerable time and financial savings can be experienced. There is a small group of patients for whom hemodialysis may be considered unsuitable because of medical reasons (such as blindness or malignancy) but in whom prolongation of life is still deemed desirable for various reasons. These patients may do quite well on chronic peritoneal dialysis.

There is some controversy about the use of peritoneal dialysis as the primary treatment choice in treating the patient with diabetic nephropathy. Yet, there is some suggestion that the use of peritoneal dialysis in diabetics actually decreases the visual loss and accompanying retinopathy seen in diabetics (5). It has been found that diabetic patients do experience significant reduction in clearance and an overall high incidence of catheter failure (6). Despite these problems, peritoneal dialysis is considered a reasonable alternate mode of therapy for the diabetic patient.

There are, however, some absolute contraindications to peritoneal dialysis. These are a diffusely infected abdominal wall and diffuse intraabdominal adhesions from either an infection or a malignant process.

Abdominal surgery is in itself no contraindication to peritoneal dialysis, especially if hemodialysis is not readily available. However, it is generally advisable to wait two to three days after abdominal surgery before instituting peritoneal dialysis. Failure to postpone dialysis for 48 to 72 hours could result in diaphragmatic, retroperitoneal, or peritoneal leakage. The patient with abdominal drains in place may pose a very messy situation in undertaking peritoneal dialysis. While it is possible to peritoneally dialyze such a patient, the risk for infection from all the ports of entry make such an adventure somewhat infeasible. Yet, in the absence of accessibility to hemodialysis, peritoneal dialysis can be performed for these patients.

In certain situations, hemodialysis may be preferred over peritoneal dialysis. Such situations include active adolescents or young adults, especially males with tight abdominal walls and well-developed muscle mass. The very large, muscular patient also may do better on hemodialysis. On the other hand, obese patients (without large muscle mass) often have poor vessels and difficulty with vascular access. These patients may benefit from peritoneal dialysis. Finally, patients with extensive abdominal adhesions will usually have an ineffective peritoneal surface area and should be placed on hemodialysis.

Whatever mode of dialytic therapy is chosen, the nurse must offer the patient support and guidance. The nurse's ability to convey a sense of belonging, a sense of being cared about, is extremely important. So, too, must the nurse convey a sense of his or her own knowledge and ability, so that the patient becomes confident in the dialytic therapy chosen. Failure by the nurse to do so may seriously jeopardize the patient's chances for long-term survival.

Nurses may or may not play an active role in deciding the mode of dialytic therapy for patients. The choice is made after considering not only a patient's physical and medical status, but also his individual strengths and weaknesses. Social situations can change when a catastrophic illness strikes, and the patient's support system must be considered. A patient may be thought to have a strong family support system until serious illness strikes. The stresses and strains of acute illness followed by chronicity may be the final straw in dividing marriages. Chronicity is very difficult to cope with, and most renal patients also experience some changes in their personality because of the uremia. Not feeling well, lacking energy, and experiencing a lessening of self-image, may cause patients to become short-tempered and verbally strike out at those nearest to them. Some family members cannot or will not tolerate mood changes and may separate themselves from the patient, thus further eroding the patient's self-worth. It is here that nursing intervention is crucial in supporting the patient and enabling him to continue onward in life. The family, too, will need some understanding of what is happening. Because age can affect the ease with which patients learn day-to-day self-care, it must be taken into consideration when evaluating alternative modes of therapy.

ACCESS

Peritoneal dialysis was widely used for acute renal failure in the late 1940s and the 1950s. Little was understood about the clearance of peritoneal dialysis or the amount of dialysis fluid to be used. Repeated punctures, which were accomplished by using a rubber catheter inserted in the peritoneal cavity with a large trocar, were necessary to initiate dialysis in the early days. A later advancement was the use of a rigid catheter. After sterile fluid became commercially available, peritoneal dialysis expanded, but repeated access to the peritoneal cavity still posed a problem.

The most popular device for access to the peritoneal cavity for chronic peritoneal dialysis today is the double-cuffed Tenckhoff catheter. The Silastic catheter enters the peritoneal cavity below the umbilicus and tunnels through subcutaneous tissue to exit externally on either side of the abdomen. A portion of the catheter (5 cm) remains external for ease in connecting to dialysate lines. (See Figure 8.2.)

Several efforts have been successfully developed into patient-practical devices for chronic peritoneal dialysis. All have aimed at overcoming specific problems associated with either repeated punctures or the early attempts at permanently implanted catheters.

Strict aseptic technique must be employed whenever the patient is connected to dialysate lines. Infection, the leading cause of catheter failure, presents the major problem of concern for medical management as well as for nursing care (7). For this reason Tenckhoff devised the double-cuffed chronic peritoneal dialysis catheter. (See Figures 8.3 and 8.4.) The catheter, which is designed to provide a pathway for the fluid to travel in and out of the peritoneal cavity, is equipped with Dacron velour cuffs that serve as barriers to infection. One cuff rests upon the fascia covering the peritoneal membrane and the other is positioned subcutaneously beneath the skin. Tissue overgrowth into and around these cuffs is accomplished within a few weeks and provides a significant barrier to infection arising from the catheter exit site. If, however, an infection should develop, the idea is that it will be limited to the tissue area between the cuff barriers rather than descending into the peritoneal cavity.

The Deane prosthesis is a plastic disc with an attached plastic rod that

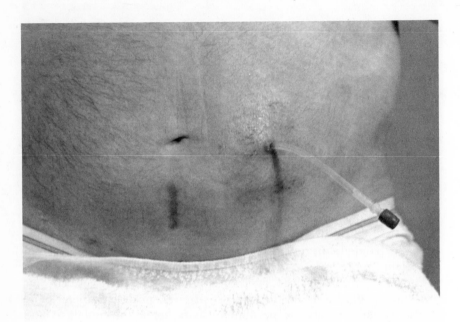

Figure 8.2. Permanently implanted Silastic catheter with external portion covered with rubber cap. Cap is removed under aseptic conditions for peritoneal dialysis to take place. Midline scar indicates point of entry of the catheter into the peritoneal cavity.

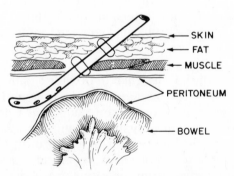

Figure 8.3. Illustration of double-cuffed catheter. One cuff rests on the fascia covering the peritoneum; the other rests just beneath the skin. The section between the two cuffs is tunneled subcutaneously so that the catheter exits the abdominal wall some distance from the point of entry into the peritoneal cavity. The two cuffs provide a barrier to infection.

216

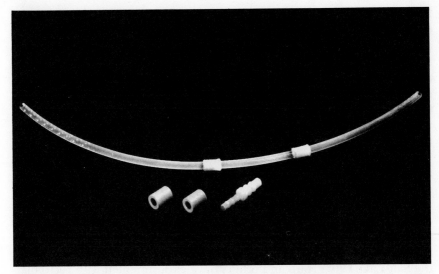

Figure 8.4. Tenckhoff's double-cuffed catheter. The plastic adapter fits into the end of catheter and permits connection for the dialysis procedure. The rubber cap is sterile and covers the connector between dialyses. (Photo courtesy of and used with permission of Physio-Control, Redmond, Wash.)

can be inserted following dialysis into the tract through the abdominal wall left by the catheter. The "button" is then left in place until the next dialysis. At that time, the skin is prepped and another rigid peritoneal catheter is inserted for dialysis. The advantages are no puncture and no permanent catheter for infection or obstruction to overtake. However, the sinus tract does not always remain intact between time of catheter removal and insertion of the prosthesis; thus another puncture is required. While utilized by some centers for maintaining peritoneal access, the Deane prosthesis has not met with universal acceptance.

One of the problems experienced with peritoneal dialysis catheters is the siphoning of omental and peritoneal contents onto the drainage holes. In some instances the tip of the catheter has been known to drift upward against the diaphragm, thus reducing its efficiency. The Goldberg catheter has been developed to obviate some of these problems. It consists of an inflatable cuff or balloon that enables the catheter to settle into the abdominal gutter. The large holes maximize fluid exchange, while the balloon minimizes suction of the omentum onto the holes. A subcutaneous cuff around the catheter is sutured beneath the skin as a barrier to infection.

A relatively novel approach to achieving access to the peritoneal cavity has been developed by the group at the University of Utah in Salt Lake City. It consists of a subcutaneously implanted siliconized segment with an arm extending from each end into the peritoneal cavity. (See Figure 8.5.) A spring keeps the transverse lumen expanded, and no portion remains external. Rather, dialysis is achieved by puncturing the subcutaneous segment with one or two needles for dialysate to flow in and out. Because a divider is present in the center of the segment, a more rapid exchange of dialysate can take place with the two-needle method (See Figure 8.6.) A needle placed on either side of the divider permits a rapid exchange of dialysate to take place. This device virtually eliminates the problem of infection via the lumen of the access device (8). While earlier versions presented some problems of excessive fibrinous encasement of the extension arms, these have since been corrected (9). This concept of an internal peritoneal dialysis access device may well be the answer in the future.

In conjunction with the subcutaneous catheter for peritoneal dialysis, the Salt Lake City group and others have experimented with recirculat-

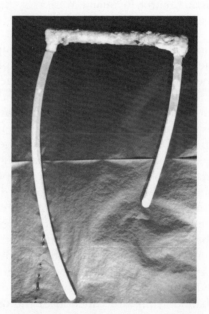

Figure 8.5. Photograph of excised subcutaneous catheter with extensions. (Used through the courtesy of and with the permission of W. J. Kolff, Institute of Biomedical Engineering, University of Utah, Salt Lake City.)

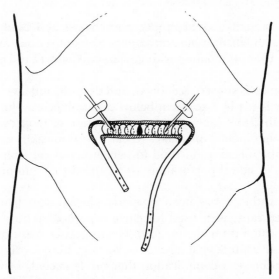

Figure 8.6. Schematic of subcutaneous catheter implanted with the two arms extending into the peritoneal cavity. One or two needles then puncture the catheter, held patent by a coiled spring, for dialysis to take place. The two-needle technique allows a more rapid exchange.

ing the peritoneal fluid through a hollow fiber dialyzer and charcoal adsorbent column in an attempt to increase the efficiency of dialysis. While work in this area is still embryonic, it is being conducted on several fronts (8) and may yet supply the answer for improved efficiency of peritoneal dialysis.

Patient teaching is extremely important for long-term survival of whatever type of access device is chosen for the patient about to begin chronic peritoneal dialysis. Nursing care begins with patient teaching before the operative procedure ever takes place. By explaining and reemphasizing the need for absolutely impeccable cleanliness, the nurse can prepare the patient for changes in hygienic habits that he must make. For reasons that are not completely understood, good bowel and bladder habits are crucial to proper functioning of the catheter. A patient's awareness of the sensations that he will experience as the catheter is being surgically implanted under local anesthesia will prepare him to assist in its proper placement. His being able to describe the sensation felt when the catheter tip is striking the bladder or the rectum can assist the physician in the proper direction for optimum placement. For this reason, and to prevent an accidental physiologic response to such stimuli, the patient should empty both bowel and bladder prior to surgery. In many institutions, catheter placement is done at the bedside in operating room simulation with gown, mask, glove. and a large sterile field.

The abdomen is shaved, scrubbed, and draped, and a vertical midline skin incision is made 3 to 5 cm below the umbilicus. The abdomen is "primed" with 2 to 4 liters of warmed dialysate or dextrose in saline to distend the abdomen. This makes trocar insertion easier and safer, and it suspends the intestines in fluid to permit better catheter positioning. The chances of bowel perforation are reduced to a minimum with this technique.

Once the catheter has been properly placed—and in most cases a double-cuffed catheter is used for chronic peritoneal catheter—dialysis must be instituted immediately (10). Nursing assessment of the patient should include routine vital signs as well as watching for signs of complications. Bleeding is a complication that rarely occurs; when it does, it generally stops spontaneously. Heparin, 100 to 400 U/liter, is added to the dialysate to prevent fibrin formation in the catheter; it does not contribute to bleeding. Pain, irritation, or other discomfort may be of concern to the patient. There really should be no pain except at the incision site, but the patient may experience pain or discomfort in the deeper pelvic structures (vagina, penis, rectum, bladder). This may be either because the intraabdominal catheter segment is too long or because of local irritation. Having the patient move around will usually provide immediate relief. Usually all symptoms disappear spontaneously from within a few days to two weeks, probably because the catheter has settled into its relocated place. Leakage rarely occurs, and then only during the immediate postimplantation period when there has been insufficient time for tissue ingrowth into the cuff. Leakage invites infection and interferes with tissue ingrowth, as well as causing skin irritation at the exit site. Small dialysate exchange volumes during the first week following implantation should prevent overdistension and thus the occurrence of leakage.

Patient teaching occurs through all of this, as the nurse explains to the patient what is going on, why, and what can be done about it. As strict aseptic technique is being carried out, the patient can be taught it in observing the initiation and termination of dialysis procedures, as well as catheter care and dressing changes. Many maneuvers can be learned during the first week to correct some of the strange sensations and minor discomforts that may accompany the body's physiologic adjustment to the foreign body (catheter) recently implanted in the peritoneal cavity. The patient's knowledge about and understanding of the changes taking place within the body will reduce apprehension and contribute to an overall smooth recovery.

A crucial, and usually very difficult, concept to get across to the patient is the absolute necessity for impeccable cleanliness. The exit site of the transcutaneous catheter is an extremely vulnerable portal of entry for infection. It is here that strict cleanliness in catheter care is a must to insure long-term catheter survival.

Routine care consists of daily cleansing of the catheter exit site as well as of the catheter itself and surrounding skin area. Betadine is usually the cleansing agent of choice. If, however, the patient is allergic to Betadine, other antiseptic agents may be used. Only sterile applicators and 4 × 4s should be used in the cleansing and dressing procedure. Starting at the exit site and working in circular motions outward is the technique easiest for patients to comprehend. The area is then dried and dressed with sterile gauze squares folded on either side of the catheter, with the catheter curled on top and covered by an additional gauze square. Nonirritating tape should be used, and sufficient exposure provided to permit the skin to breathe. Accumulation of moisture causes skin irritation, breakdown, and finally infection.

Approximately two to four weeks following catheter implantation, the exit site should be clean, dry, free of redness and tenderness, and virtually crust free. Any state other than this should lead one to suspect an infection. By now, wound healing should be completed, and the patient should be able to engage in virtually unlimited activities. Showers are preferred to baths, and soap and dirt accumulating during the shower must be rinsed off at the end. The exit site is patted dry, then recleaned with Betadine and dressed as usual. Some patients even engage in swimming, although it is not encouraged, primarily because little is known about infection via this route.

Self-examination for catheter infection should become a matter of routine for the patient. Self-examination involves close inspection for redness, swelling, unusual bulging of the catheter exit site or tunnel, and any bleeding, crusting, or discharge. The patient should also adopt the habit of weekly palpation of the subcutaneous catheter and its cuff. It should be possible to pick up the cuff and its surrounding tissues between the thumb and index finger and gently squeeze it without causing any pain. Pain or any other adverse sign could be an early warning of infection, and the patient should seek immediate medical help.

Because such routine examination is performed so close to the exit site, it should be performed with clean and preferably gloved hands. The conclusion of dialysis affords an ideal time to do this, since the area is clean and the patient still has gloves on.

HOME DIALYSIS

Peritoneal dialysis treatments are time consuming—requiring approximately 40 hours per week. This is one of the reasons that emphasis was placed on home dialysis early on by the Seattle and the Toronto groups (11,12,13). Boen introduced the concept of an automated system for the delivery of dialysate to the peritoneal cavity in 1963, and the following year this system was used in the home in Seattle (1). The closed-system concept significantly reduced the incidence of peritonitis and made self-dialysis a practicality for the patient undergoing chronic peritoneal dialysis (14,15).

There are, of course, several advantages to home peritoneal dialysis, not the least of which is the time factor. Other advantages are the same as for hemodialysis, including some of the psychosocial ramifications. Being able to perform self-dialysis at home gives the patient the responsibility for managing his own therapeutic regimen. The patient can maintain a flexible dialysis schedule so as not to disrupt plans for anniversary celebrations, children's school activities, or other special occasions. There need not be a sensation of being boxed into a specific schedule.

Peritoneal dialysis, while it is time consuming, is also extremely safe and can be performed at night during sleep. There is no danger of life-threatening air embolism that requires the patient to be awake and constantly monitoring the dialysis procedure. A 40-hour week of dialysis can be divided into 8 hours 5 times/week or 10 hours 4 times/week. Patients requiring only 36 hours of dialysis may be able to dialyze 12 hours thrice weekly. However, 12-hour periods may be too tiring for children and too impractical for persons trying to continue working.

DELIVERY SYSTEMS

Presently two major closed systems are used to deliver sterile fluid to the peritoneal cavity. A proportioning system delivers sterile water and concentrate in a ratio to produce the desired mixture of dialysate. This produces 40 liters of dialysate per each 2-liter bottle of concentrate, sufficient for one dialysis. The two proportioning peritoneal delivery systems currently being manufactured in the United States utilize reverse osmosis units to produce essentially pyrogen-free water for mixing with the concentrate. The cycling system uses commercially prepared dialysate that flows into the peritoneal cavity.

For peritoneal dialysis, system PDS/RO 300 manufactured by Physiocontrol (see Figure 8.7) uses an ultraviolet lamp as a back-up

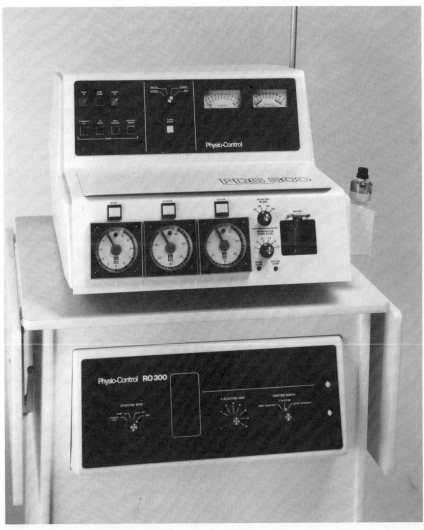

Figure 8.7. Peritoneal dialysis system. PDS/RO by Physio-Control has the dialysis control console above with the reverse osmosis water treatment system below. (Photo courtesy of and used with permission of Physio-Control, Redmond, Wash.)

223

sterilizing unit to assure that pure water is delivered to the mixing chamber where concentrate and water mix. The "Inflow" timer can be set to deliver the desired amount of dialysate. The timer labeled "Diffusion" determines the length of time dialysate remains in the peritoneal cavity, while "Outflow" is the amount of time allotted for the dialysate to empty from the patient. Once each timer has completed its "time," it then moves automatically to the next phase of the cycle—thus the term *automated peritoneal dialysis* or *APD*.

Drake Willock manufactures an automated peritoneal dialysis system similar to the one mentioned above. This device also produces pyrogen-free water via a reverse osmosis column but does not utilize ultraviolet light as an additional sterilizing agent. Also designed for use in the home, this machine utilizes alarm systems similar to those in the machine mentioned previously. The timing mechanism is basically the same for both machines; it operates much like the timer on an automatic dishwasher. Figure 8.8 shows this machine, with concentrate bottle hanging and with water and concentrate lines in place in the pumps.

The other type of delivery system being used today is the "cycler" manufactured by American Medical Products. (See Figure 8.9.) This device functions by "cycling" one- or two-liter bottles or bags of dialysate through the system. Directly beneath the bottles is the heater that warms the dialysate. The two dials control inflow and outflow to and from the patient. All of the effluent is collected in a large drainage bag, so that no water source or drain is needed to operate this device.

While this device is used by many people for home dialysis, the added factor of multiple puncture points at the dialysate bottles must be taken into consideration. This offers many more possible portals of entry for viral or pathogen invasion, thus nullifying the beneficial effect achieved with a closed system.

Cost must be considered in any home dialysis program. For the proportioning machines, the cost of the delivery system itself is significant, yet somewhat comparable to that of delivery systems utilized for hemodialysis. In addition, patient supplies for sterile tubing, tape, dressings, and the like will add an additional $15 to $20 per dialysis. Concentrate costs approximately $25 per two-liter bottle; thus, the cost per dialysis would be $40 to $45, comparable to that of hemodialysis. While the cycler represents a much lower initial investment (less than one-third the cost of the proportioning units), the difference is more than made up by the cost of the dialysate at approximately $3 per two-liter bottle; the cost of supplies plus dialysate for 40 liters ranges from $75 to $80 per dialysis (11).

Each machine has features that appeal to specific patients with specific

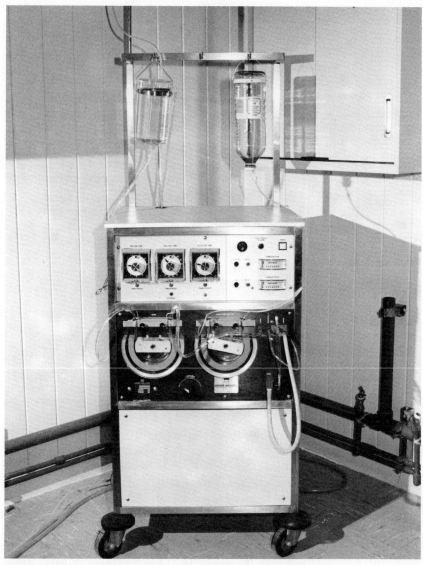

Figure 8.8. Drake Willock APD machine. Reverse osmosis column is located at the back of the machine.

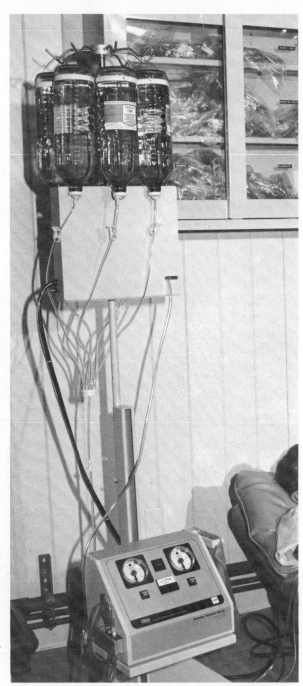

Figure 8.9. Peritoneal dialysis cycler manufactured by American Medical Products warms the dialysate before delivering it to the patient. This machine can handle up to 16 liters of dialysate (eight of the two-liter bottles).

226

needs, and these must all be considered before choosing a delivery system for a patient.

HOME TRAINING

Teaching the patient to perform self peritoneal dialysis at home can usually be accomplished within three weeks. Even if the patient will not be dialyzing a full 40 hours per week, dividing the total number of dialysis hours into the five-day week will give the patient five opportunities each week for learning initiation and termination procedures.

The patient is taught how to take and record vital signs very early. Usually an apical pulse is taken, thereby permitting the patient to learn what his normal heart sounds like and to detect any arrhythmias. Weight, temperature, blood pressure, and pulse are recorded before and after dialysis. Interdialytic weight gain is the best indicator for excessive fluid, and an excessive weight gain may indicate to the patient the need to use a higher dextrose concentration in the dialysate in order to remove the fluid. If the patient were using the proportioning system for home dialysis, it may be necessary to go to the concentrate containing 50% dextrose (see Table 8.2) in order to produce 2.5% dextrose dialysate to achieve the desired osmotic fluid removal. A daily fluid accumulation of one pound (500 cc of fluid equals one pound of weight) per day is considered safe. By most standards more than a two pound-per-day weight is excessive.

Procedures for readying the equipment for dialysis are learned along with the dialysis procedures, so that the patient is constantly exposed to all aspects of the therapeutic regimen. Normal kidney function as well as the patient's own particular type of kidney disease are discussed, with emphasis on how the renal replacement therapy of peritoneal dialysis performs the work of the now defunct kidneys.

Table 8.2. Composition of McGaw Concentrate for Peritoneal Dialysis

Concentrate (gm)		Diluted 1:20 to Provide	
Hydrous dextrose	50.0	Dextrose	2.5 gm%
Sodium acetate	9.4	Sodium	130.0 mEq/L
Sodium chloride	11.2	Calcium	3.5 mEq/L
Calcium chloride	0.51	Magnesium	1.0 mEq/L
Sodium bisulfite	0.10	Chloride	100.0 mEq/L
Magnesium chloride hexahydrate	0.20	Acetate	34.5 mEq/L

Asepsis

Since strict aseptic technique is probably the most difficult as well as most important of the maneuvers for the patient to learn, it is constantly emphasized, retaught, and reinforced in the patient. A five-minute scrub with Betadine immediately before connecting the patient line (dialysate tubing) to the patient's catheter is crucial, and it must be carried out utilizing all the principles of asepsis.

Asepsis, gloving without contamination, and remaining gloved and maintaining sterility are all very new and very difficult concepts for the patient. It may be necessary, as well as beneficial, to have the patient practice gloving several times either during dialysis or at the end of the day when dialysis has been terminated. It takes some practice (as we all know) to become adept at putting on sterile gloves. Some benefit may be derived from obtaining a mannequin torso from a department store and implanting a peritoneal catheter into its abdominal wall. This would provide the patient with a catheter to safely practice on, without fear of injuring his own catheter or inducing pathogens. Learning the technique of scrubbing up the catheter and gently working off the rubber cap while scrubbing, yet without tugging on the short length of catheter at the same time, can be a little tricky. A model or "dummy" to practice on may hasten the patient's development of confidence and skill, as well as prevent self-induced peritonitis.

Determining Dialysis Times

In our institution, we also teach patients to adjust the various dialysis times to meet their own specific needs. Patients dialyze 40 hours per week. For example, a patient dialyzing on a proportioning machine for 10 hours would have 40 liters or 40,000 cc of fluid instilled and drained over a 10-hour period, or 4000 cc/hour. If the pump is set to deliver 500 cc/min, and the patient normally uses a 2000-cc exchange, the "Inflow" timer is set at four minutes or 2000 cc. At 2000 cc of dialysate per exchange, and needing to exchange 4000 cc per hour, the patient would need two exchanges per hour. If the patient "inflows," or fills the peritoneal cavity in four minutes to accomplish an inflow of 2000 cc, the length of time to outflow or empty will be pretty well determined by the ease with which the patient empties. Suppose it took the patient 10 minutes to empty; adding another 20% to the time to allow for ultrafiltration would give an outflow time of 12 minutes. Inflow of four minutes, outflow of 12 minutes, leaves only the "dwell" or diffusion time as the variable. To accomplish two exchanges per hour, the total exchange should take 30 minutes, thus leaving a swell time of 14 minutes.

However, by using less fluid per each exchange, it is possible to get many more exchanges per hour, thus enhancing fluid removal. Smaller volumes with more frequent exchanges may actually be more efficient, too (16). In adjusting times to meet patient needs and fill the predetermined length of dialysis, the patient will still receive 40 liters of dialysis. By maintaining a closed system and not interrupting it to add an additional bottle of concentrate, we can protect the patient against an intrusion by pathogens, as well as prevent unnecessary waste of unused or leftover concentrate.

A step-by-step formula for calculating times using an automated device for peritoneal dialysis is as follows:

1. $\dfrac{\text{Dialysis time in hours}}{40{,}000 \text{ cc}} = \text{cc/hr}$

2. $\dfrac{\text{cc/hr}}{\text{inflow in cc}} = \text{no. of exchanges/hr}$

3. $\dfrac{60 \text{ min}}{\text{no. of exchanges}} = \text{length of each exchange in minutes}$

4. Determine inflow time from amount delivered per hour.
5. Determine length of first outflow and add 20% to that time.
6. Difference between total of inflow and outflow time and total exchange time is the dwell time (8,17).

Peritonitis

Infection, especially peritonitis, is of prime concern to the patient undergoing peritoneal dialysis. Therefore, the patient needs to be taught the signs and symptoms of peritonitis and the appropriate measures to take.

Classic peritonitis manifests itself clinically with fever, abdominal pain, cloudy outflow, and rebound tenderness. Fibrin formation tends to occur, and protein losses are enhanced. The immediate treatment for peritonitis is continual peritoneal dialysis with no dwell time. Cultures will determine the causative organism, if one can be found, and the appropriate antibiotics prescribed.

Protocols for drug therapy vary from institution to institution and may employ oral antibiotics, intraperitoneal antibiotics, or a combination thereof. Some institutions, notably Toronto and Tulsa, use prophylactic cloxacillin to prevent peritonitis.

In Seattle, the protocol is to initially gram stain and culture the peritoneal fluid. This is followed by 48 to 72 hours of continuous peritoneal dialysis and the appropriate antibiotic. Cephalosporin and gentamycin are added to the dialysate, as well as heparin to decrease the fibrin formation. This is followed by four to five days of daily dialysis with antibiotics, then two months of oral and intraperitoneal antibiotics. One week after the antibiotics have been stopped, the peritoneal fluid is again cultured (18).

A culture is easily obtained from the peritoneal catheter. Using sterile technique, simply prep the rubber cap with Betadine, insert a needle attached to a 3-cc syringe, and aspirate the fluid. Care must be taken to run the needle through the cap in a straight line or the catheter itself can be punctured, thus providing a direct portal of entry for unwanted organisms.

Aseptic or mechanical peritonitis also occurs in patients for reasons that are not understood. The symptoms will be the same, with abdominal pain, rebound tenderness, and cloudy outflow resolving much more rapidly than in infectious peritonitis. While the symptoms may abate with continual dialysis alone, it is generally recommended that antibiotics be given initially until it can be determined if the peritonitis is bacterial or mechanical.

For the patient, the first sign of peritonitis may be cloudy outflow with some fibrin threads noted. Indeed, some may never experience any other symptoms. At the first sign of peritonitis, be it cloudy outflow or pain, the patient should add heparin to the dialysate. We routinely add 4000 units of heparin to the concentrate bottle, which provides 100 units of heparin/liter of dialysate. This is not much, but it seems to be sufficient in preventing fibrin formation and build-up and subsequent clotting of the catheter. This small amount of heparin does not contribute toward patient bleeding.

What sometimes happens is that the patient has a day or two when cloudy outflow is noted after the first few exchanges. Then fibrin strings are noted in the outflow dialysate, which may be coming more cloudy. Often this occurs before the patient experiences pain and/or fever. Part of the patient teaching involves impressing upon him the need for close monitoring, especially of initial dialysate outflows. Some institutions teach patients to culture the outflow, and to institute various techniques according to a preestablished protocol. They may add specific antibiotics to the dialysate, increase the frequency and length of dialysis, and continue monitoring their course at home. Other institutions will have the patient report to the center at the first sign of peritonitis, where cultures are taken and in-hospital treatment of peritonitis is begun immediately.

Whatever the procedure is, the nurse must make sure that the patient fully understands the ramifications of peritonitis and what the patient can and should do in the event that it does occur.

Diet and Medications

For the patient with end stage renal disease, diet and medications are essential components of the therapuetic regimen. Multiple vitamins, especially the water-soluble ones lost through dialysis, must be supplemented daily. Renal patients are folate depleted and require a minimum of folate each day, as well as iron supplements for those patients with low iron stores. And, because renal patients can no longer excrete phosphorus through the kidneys, phosphate binders are crucial to preventing metastatic bone disease.

But diet is the renal patient's most important medication. The patient undergoing peritoneal dialysis loses protein during dialysis, as much as 30 to 70 grams per week. However, protein loss is much greater when hypertonic dialysate is used. Infection in patients produces a higher catabolic rate, thereby also increasing protein loss. At the same time, most patients also have a decrease or even a loss of appetite during periods of infection. These factors may all result in negative nitrogen balance. Malnutrition can develop in a patient after excessively high protein losses due to peritonitis.

Tenckhoff recommends a protein intake of 1.5 gm/kg body weight for the patient undergoing chronic peritoneal dialysis (2,12). We place our patients on a 100-gm high-biological-value protein and 20-gm low-biological-value protein diet. Because there is no potassium in the concentrate we use, there is no actual potassium restriction, but patients are instructed in and learn an awareness of high-potassium foods. The quantity of protein may be difficult for some patients to ingest, especially the very young with finicky eating habits, and the elderly who simply are not very interested in eating. Persons living on fixed incomes may find it a financial hardship to consume the protein they need. However, high-quality protein is not just meat, but includes fish, eggs, and milk. Chicken may be more economical than beef, and fish from the patient's favorite fishing hole can offer a variety in the menu, as well as provide the essential amino acids. Grilled cheese sandwiches are usually met with much delight by renal patients and can be an excellent source of high protein. A milkshake made with one or two raw eggs together with milk and ice cream in a blender offers a tasty source of high-quality protein as well as calories.

The nurse should be aware of the special problems or situations that may prevent a patient from adhering to the necessary diet. By making the dietitian aware of these problems, the nurse can function as a member of the nephrology team and call upon the various disciplines available to assist the patient. In some circumstances the social worker and dietitian, working in concert, can enable the patient to more easily adapt to the changes required in working out a therapeutic regimen.

Problem Solving

Pain on Inflow

Included in the patient's training program will be general information for the problem solving of situations arising during the course of a peritoneal dialysis. For example, pain on inflow of dialysis may occur during the first exchange or two because of irritation. This may disappear after the first week or so, when the patient adjusts to dialysate inflowing. This is particularly true if the patient experiences continual pain in the area of the bladder or rectum, arising because the intraperitoneal segment of the catheter is poking those areas. After the catheter has settled into place, the pain will usually disappear. Immediate relief can usually be achieved by simply changing position in bed during dialysis, thereby changing the intraperitoneal position of the catheter. Cold dialysate will sometimes cause pain on inflow and can be corrected by flushing out the dialysate left in the line before connecting to the patient, or by making sure that the dialysis cycles are not so long as to cause the warmed dialysate to cool prior to instillation into the peritoneal cavity. Another cause of pain on inflow has been found to be the pulsatile nature of dialysate inflow. The installation of a pulse dampener to convert dialysate inflow to a steady stream eliminated this type of pain (19). Finally, pain between the shoulder blades toward the end of dialysis is usually due to stretching and irritation of the diaphragm. This may disappear after the patient adjusts to the quantity of fluid required for each exchange. Meanwhile, decreasing the amount of dialysate per exchange will afford the patient some relief and enable him to sleep. Because of the individuality of patients, there is tremendous variation in their ability to tolerate the acidic dialysis solutions. Most patients tolerate a solution pH of 5.5 to 5.7 without any discomfort. If, however, dialysate pH is suspected as the cause of the pain (such pain characteristically starts with the inflow and may dissipate during the dwell time), the addition of alkalinizing substances to the dialysate will furnish an instant cure.

We had one patient who hiccupped at the start of each outflow. Apparently the sudden surge of dialysate inflow irritated the phrenic nerve, and he responded accordingly. This response disappeared as the patient adapted to peritoneal dialysis, but it reminded us that each patient may respond differently to the same stimulus.

Skin Care

Problems can occur in stressing the importance of cleanliness in catheter care, and the patient should also be taught to avoid skin irritation and subsequent skin breakdown. Vigorous scrubbing, or failure to remove all

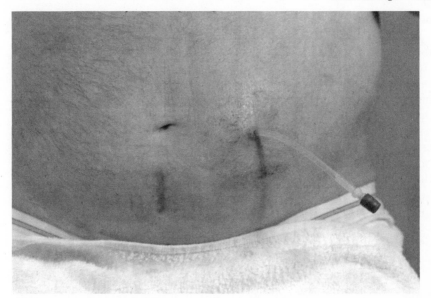

Figure 8.10. Note area of irritation surrounding catheter. This was caused by completely sealing the dressing with tape and not providing "breathing room." Area of irritation is size of dressing.

the soap, may cause skin irritation. (See Figure 8.10.) Skin maceration will occur, too, if the dressing over the catheter is completely covered with tape. Failure to provide "breathing room" for the area under the dressing will result in moisture accumulation and subsequent skin maceration. While some patients note a "toughening" of the skin with Betadine, others may develop a sensitivity with local skin irritation. It may be necessary to change antiseptic cleansing agents, or the patient may have to try other maneuvers until the area heals. The use of Vaseline or such substances may only make the condition worse. Some patients have used a period of air exposure to allow the skin to dry and then heal. Others have applied cocoa butter to the skin. If the skin breakdown is severe, antibiotic ointments may be needed to prevent local infection. Whatever may work for one patient to promote healthy skin surrounding the peritoneal catheter exit site may not work for the next patient.

Failure to Outflow
Another problem to teach the patient about is failure to outflow, which may produce some agonizing moments for the patient undergoing chronic peritoneal dialysis. If this occurs shortly after the catheter has

been implanted, it may be due to a kink of the subcutaneous segment. If, however, it occurs after the patient has gone home on dialysis, several factors may play a role. One of the easiest to solve, and the least understood, is the full colon. Colonic evacuation in instances of poor peritoneal outflow will often relieve the situation; therefore, it is a good habit for the patient to have a bowel movement before beginning the dialysis procedure if at all possible. If the patient has problems with constipation, then stool softeners, a high-fiber diet, suppositories, and/or enemas may be used to rectify the situation. Occasionally failure to drain or a sluggish outflow will be due to the patient's level being lower than the drain level, negating a gravity outflow. By raising the bed (it may not be possible to change the level of the drain), gravity outflow may be increased. Occasionally, a patient utilizing the proportioning automated peritoneal dialysis delivery system will encounter some difficulty with outflow at the beginning of dialysis. This can sometimes be corrected by pushing "Inflow," then immediately going to "Outflow" at the start of the outflow phase of the cycle. Should this problem persist, however, dye injection x-rays may be necessary to determine if catheter obstruction is present. If the catheter appears normal and no peritonitis is present, then functional obstruction of the catheter should be presumed. Functional catheter obstruction has been remedied with bowel stimulation, ambulation, or simply a 12- to 24-hour waiting period before resuming dialysis (2).

Bloody Effluent

Another problem that may occur and be of concern to the patient is bloody effluent. Bloody effluent that occurs in the early post-catheter-implantation period is usually of no consequence. It usually subsides within days. Occasionally a patient will note some pink-tinged effluent, but it will usually disappear after a few exchanges. The cause is unclear; it may be due to irritation or pulling on the catheter. A small amount of bloody effluent can also be seen a few days just before the vaginal bleeding associated with menstruation in women. This, too, subsides, and is of no consequence. The excessive menstruation seen in women on hemodialysis does not occur in women undergoing peritoneal dialysis.

Other Problems

Some so-called side effects of peritoneal dialysis may be manifested in varying degrees in individual patients.

Thirst, as mentioned earlier, can be a common complaint in patients undergoing peritoneal dialysis, especially if the patient is requiring higher dextrose concentrations in order to reduce the extracellular volume. In attempting to satisfy the thirst, the patient drinks more fluid, requires higher dextrose concentrations to remove the excessive fluid, and actually causes more thirst. The only solution is for the patient to reduce interdialytic weight gain, thus reducing the need for higher dextrose concentrations in the dialysate to remove the excessive fluid.

Ascites arises from irritation of the peritoneal membrane by the hypertonic and acid dialysis solutions. Higher dextrose concentrations can also contribute. (See Figure 8.11.) The ascites may be slight and pose only minor problems for the patient, the primary one being the difficulty in getting clothing to fit. Or it may be severe enough to cause respiratory embarrassment, particularly if the patient is discontinued suddenly from peritoneal dialysis to hemodialysis or for a transplant. The ascitic fluid will usually have the appearance of plasma and be virtually cell free and sterile. Severe ascites will usually resolve after several weeks to months, some cases with treatment, some without.

Anemia, a complication of chronic renal failure, may be less of a problem in the patient undergoing chronic peritoneal dialysis than in the patient on hemodialysis, because there is no blood letting with peritoneal dialysis. It is possible to avoid frequent venipunctures in peritoneal dialysis patients by aspirating a few milliliters of ascitic fluid aseptically through the catheter cap predialysis. This fluid can be used to determine electrolytes, phosphorus, BUN, and creatinine. Since ascitic fluid calcium levels are lower than serum calcium levels, a multiplication factor of 1.21 will usually correct ascitic fluid levels to serum levels of calcium (2). Whenever possible, ascitic fluid sampling should be done to eliminate blood letting and subsequent blood loss.

SUMMARY

Peritoneal dialysis is a reasonable alternative to hemodialysis for many patients with end stage renal disease, and it should offer the patient for whom it is chosen a reasonably healthy and reasonably long life.

Peritoneal dialysis has come a long way from its humble beginning. The oldest form of renal replacement therapy for the patient with end stage renal disease, it is only now enjoying renewed acceptance as the primary treatment choice for chronic dialytic therapy. The advantages of unattended, overnight dialysis, no venipunctures, and virtually unlimited diet, make this mode of therapy quite attractive. Recent advances with the proportioning units for delivery of dialysate, and promising work with peritoneal access, combine to make this the most exciting area in the field. Ultimately, more and more patients will be utilizing this

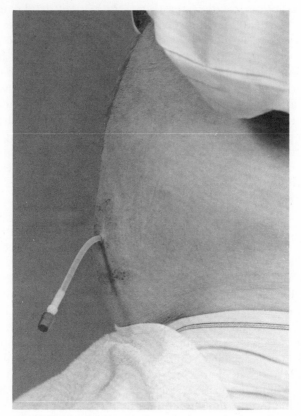

Figure 8.11. Ascites in patient undergoing chronic peritoneal dialysis.

form of therapy, and nursing will continue to assume the major proportion of patient teaching. Through multidisciplinary approaches to patient care, nursing's impact upon patient teaching and upon the patient's total care will be even more important.

REFERENCES

1. M Clark: Peritoneal dialysis in the home. Annual Meeting of American Association of Nephrology Nurses and Technicians, Seattle, 1977.
2. H Tenckhoff: *Chronic Peritoneal Dialysis.* Seattle, Univ of Washington, 1974.
3. K D Nolph, A J Ghods, J Van Stone, P A Brown: The effects of intraperitoneal vasodilators on peritoneal clearances. *Trans Amer Soc Artif Int Organs,* Vol XXII, 1976.

4. _____ : Open forum on peritoneal dialysis. *Dialysis and Transplantation* 2 (4), 1973.

5. B Von Hartitizch, T R Medluck: Chronic peritoneal dialysis—a regime comparable to conventional hemodialysis. *Trans Amer Soc Artif Int Organs,* Vol XXV, 1976.

6. F O Finkelstein, A S Kliger, C Basil, et al.: Chronic peritoneal dialysis in diabetic patients with end stage renal disease. *Proc Cl Dialysis and Transplant Forum,* 1975.

7. J Rubin, D G Oreopoulos, T T Lid, et al.: Management of peritonitis and bowel perforation during chronic peritoneal dialysis. *Nephron* 16, 1976.

8. A Gordon, A J Lewin, M H Maxwell, et al.: Augmentation of efficiency by continuous flow sorbent regeneration peritoneal dialysis. *Trans Amer Soc Artif Int Organs,* Vol XXII, 1976.

9. R L Stephen, E Atkin-Thor, W J Kolff: Recirculating peritoneal dialysis with subcutaneous cathether. *Trans Amer Soc Artif Int Organs,* Vol XXII, 1968.

10. H Tenckhoff, H Schechter: A bacteriologically safe peritoneal access device. *Trans Amer Soc Artif Int Organs,* Vol XIV, 1968.

11. D G Oreopoulos, M Jones, H Devine, et al.: Three years' experience with home peritoneal dialysis. *Proc Cl Dialysis and Transplant Forum,* 1975

12. H Tenckhoff, C R Blagg, K F Curtis, et al.: Chronic peritoneal dialysis. *Proc EDTA,* Vol X, 1973.

13. S Counts, R Hickman, A Garbaccio, et al.: Chronic home peritoneal dialysis in children. *Trans Amer Soc Artif Int Organs,* Vol XIX, 1973.

14. J Bergstrom, M Marklund, S Olofsson, et al.: An automated apparatus for peritoneal dialysis with volumetric fluid balance measurement. *Dialysis and Transplantation* 2 (4), 1976.

15. D G Vidt: Home peritoneal dialysis—alternative to chronic hemodialysis. *Cleveland Clinic Quarterly* 42 (3), 1975.

16. K D Nolph, A J Ghods, P Brown, et al.: Factors affecting peritoneal dialysis efficiency. *Dialysis and Transplantation* 6 (2), 1977.

17. S T Boin: Overview and history of peritoneal dialysis. *Dialysis and Transplantation* 6 (2), 1977.

18. T Mabry, G Acchiardo, G Trapp: Psychological aspects of dialysis from the personal viewpoint. *Dialysis and Transplantation* 6 (11), 1977.

19. P Ivanovitch, K M Jones, A Borspang: Pulse dampener for elimination of automated peritoneal dialysis pain. *Dialysis and Transplantation* 5 (1), 1976.

BIBLIOGRAPHY

Atkins R C, Mion C, Despaux, et al.: Peritoneal transfer of kanamycin and its use in peritoneal dialysis. *Kidney International,* Vol 3, 1973.

Black H R, Finkelstein F O, Lee R V: The treatment of peritonitis in patients with chronic indwelling catheters. *Trans Amer Soc Artif Int Organs,* Vol XX, 1974.

Blumenkrantz M J: Maintenance peritoneal dialysis as an alternative for the patient with end stage renal failure. *Clinical Digest* 6 (14), 1977.

Blumenkrantz M J, Kamdar A, Coburn J W: Peritoneal dialysis for diabetic patients with end stage nephropathy. *Dialysis and Transplantation* 6 (2), 1977.

Blumenkrantz M J, Shepiro D J, Miller J H, et al.: Chronic peritoneal dialysis for management of chronic renal failure. *Proc Cl Dialysis and Transplant Forum,* Nov 1973.

Finkelstein F O, Kilger A S, Basil C, et al.: Sequential clearance and dialysance measurements in chronic peritoneal dialysis patients. *Nephron* 18, 1977.

Ginette J B, Dean N: Repeated peritoneal dialysis by the catheter placement method: description of technique and a replaceable prothesis for chronic access to the peritoneal cavity. *Proc EDTA,* 1967.

Goldberg E H, Hill W: A new peritoneal access prosthesis. *Proc Cl Dialysis and Transplant Forum,* Nov 1973.

Gutman R A, Shelburne, J D: An outbreak of cryptogenic peritonitis: implications for reverse osmosis production of biologically safe water. *Dialysis and Transplantation* 6 (3), 1977.

Henderson L W: The problem of peritoneal membrane area and permeability. *Kidney International,* Vol 3, 1973.

Lee R V, Black H R, Finkelstein, F O: Treating peritonitis in patients with indwelling peritoneal catheters. *Dialysis and Transplantation* 3 (6), 1974.

Lewin A J, Gordon A, Greenbaum M A, et al.: Sorbent based regenerating delivery system for use in peritoneal dialysis. *Proc Dialysis and Transplant Forum,* Nov 1973.

McDonald H P, Gerber H, Mishra D, et al.: Subcutaneous dacron and teflon cloth adjuncts for silastic arteriovenous shunts and peritoneal dialysis catheters. *Trans Soc Artif Int Organs* Vol XIV, 1965.

Oreopoulos D G: Maintenance peritoneal dialysis, in *Stragegy in Renal Failure,* Eli Friedman (ed.), New York, John Wiley & Sons, Inc, 1978.

Rodriguez H J, Walls J, Slatopolsky E, et al.: Recurrent ascites following peritoneal dialysis. *Ann Int Med* 134 (8), 1974.

Rae A: Peritoneal dialysis access. *Dialysis and Transplantation* 6 (2), 1977.

Sherrard D J, Curtis F K, Lindner A, et al.: Peritoneal dialysis: a feasible alternative. *Proc Cl Dialysis and Transplant Forum,* Nov 1973.

Swamy A P, Cestero R V M, Campbell R G, et al.: Dialysate glucose and hyperlipidemia. *Dialysis and Transplantation* 6 (1), 1977.

Tenckhoff H: Peritoneal dialysis today: a new look. *Nephron* 12, 1974.

Tenckhoff H: Solutions and equipment. *Dialysis and Transplantation* 6 (2), 1977.

Tenckhoff H, Curtis F K: Experience with maintenance peritoneal dialysis in the home. *Trans Amer Soc Artif Int Organs,* Vol XVI, 1970.

Vidt D G, Somerville J, Schultz R W: A safe peritoneal access device for repeated peritoneal dialysis. *JAMA* 214 (13), 1970.

9

The Patient Receiving
a Renal Transplant

Judith Heffron Taylor, R.N., M.S.N.

Susan A. Hopper, R.N., M.S.N.

Penny Pierce, R.N., M.S.N.

*"To Remember Me . . ."**

The day will come when my body will lie upon a white sheet neatly tucked under four corners of a mattress located in a hospital busily occupied with the living and the dying. At a certain moment a doctor will determine that my brain has ceased to function and that, for all intents and purposes, my life has stopped.

When that happens, do not attempt to instill artificial life into my body by the use of a machine. And don't call this my deathbed. Let it be called the Bed of Life, and let my body be taken from it to help others lead fuller lives.

Give my sight to the man who has never seen a sunrise, a baby's face or love in the eyes of a woman. Give my heart to a person whose own heart has caused nothing but endless days of pain. Give my blood to the teen-ager who was pulled from the wreckage of his car, so that he might live to see his grandchildren play. Give my kidneys to one who depends on a machine to exist from week to week. Take my bones, every muscle, every fiber and nerve in my body and find a way to make a crippled child walk.

Explore every corner of my brain. Take my cells, if necessary, and let them grow so that, someday, a speechless boy will shout at the crack of a bat and a deaf girl will hear the sound of rain against her window.

Burn what is left of me and scatter the ashes to the winds to help the flowers grow.

*Reprinted with permission from the November 1976 *Reader's Digest*. Copyright © 1976 by The Reader's Digest Association, Inc.

If you must bury something, let it be my faults, my weaknesses and all prejudice against my fellow man.

Give my sins to the devil. Give my soul to God.

If, by chance, you wish to remember me, do it with a kind deed or word to someone who needs you. If you do all I have asked, I will live forever.

—Robert N. Test in Cincinnati *Post*

Renal transplantation and maintenance dialysis share the responsibility for sustaining the life of a person with end stage renal disease (ESRD). Transplantation is no longer an experimental procedure but an accepted and established mode of therapy for renal failure. It is the health team's desire to offer the person with ESRD the chance to choose a life that offers the quantity and quality best suited for him—whether it be hemodialysis, peritoneal dialysis, transplantation, or a combination.

The major obstacle to transplantation is the body's ability to recognize and reject foreign tissue, rendering the kidney nonfunctional. This immunological mechanism that destroys transplanted tissue is a major hazard to the success of kidney transplantation. The fundamental principle that has made clinical renal homotransplantation a practical possibility is that most rejection episodes can be successfully reversed with little loss of organ function.

Transplantation is not a gift of life; the person on dialysis is alive. Nor is it a reward or a saviour from dialysis, as some people view it. Transplantation is merely a trade of one form of therapy for renal failure for another—one of no guarantee and much uncertainty. ESRD has no "cure," only different and complicated modes of treatment.

The purposes of this chapter are:

1. To discuss the history of renal transplantation.
2. To discuss the principles of immunolgy as related to renal transplantation.
3. To describe methods of organ procurement and preservation.
4. To outline the criteria for organ donor and recipient selection.
5. To describe the surgical aspects of transplantation.
6. To discuss complications of renal transplantation.
7. To discuss the immediate and long-term medical and nursing management of the renal transplant patient.

HISTORY OF TRANSPLANTATION

Transplantation of organs and tissues for various reasons has been performed for over 5000 years. Records from Hindus and Egyptians reveal that skin transplants were performed to replace noses destroyed by syphilis. Celsus and Galen wrote of successful transplanting of tissue from one part of the body to another. Such transplant efforts continued to be described throughout history.

In modern medical history, John Hunter, founder of scientific surgery, performed both experimental and clinical transplantation in the 1700s. From that time on, transplantation efforts continued, with skin grafting performed in the late 1800s. Techniques for transplantation of organs and vessels were developed at the beginning of the twentieth century. The pioneer physician in this area is commonly thought to be Alexis Carrel. His associate, Dr. Charles Guthrie, however, did much of the work, transplanting the head of a dog in 1908 and publishing a report on transplantation of numerous organs (heart, lungs, kidneys, thyroid, ovaries) in 1912. Carrel, who received much publicity regarding these transplant efforts, received a Nobel prize for this experimental work. Also of interest in Carrel's work was his development of an extracorporeal pump for human organs in conjunction with Charles Lindbergh; this work is described in medical literature, as well as in Lindbergh's biography. Undoubtedly, this machine served as the model for present-day cardiac bypass and organ preservation equipment (1).

During World War II, another aspect of transplantation—rejection—was studied via the use of skin grafts. Such grafting was attempted from healthy persons to those who received extensive injuries and burns as a result of the fighting. Several investigators studied the problems associated with skin grafting. Peter Medawar of the Glasgow Royal Infirmary became the best known for his studies on rejection of transplanted skin. His work on rapidly rejected second grafts indicated that an actively acquired immune reaction was involved, a hypothesis supported in later years in research with mice. In the 1950s Professor T. M. Burnett in Australia also described the formation of antibodies as a response to foreign protein matter. The combined work of Medawar and Burnett formed the beginning of the modern science of immunology. For their investigation they were jointly awarded the Nobel Prize in 1960 (1). Jean Dausset, a French immunologist, proposed that leukocyte or platelet antigens, which he had identified using antibody sera from multiparous women and patients who had received blood transfusions, were histocompatibility antigens (2). Many researchers began work on the identification of these antigens, and that work continues today, with more antigens being identified yearly. Concomitant with this research, clinical experimentation with renal transplantation continued. Both France and America have been claimed to be the country in which the first renal transplant was performed (1,2). There is evidence, however, that indicates the performance of a renal transplant in 1947 when a kidney was attached to vessels in the arm of a uremic male; although the kidney was rejected quickly, the man did recover from acute renal failure, tided over by the kidney transplant. Investigation of clinical renal transplantation may well have declined with the development of the artificial kidney machine, which provided critically ill patients with hope of successful replacement of renal function.

The first clinically successful renal transplant reported in the American medical literature was performed at Peter Bent Brigham Hospital in December 1954 between identical twins. This transplant, performed by Dr. Joseph Murray and Dr. J. Hartwell Harrison, was based on much investigative work by Dr. David Hume (1). Both Dr. Murray and Dr. Hume had performed multiple human renal transplants before that time, but no attention had been paid to the immunologic factors that were just beginning to be identified. In France, Dr. Jean Hamburger selected donor-recipient pairs on the basis of leukocyte typing, as done by Jean Dausset. Based on the work of these physicians (Hamburger, Hume, Murray), the era of modern transplantation had begun. Since that time (the late 1950s), renal transplantation has become a clinically accepted form of treatment for end stage renal disease. The search for better techniques has been a difficult one; however, 30,000 persons have received this form of treatment for their renal failure. Obviously, work is continuing in the various areas that have made renal transplantation possible. By no means have all the questions been answered that would make renal transplantation the perfect solution for end stage renal disease.

TRANSPLANTATION IMMUNOLOGY

The immunologic factors involved in organ transplantation continue to be the greatest barrier to total success in this treatment modality.

A basic review of genetics is helpful in understanding transplant immunology. Every human ovum and spermatozon has 23 chromosomes; when they are joined at the time of fertilization, 46 chromosomes are present; these are the new person's total chromosomal inheritance. Genes are part of the chromosome structure and are the functional sites of heredity. Genes carry the genetic code for protein and enzyme synthesis. Because the nucleus of a single human cell carries an estimated 30,000 gene pairs, the number of combinations is almost endless. But since these chromosomes and genes are inherited, similarity within a family is quite possible.

This compatibility of tissue based on inheritance is easily exemplified by the process of blood typing. The ABO typing that is classically performed to ensure compatibility of blood transfusions identifies antigens on red blood cells. In the same fashion, compatibility of other tissue can be identified. All types of studies that measure tissue compatibility between donor and recipient are known as *histocompatibility* tests.

Dausset, in studying the sera of individuals who received organ transplants, identified antibodies directed against antigens of the donor. He suggested that the antibodies were formed in response to histocompatibility antigens. These antigens, once called human leukocyte antigens, have become the principal histocompatibility system identified. A single complex genetic region of the 6th chromosome (which in man has been designated HLA) controls these histocompatibility antigens. On the HLA region four have been identified, with individual antigens being coded by genes on these loci. The histocompatibility antigens are present on the cell surface of almost all the cells of the body. Since Dausset's identification of the first antigen in 1958, researchers around the world have continued to identify others. At the 1977 world workshop of tissue typing, the chart of Nomenclature for Factors of the HLA System—1977 (Figure 9.1) was developed to update the list of identified antigens.

Based on the genetic inheritance previously described, every individual inherits one HLA region (a haplotype consisting of an A, B, C, D gene coding for respective antigens) from each parent. Diagrammatically, this inheritance is illustrated in Figure 9.2 (each letter represents a haplotype). This discussion will deal only with the two serologically important genes, the A and B. The D locus is defined by lymphocyte reactivity in the mixed lymphocyte reaction. (See below.) Thus every offspring shares two of four A and B antigens with each parent (except in rare cases when parents share antigens and thus are of the same haplotype). Among offspring, therefore, each has a one-in-four possibility of being the same HLA type. (See Figure 9.2.) The HLA identical match offers the best chance for transplant success based on the identity of tissue and cellular composition.*

HLA typing is done by a method of lymphocytotoxicity testing. The HLA antigen is identified by exposing lymphocytes to antisera with known antibodies. If the lymphocytes carry a cell surface antigen recognized by these antibodies in the serum, the lymphocytes are lysed. It is

---

Note: The identical twin receiving a transplant from the other twin is an immunologically perfect match, since both share exactly the same chromosomes and genes. Such transplants may be referred to as isografts, indicating that the donor and recipient are genetically identical. All other transplants are called homografts and allografts, indicating that the donor and recipient are of the same species. Xenografting, the use of organs from other species, such as baboons and chimpanzees, has been attempted but has proved unsuccessful. Thus, no discussion of xenografts is included here.

NOMENCLATURE FOR FACTORS OF THE HLA SYSTEM—1977

Designations are assigned by W.H.O. Committee on leukocyte nomenclature. New   designations are italicized. The broad specificities are shown in parentheses following particular splits (such listing is optional).

Locus A	Previous	Locus B	Previous	Locus C	Previous
A1		B5		CW1	
A2		B7		CW2	
A3		B8		CW3	
A9		B12		CW4	
A10		B13		CW5	
A11		B14		*CW6*	*T7*
A25(10)	AW25	*B15*	BW15		
A26(10)	AW26	*B17*	BW17	**Locus D**	*Previous*
A28		B18			
A29		B27		DW1	
AW19		*B37*	BW37	DW2	
AW23(9)		*B40*	BW40	DW3	
AW24(9)		BW16		DW4	
AW30		BW21		DW5	
AW31		BW22		DW6	
AW32		BW35		*DW7*	LD107
AW33		BW38(16)		*DW8*	LD108
AW34		BW39(16)		*DW9*	TB9, OH
AW36		BW41		*DW10*	LD16
AW43		BW42		*DW11*	LD17
		BW44(12)	B12(not TT)		Previous
Locus B	**Previous**	*BW45*(12)	TT*	**Locus DR**	(workshop)
		BW46	HS, SIN2	*DRW1*	WIA1, Te6
BW4	W4, 4a	*BW47*	407*, MO66,	*DRW2*	WIA2, Te4
BW6	W6, 4b		CAS, BW40C	*DRW3*	WIA3, Te5
		BW48	KSO,JA,BW40.3	*DRW4*	WIA4, Te1.1
		BW49(21)	BW21.1, SL-ET	*DRW5*	WIA5, Te5.2
		BW50(21)	BW21.2, ET*	*DRW6*	WIA6, Te10
		BW51(5)	B5.1	*DRW7*	WIA7, Te3
		BW52(5)	B5.2		
		BW53	HR		
		BW54(22)	BW22j,SAP1,		
			SN1,J1		

Figure 9.1. Nomenclature for factors of the HLA system, 1977.

then possible to identify the specific antigen against which the specific antibody is reacting. In typing for renal transplantation, lymphocytes of both the potential donors and recipients are exposed to the antisera. Thus, all individuals are typed at one time against a standard antisera. This antisera is internationally standardized, allowing for testing for the above listed HLA antigens. Sharing systems are available and are utilized

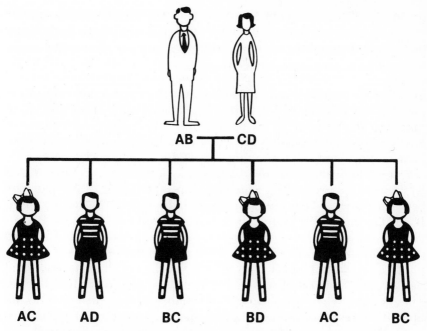

Figure 9.2. Diagram of inheritance of HLA antigens in family group.

for serum with rare antibodies. Antisera is obtained from persons who have had multiple blood transfusions or multiple pregnancies and who, therefore, have formed antibodies against HLA antigens.

Once an individual has been HLA typed, this study need not be repeated, since one's genetic identity does not change. However, it may be repeated before transplantation if the testing has not been recently performed, since new antigens are being identified yearly. Following an updated study, the genetic identity of the donor and recipient can be compared to allow the selection of the most compatible pair for transplantation purposes.

Studies other than this histocompatibility testing have also contributed to successful graft survival. These studies include white cell crossmatching, which resembles the white cell crossmatching performed to ensure compatible blood transfusions. Donor lymphocytes are mixed with recipient serum in the presence of complement to test for cell agglutination or lysis, which would indicate the presence of preformed circulating antibodies in the recipient. The antibodies identified in this way have been formed following blood transfusions, pregnancies, previous transplants, or infections (3). If the recipient has antibodies against the donor lymphocytes (a positive crossmatch), the graft would be rejected immediately if a transplant were performed (3). Thus, a negative crossmatch is essential between donor and recipient before transplantation. Because presence of these antibodies varies in the serum, specimens may be drawn on a regular basis to screen for the possible development of new antibodies. Some of these antibodies may be present in detectable amounts only for short periods; thus, regular screening increases the possibility of detecting low titers of antibodies. Such specimens can also be retained for use at a later time in a crossmatch study. Furthermore, when persons are awaiting cadaveric transplants, a specimen is always available for testing against donor lymphocytes.

A third study that has gained importance in recent years is the mixed lymphocyte culture (MLC), which measures the degree of compatibility between the HLA-D loci in both donor and recipient (5). Unlike the A, B, and C antigens, the D antigen cannot be identified by antisera. D locus disparity is measured by lymphocyte reactivity in the MLC, in which cell-surface differences are tested by the proliferative response of lymphocytes in vitro. The MLC requires a five-day incubation period and measures the amount of stimulation that these two sets of lymphocytes will undergo. When lymphocytes are stimulated, they enlarge and multiply. This response is measured by the incorporation of radioactive thymidine (which is added to the culture) into the responding cells.

Because this study entails a five-day culture period, it can be employed only in the testing of living related donors and not with cadaver transplantation (except in a retrospective study), where donor kidneys can be preserved no longer than three days.

The work being done in this area of immunology is continuous, with new testing techniques being developed and new antigens being identified. The ultimate secrets of immunology, those that would allow selection of perfect donor-recipient pairs, have not yet been discovered. Work is also being conducted to shorten the time required for a reliable MLC study so that it can be employed prospectively in cadaveric transplantation.

TRANSPLANT REJECTION

All studies to match a donor and recipient have a single purpose—to prevent a reaction that would result in the destruction of the transplanted organ. This reaction is known as "rejection," and its prevention remains a major problem in renal transplantation.

Rejection may take several forms, depending upon the immunological process that has been activated. The human immune response to a foreign antigen is a complex one. Two types of lymphocytes are involved. B-lymphocytes (so called because they arise from the Bursa of Fabricus in the chicken and a yet unknown source in humans) form antibodies (humoral immunity), and T-lymphocytes (so called because they are thymus dependent) produce cell-mediated immunity (7). Figure 9.3 illustrates the formation of these cells from bone-marrow stem cells. In the human body, either or both of these cells cause death of viable tissue, such as death of a transplanted kidney. All types of rejection (hyperacute, accelerated, acute, and chronic) are caused by interaction of these two types of cells.

Humoral immunity is dependent on B-lymphocytes, which form antibodies when they recognize antigens; production of antibodies occurs within 48 to 72 hours of contact. Subsequent contact stimulates a secondary response within 24 to 48 hours. Active and passive immunity (as occurs following the immunization process) are two types of humoral immunity. The humoral immune response also may trigger activation of the complement and Kallikrein systems, leading to activation of the coagulation cascade and deposition of platelets and fibrin at the site of reaction (8). Hyperacute and accelerated rejection involve humoral immune responses. In such situations a reaction occurs between antigens found in the transplanted organ and circulating antibodies in the recipient's serum. Within a few hours, destruction of tissue results from the antigen-antibody reaction and the stimulation of the complement and coagulation effector systems. The end result is diffuse deposition of antibody, complement, and fibrin, resulting in the thrombosis and necrosis of the kidney (3,8,9).

Accelerated rejection shows a similar pattern, although occurring more slowly, probably due to the formation of antibodies as a secondary response following contact with an antigen to which the recipient is already sensitized.

Neither of these rejection mechanisms can be suppressed or reversed by medication or other types of treatment. Antibody production continues as long as the foreign body is present. Prevention of such rejection phenomena can be accomplished to a large extent by performing crossmatch studies before transplantation. In such situations, a positive crossmatch predicts this antigen-antibody reaction. Some accelerated rejections will occur following a negative crossmatch in which the quantity of antibody is too low to be detected by the test.

In the acute rejection process, the T-lymphocytes are responsible for a cellular immune response. In this response of delayed hypersensitivity, the T-lymphocyte is sensitized by contact with a specific antigen. After several contacts with the antigen, the T-lymphocyte releases various

MATURATION PATHWAYS OF PRINCIPAL CELLS
IN THE IMMUNE RESPONSE

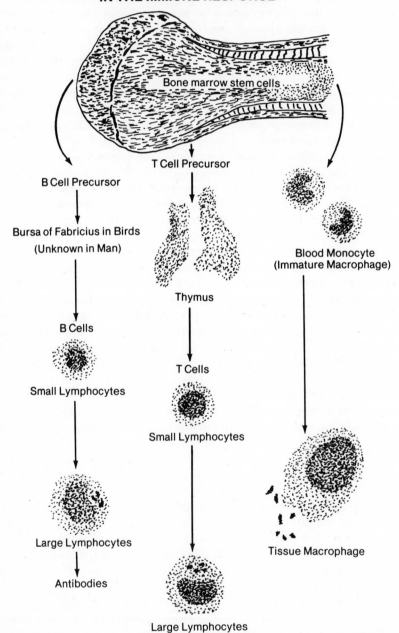

Figure 9.3. Formation of B and T lymphocytes in the immune response.

chemical factors, which cause death of cells carrying these antigens. The released chemical factors, known as lymphokines, include chemotactic factor, migratory inhibition factor, blastogenic factor, and transfer factor (7). The sensitized lymphocytes convert other T-lymphocytes to "killer" cells, which can destroy other cells on direct contact. The lymphockines amplify this reaction by recruiting more "killer" cells and by modifying other cell-mediated reactions (7). This reaction occurs in the acutely rejected kidney and may lead to necrosis of the graft (3). (See Figure 9.4.) In this type of immune reaction, several therapies can be employed to slow or halt the cell-mediated rejection response. Drug therapy has been most effective in disrupting this reaction and is discussed later in this chapter (10).

The fourth type of rejection, chronic rejection, is most likely a combination of humoral and cell-mediated responses. B-lymphocyte antibody production is enhanced by interaction with T-lymphocytes. In chronic rejection, changes occur both in cellular and endothelial capillary tissue within the kidney. Such damage is irreversible and leads to failure of the graft, primarily by ischemia. This process does not respond to any therapeutic maneuver.

The revelation of the secrets of the body's immunological character through continued research has made human renal transplantation a successful reality. Yet many aspects of this system are still undiscovered; their identification may eliminate the processes of rejection that presently prevent organ transplantation from being totally successful.

While we wait for these answers to be found, other exciting aspects of the immune system are also being investigated—its role in the transplantation of other organs and tissues, its role in neoplastic disease, and the correlation that some factors of the immune system have in hereditary disease (8,11).

The hope for the future is that other diseases will be cured or eradicated because the mysteries of the human immune system will have been revealed. At that time, too, this last barrier to successful renal transplantation will be removed and transplantation will indeed be the perfect cure for end stage renal disease.

SOURCES OF DONOR KIDNEYS

For the treatment of ESRD, there are two sources of kidneys. Living related donors who are immediate family members can offer a kidney for transplantations. Sibling to sibling, parent to child, or child to parent offer the best success for transplantation. Today about 30% of trans-

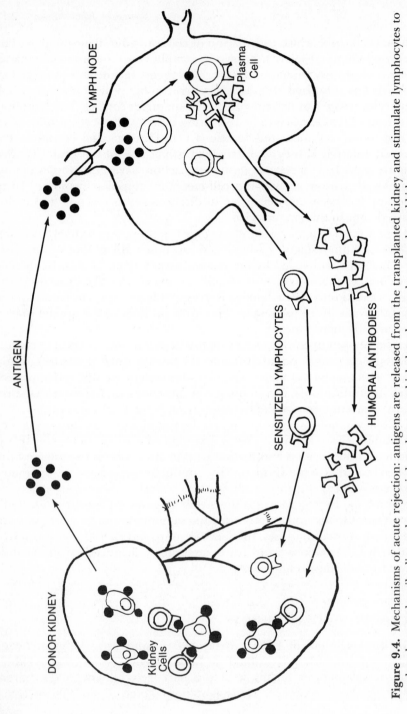

Figure 9.4. Mechanisms of acute rejection: antigens are released from the transplanted kidney and stimulate lymphocytes to produce humoral antibodies and cytotoxic lymphocytes, which then destroy the transplanted kidney.

LYMPH NODE

Plasma Cell

ANTIGEN

SENSITIZED LYMPHOCYTES

HUMORAL ANTIBODIES

DONOR KIDNEY

Kidney Cells

plants are performed between living relatives. The majority of kidney transplants performed are from cadaveric donors. Kidneys may be matched according to size, but race, age, and the like are not determinants to the transplantability of the kidney.

Living nonrelated kidney donors have been used in the past, but because of the ethics of this type of donation, they are strongly discouraged. Volunteers from the community, prison inmates, or persons who would sell their kidneys have been severely criticized for their motives. More important is the fact that grafts of this type of kidney have not been more successful than those of cadaveric kidneys.

ORGAN PROCUREMENT AND PRESERVATION

For a living related donation, preservation is not a problem, since the surgery for the donor and recipient occurs simultaneously and in close proximity. Preservation presents a problem for the cadaveric donor, however, owing to the time necessary for removal of the organs, obtaining the suitable recipient, transportation to the transplant center, preparation of the recipient, and initiation of surgery. Irreversible cellular damage occurs after approximately 60 to 70 minutes of warm ischemia time (WIT) and 36 hours of cold ischemia time (CIT). The use of hypothermia and perfusion can sustain the retrieved kidney without the occurrence of irreversible damage.

Once effective circulation to an organ ceases, it undergoes certain catabolic changes and degeneration of its cellular ultrastructure. These changes usually are reversible at first, but after a period of time irreversible changes occur. As the oxygen supply to the kidney is interrupted, the cells and blood in the renal vascular system begin to undergo ischemic changes. Hypoxia causes metabolic acidosis. Insufficient oxygen causes a shift from aerobic metabolism to anaerobic glycolysis and the production of lactic acid with a buildup of hydrogen ions in the intracellular fluid. Anaerobic metabolism (no ATP is formed by the mitochondria) causes an increase in the cellular permeability; lytic enzymes are released by lysosomes, and the catabolic waste products destroy surrounding tissue (12).

Tubular epithelial cells (most sensitive to a decrease in Po_2) die and slough, blocking the tubules. In the vascular system, red blood cells agglutinate, causing minute renal vessel thromboses and necrosis. Total loss of the nephron is a result of absence of blood flow through the renal vessels, causing ischemic changes as well as blockage of the tiny tubules. The determinant of the reversibility of the anoxic changes that occur in the kidney is the duration of oxygen deprivation and production of metabolic waste toxins. This time is referred to as the warm ischemia time (WIT).

If the metabolic rate can be reduced, the rate of cellular ischemic changes can be slowed. Hypothermia decreases the basal metabolic rate (BMR), thus decreasing the oxygen need of the cell and production of waste products. Cold ischemia time (CIT) is the length of time the kidney is hypothermic. The fundamental objective of preservation is to keep the organ viable outside its natural environment. To minimize catabolic tissue damage, the following may be employed in organ preservation:

1. Minimize warm ischemia time.
2. Decrease metabolic needs of the cell by bypothermia and direct inhibitors.
3. Maintain optimal temperature.
4. Supply needed nutrients and oxygen.
5. Remove waste products.

The optimal goal of organ preservation would be the establishment of long-term organ banks. Currently it is impossible to keep a kidney viable for longer than about two days.

Static Storage Hypothermia

The kidney is flushed in situ through the aorta or, after retrieval, through the renal artery with a cold synthetic intracellular-like solution until cool to the touch and uniformly blanched. This rinses the blood from the renal vessels to prevent clot formation and subsequent damage to the cells. Metabolic inhibitors can be mixed with the electrolyte and colloid solution to supplement the hypothermic effect on the metabolic rate. The kidney is then submerged in this sterile washout solution and packed in ice. It can remain viable in this type of cold storage for approximately 12 to 24 hours.

Pulsatile Perfusion Hypothermia

After an initial perfusion with a cool solution, the retrieved kidney is placed in a pulsatile perfusion machine. Dr. Folkert O. Belzer first used a pulsating machine in 1967. The objectives of pulsatile perfusion are:

1. Hypothermia can be maintained as the organ is perfused with a plasma protein fraction and albumin solution.

2. Oxygen and nutrients can be supplied to the organ.

3. Waste products can be removed.

4. The pulsating, rather than continual, perfusion can reduce vasoconstriction, endothelial swelling, microemboli formation, and platelet adherence, all of which would cause damage to the organ cells.

The kidney can remain viable, sustaining no permanent damage, for 48 to 72 hours on this perfusion machine.

As yet, freezing has proved unsuccessful in the preservation of organs, owing to water crystal damage to the cell membrane.

Preservation cannot reverse previous cellular ischemic lesions. The total preservation time (WIT plus CIT) must be taken into account to avoid the tragic possibility of transplanting a nonviable organ.

The Cadaveric Donor

Careful evaluation of the cadaveric donor is essential to the morbidity and mortality of the kidney recipient as well as to the success of the transplanted kidney.

Donor selection criteria are generalized as follows:

1. Age: 5 to 65 years.

2. No systemic infections.

3. No cancer (except primary central nervous system carinoma, which is unable to metastasize across the blood-brain barrier).

4. No history of renal disease or high blood pressure.

5. No systemic diseases or lupus erythematosus.

6. Adequate renal function as determined by blood levels of creatinine and urea nitrogen, urine volume, urinalysis, and urine cultures.

Once the donor has been determined legally dead (two flat EEGs, 24 hours apart, confirming irreversible brain damage) by the primary physician and the consent form has been signed by the nearest relative, all activity should be centered around preserving the viability of the kidney. (See Figure 9.5.) Circulation and ventilation can be maintained by external cardiac massage and the use of an Ambu bag or a respirator. There should be no episodes of prolonged hypotension or anoxia before death.

Volume expanders, heparin, and vasodilators (propranolol and others) can be used to prevent vasoconstriction, blood stasis, emboli formation, and platelet adherence. Sodium bicarbonate may be used to prevent acidosis. The glomerular filtration rate and urinary output can

---

UNIFORM DONOR CARD

OF _____
                              name of donor

In the hope that I may help others, I hereby make this anatomical gift, if medically acceptable, to take effect upon my
death. The words and marks below indicate my desires.

I give: (a) ☐ any needed organs or parts
          (b) ☐ only the following organs or parts

_____
              Specify the organ(s) or part(s)

for the purposes of transplantation, therapy, medical research
or education:
          (c) ☐ my body for anatomical study if needed.

Limitations or
special wishes, if any: _____

Signed by the donor and the following two witnesses in the
presence of each other:

_____   _____
    Signature of Donor   City and State

_____   _____
      Date Signed   Date of Birth of Donor

_____   _____
        Witness   Witness
THIS IS A LEGAL DOCUMENT UNDER THE UNIFORM
ANATOMICAL GIFT ACT OR SIMILAR LAWS
For further information consult your physician or
AMERICAN KIDNEY FUND
P.O. Box 3586, Washington, D. C. 20007

Figure 9.5. Example of a donor card used to express one's desire to donate the kidneys on declaration of death.

be maintained by adequate fluid balance and the use of diuretics (furosemide and mannitol).

The transplant team takes the responsibility for removal of the organs (the primary physician is never involved.) The nephrectomy can take place in the person's room or in the operating room. The kidney with artery, vein, and ureter is removed in one section. The kidneys are transported using either static storage or pulsatile hypothermia to the waiting recipient.

A computerized system for storing waiting transplant recipient tissue types aids in the sharing of retrieved cadaver organs throughout the entire United States and the world. Thus, it is feasible for available kidneys to be delivered to the most suited or most needy recipient either locally, nationally, or internationally.

The increased number of available cadaver kidneys has resulted from the public's increased awareness of the desperate need for kidneys, as well as from the education of the medical community.

Evaluation of the Living Related Donor

The use of a biologically related kidney for transplant increases the success of the graft (90 to 98%) as well as decreasing the time the patient may require dialysis posttransplantation. Once the willingness to donate an organ is expressed, the donor must undergo an extensive evaluation so as not to jeopardize his health by this voluntary loss of a kidney. In addition, psychological and sociological suitability are scrutinized. This entire evaluation usually requires a two-day hsopitalization.

The donor must be an adult between the ages of 18 to 50 years and in good general health. A complete history and physical, chest x-ray, and electrocardiogram are done to rule out clinical problems that would make donation impossible. Blood tests for chemistries, hematology, and coagulation must be within normal limits. Urinalysis should be normal, and creatinine clearance must be greater than 100 cc per minute. Urine cultures must be negative. If the cultures are positive, the donor is treated with the appropriate antibiotic therapy until serial cultures are negative. Nursing technique and patient teaching in obtaining careful and complete samples are stressed.

Radiological Studies

Intravenous Pyelogram (Urogram, IVP). The injection of dye into a vein in the forearm outlines the kidney collecting system (calyx, pelvis, ureteropelvic junction, ureter, and bladder).

Arteriogram (Aortography). The injection of dye into the femoral artery reveals the blood supply to the kidney, renal branches, and their arrangement. Nursing responsibilities include observation of the puncture site for bleeding or hematoma formation, and assessment of circulation of the ipsilateral leg by checking skin color, temperature, and pedal pulses.

Choice of Kidney

Several considerations determine the choice of the potential donor's kidney for transplantation. Ureteral junction abnormalities or duplication of renal artery and vein will not prevent the use of the kidney. It makes the operation considerably longer because of the greater possibility of technical complications. If both kidneys have adequate function, the single-artery kidney is preferred. The left kidney is usually taken because of the longer length of the renal vein on that side. The right kidney is taken in childbearing women, owing to the greater risk of urological problems (hydronephrosis and pyelonephritis) to that kidney caused by the pressure of the pregnant uterus. If one kidney presents with a slight abnormality or if equal function is not found in both kidneys, primary interest is with the donor, and the poorer kidney will be taken for the recipient. If at any time during the evaluation the donor desires to withdraw, then his decision remains confidential. The recipient will be told that the donor is not suitable to give a kidney, and the recipient's name can be put on the cadaveric kidney waiting list.

The health team evaluates the workup and informs the donor of the results. The decision to donate is then confirmed and a date for surgery is arranged. A teaching manual is given to the donor at this time to explain the donor nephrectomy, hospitalization procedures, and what can be expected of life with one kidney.

TRANSPLANT RECIPIENT SELECTION

The desire or need for a renal transplant is individually assessed on the basis of physical, social, and psychological studies. There are few conditions in which transplantation is absolutely contraindicated, though certain physical and psychological problems increase the risks of surgery and immunosuppressive therapy. Many conditions can be treated or surgically corrected before transplantation, eliminating many of the operative risks. Thus, contraindications to transplant are few and usually relative to the patient's overall clinical status.

As the patient approaches the time when conservative management is not adequate to sustain life, hemodialysis and transplantation may be offered. The entire health care team, patient, and family discuss the desire for and risks involved in transplantation versus hemodialysis. The standard requirement for the transplant candidacy is that the patient have irreversible end stage renal disease (ESRD) and life cannot be maintained without further therapy.

Assessment of the Transplant Candidate
Primary Disease
Polycystic kidney disease, pyelonephritis, and urinary tract infections are indications for a bilateral nephrectomy to prevent bleeding and the spread of infection to the newly transplanted kidney. Malignant hypertension, unrelated to fluid overload, may also be controlled with a bilateral nephrectomy.

Selective bilateral nephrectomy, once routine, has been reevaluated as to its beneficial role pretransplant. The mortality and morbidity of this surgical procedure are relatively high. Also, the problems for the patient on dialysis of anemia (hematocrits less than 16–18%) and susceptibility to fluid overload are exacerbated following a bilateral nephrectomy.

With focal sclerosing, membranoproliferative, and rapidly progressing glomerulonephritis, the patient's kidneys are removed in an attempt to prevent recurrence of the primary disease. Patients with Goodpasture's syndrome have a bilateral nephrectomy to reduce the circulating antiglomerular basement membrane antibodies, which would attack the new graft.

Patients with lupus erythematosus, sickle cell disease, scleroderma, cystinosis, and amyloidosis have had good results with transplantation. Oxalosis is still a contraindication for transplantation, owing to graft loss from oxalate deposits.

Chronic glomerulonephritis and Alport's nephritis do not require a preliminary bilateral nephrectomy.

Urinary System
Lower tract abnormalities, outflow and bladder problems, frequently require surgical correction. Transplantation is contraindicated if these abnormalities cannot be corrected. If urinary bladder abnormalities prevent it from being used, an ileal loop can be constructed and the ureter successfully anastomosed to it. Voiding cystourethrogram, intravenous pyelogram, and cystoscopy are performed to assess the lower urinary tract. Transurethral resection or dilatation may be required (especially with older men) for prostatic hypertrophy or sphincter stenosis.

Pulmonary System
There is a high incidence of lung infection as a result of immunosuppressive medication. All patients should abstain from smoking before and after transplantation. Pneumonia, common following surgery, can be prevented by good nursing support, pulmonary toilet, respiratory therapy, and antibiotic therapy. Pneumocystis, "transplant lung,"

cytomegalic virus, and nocardia infections are common in transplant patients and are difficult to treat. Tuberculosis is not a contraindication and is treated indefinitely with antitubercular therapy. Most patients receive Isoniazid, a tuberculocidal agent, prophylactically. Patients with chronic obstructive pulmonary disease or other pulmonary compromise are evaluated individually because of the high risk of mortality from these conditions.

Gastrointestinal System

Peptic ulcer and intestinal diverticuli must be surgically corrected before transplant because of the increased risk of gastrointestinal bleeding or perforation with the use of high-dose steriods. Upper gastrointestional examinations and a barium enema may be ordered. Pancreatitis and pancreatic stones may require pretreatment. Chronic hepatitis and hepatic cirrhosis are a relative contraindication and are carefully evaluated, since Imuran (azathioprine), used to prevent rejection, is potentially hepatotoxic. Bilirubin, LDH, SGOT, and alkaline phosphatase should be in normal range before transplantation. A patient who is chronically HAA (Australian antigen) positive may still be evaluated for a transplant. Active hepatitis is an absolute contraindication.

Cardiovascular System

Patients with a history of myocardial infarction become a high risk and are counseled to the surgical risks. ESRD causes hyperlipidemia, which is further aggravated by the catabolic effect of steroids. Atherosclerosis may cause technical problems with anastomosis of the vessels and stenosis after surgery. Hypertension may become a problem postoperatively because of sodium and water retention due to the steroids.

Systemic and Metabolic

Contraindication to transplantation for a patient with diabetes mellitus is determined by his overall clinical condition. Steroids cause labile glucosemia, and the regulation of insulin becomes a difficult challenge. Vascular anastomosis can also be difficult in the diabetic patient. Hyperuricemia (gout) is difficult to treat because of the aggravating effect of allopurinal on azathioprine, causing a supertoxic effect on bone marrow and a sudden dangerous decrease in WBC (less than 1000 per cubic millimeter). Hyperparathyroidism can be surgically treated by removal of the parathyroid glands, thus preventing calcium from depositing in the transplanted kidney and interfering with renal function. Active or incurable malignancies are an absolute contraindication. Patients with a history of tumor are counseled to the increased risks of recurrence and are required to wait one year after treatment before being considered for transplantation.

Central Nervous System

A history of seizures does not prevent a patient from receiving a kidney transplant. The uremic neuropathies seem to get better or disappear following transplant.

Other Considerations

Owing to the general aging process, persons older than 60 years are usually excluded from transplantation. Children under the age of one to two years or 5 to 10 kg in weight present a surgical challenge and post-operative problems. If the patient demonstrates the inability to adjust to the dialysis regimen or is deteriorating on dialysis, transplantation may be offered as a treatment of last resort. Also, transplantation may be the choice of treatment for dialysis dementia, though it has not proved very successful.

Psychological Evaluation

As yet there are no standard psychological criteria for evaluating the stability of a candidate for transplantation. Factors to be considered are:

1. Psychosis. Steroids cause mental changes and can aggravate psychosis and paranoia. Transplant must be offered to these patients with caution. A psychiatric consultation may be indicated.
2. Noncompliance. Transplantation can prove very dangerous to the patient who exhibits noncompliant behavior while on dialysis. The need to follow a strict medication regimen and to provide self-care (or any problem due to lack of family support) must be scrutinized before such a patient is offered a transplant.

Socioeconomic Evaluation

Available resources for the surgery, the hospitalization, and the long-term medical therapy consisting of expensive medications and diet, as well as questions of family support and the potential for vocational rehabilitation are examined before the decision for transplantation.

SURGICAL ASPECTS OF TRANSPLANTATION
Recipient Transplant Surgery

The kidney is usually placed retroperitoneally in the anterior iliac fossa. This placement has three advantages over returning the donor kidney to the patient's normal anatomical position:

1. Surgical anastomosis of the renal artery, vein, and ureter is made easier, owing to the length needed for the closer approximation of the graft to the vessels and bladder.
2. The potential complication of peritonitis is usually averted. Post-operative observation of the graft is much easier. It is almost impossible to detect swelling of the kidney in the flank position. Kidney biopsies are easier to perform on the anterior site.
4. Reoperation, if necessary, is much easier.

The kidney must be turned over in order to place the renal artery anterior and the renal vein posterior, so that the vein can then be anastomosed first. The iliac artery and vein or hypogastric artery and vein are used. (See Figure 9.6.) A submucosal tunnel is created for the ureter, which is then implanted into the bladder (neoureterocystostomy) or is connected to the stump of the recipient's own ureter (ureteroureteral anastomosis). The tunnel acts as a one-way valve to prevent reflux of urine (which could cause infection) into the newly transplanted kidney. The recipient's own diseased kidneys may be removed at the time of the transplant or during a previous, separate operation. Before ureteral implantation the spermatic cord may be ligated in the male to prevent the ureter from kinking around it. Fertility is not affected unless the other vas deferens is occluded. Male patients are counseled to this risk before surgery.

Transplant surgery usually takes four to five hours. The patient is returned to the recovery room until he becomes stable and then to a surgical intensive care unit or to his own room.

Living Related Donor Nephrectomy

The technique of removing a kidney from a living related donor is the same as for other nephrectomies with two exceptions:

1. Greater surgical care must be taken not to injure the kidney, the ureter, or the vessels, which must be removed intact with the greatest possible length in order to insure satisfactory vascular anastomosis into the donor. Inadvertent vessel occlusion or hypotensive episodes interfere with the blood supply to the kidney, causing ischemic damages.
2. The ureter is removed intact. Most nephrectomies do not explore retroperitoneally down to the ureterovesicular junction, but cut and tie the ureter close to the kidney.

Thus the donor nephrectomy is a long, delicate surgical procedure. A

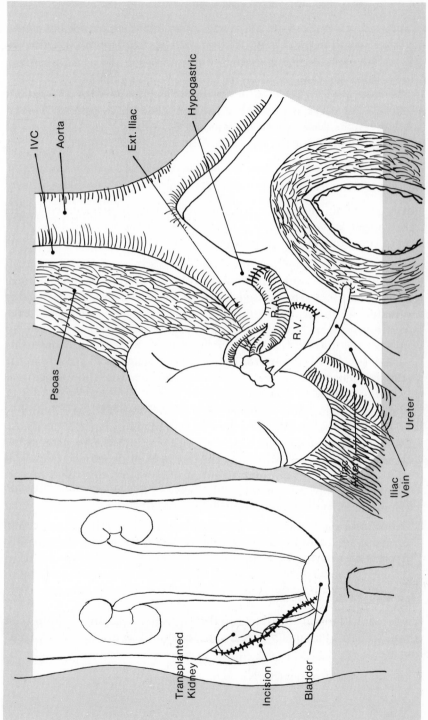

Figure 9.6. Surgical placement of renal transplant.

midline incision from xyphoid to pubis or a flank incision is used to allow for adequate exposure of the kidney. At the patient's request, other surgical procedures may accompany the donation, such as appendectomy or tubal ligation.

The postoperative care of the donor is the same as for any patient undergoing a surgical procedure for unilateral nephrectomy. Special care is given the donor, as he experiences not only physical pain, but also psychological pain due to grieving for the loss of a body part.

Patterns of Renal Function

Nursing care and medical management are largely determined by the transplanted kidney's ability to excrete waste products and fluid. The level of renal function after transplantation may be described as follows (13):

1. Immediate passage of urine and rapid restoration of normal renal performance. Early massive diuresis of approximately 100 cc or greater per hour has several effects: the urine has a decreased urea content; urinary specific gravity measurement is close to that of glomerular filtrate (1.015); and there is an inability to concentrate urine. Increased serum urea clearance is indicative of recovery as the tubular cells begin to reabsorb sodium and excrete the nitrogenous waste products.

2. Temporary anuria or oliguria lasting from five to 60 days followed by subsequent and usually slow gain in renal performance. This condition may be caused by the superimposition of rejection on acute tubular necrosis. Statistics show that the duration of prolonged oliguria is not used as an indicator of graft survival. Fluid and electrolyte restrictions are required to maintain the body's physiological equilibrium. Hemodialysis may be temporarily instituted.

3. No significant function. Irreversible changes occurring in the organ prevent adequate function. The patient is returned to his pretransplantation dialysis regimen.

Evaluation of Renal Function

Assessment of renal function for the transplant patient is done on a continual basis. Parameters the health team uses to evaluate renal function are:

1. Blood urea nitrogen (BUN).

2. Serum creatinine.
3. Urine creatinine clearance.
4. Total urinary output.
5. Fluid status: blood pressure, stable weight, and assessment for edema.
6. Renograms. Multiple renograms are ordered each week. Baseline studies are performed the first day posttransplant, and renograms are done approximately every other day until the patient is discharged. Renogram studies demonstrate:
    a. The kidney's uptake of dye (within the first five minutes).
    b. The excretion of dye into the bladder (within five to 12 minutes). (See Figures 9.7 and 9.8.)
    c. Displacement of kidney, ureter, or bladder, possibly because an external mass is applying pressure. Ultrasound studies would then be indicated.
7. Kidney biopsy. A percutaneous biopsy may be performed to document an acute or chronic rejection episode. Biopsies involve several risks and are *not* a routine procedure. Bleeding and perirenal hematoma formation are the most common complications (14). Emergency surgical correction and possibly a nephrectomy may be necessary. Observations should be made for hematuria, which is common following a biopsy. Nursing responsibilities include observation for bleeding (vital signs and wound dressings), maintaining bed rest, assessing pain at the biopsy site, and collecting urine specimens as ordered.

Postoperative Care

The nursing care of the postoperative kidney transplant patient is basically the same as for any surgical patient receiving general or spinal anesthesia. Baseline nursing assessment is essential to detect slight changes in the patient's physical condition. Nursing interventions based on these assessments prevent potential surgical complications and insure graft success.

General
With the defective wound healing and impaired defense mechanisms of the uremic patient treated with immunosuppressive drugs, the objective of nursing care postoperatively is primarily one of prevention.

This section discusses nurisng care specific to the renal transplant patient; it will not cover basic postoperative patient care.

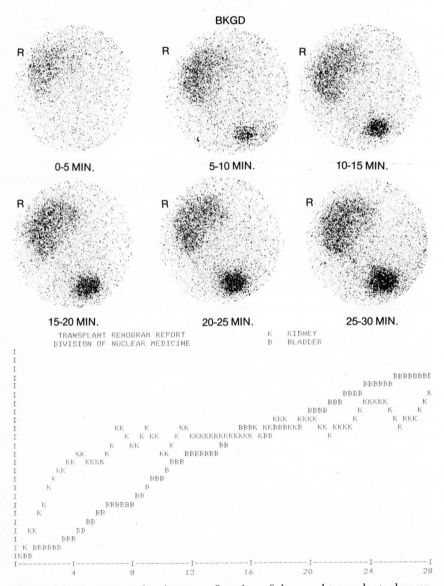

Figure 9.7. Renogram showing poor function of the renal transplant: slow uptake of dye and slow excretion into the bladder.

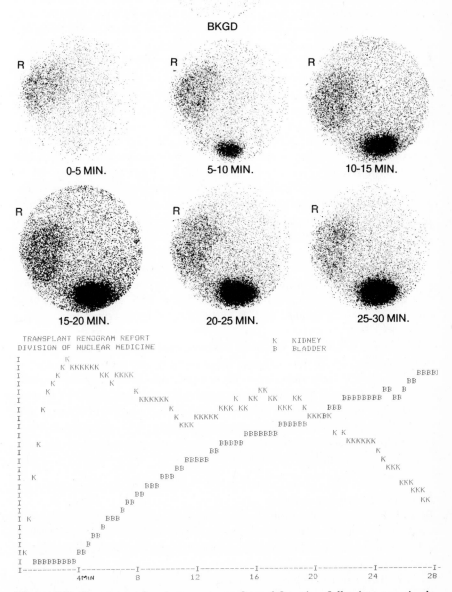

Figure 9.8. Renogram showing a return of renal function following an episode of rejection: rapid uptake of dye by the kidney and slower excretion into the bladder.

Renal System

To prevent complications, general urological management is essential for the kidney transplant patient. A Foley catheter is placed in the bladder to accurately measure urine output each hour and to allow for continual outflow of urine to keep the intravesical pressure at a low level and allow for better wound healing. The Foley catheter may be attached to a three-way overhead irrigation set (1000 ml normal saline with one ampule of genitourinary irrigant). Bladder irrigation is ordered to keep the urine pink-tinged, thus decreasing the incidence of blood clot formation. A blood clot or a kink in the tubing would cause urine to accumulate and increase the pressure within the bladder. This causes a stretching of the bladder and places a strain on the ureteral anastomosis, which could cause suture breakdown and a "blow-out" of the ureter. The catheter tubing must never be clamped for longer than 15 minutes (for obtaining urine culture and sensitivity). The Foley catheter is discontinued as soon as possible to eliminate a source of infection; males usually have the catheter for five to seven days and females for three to five days. While in place, strict catheter care is routinely performed three times daily. After removal of the catheter, the patient is encouraged to void often. This decreases the length of time the urine is static within the bladder and also prevents stretching of the bladder. Normally the patient has a small bladder because of the time of disuse following a bilateral nephrectomy or because of low urine volume. The bladder will gradually and safely increase in size within the weeks following transplantation. Spasms that occur to the surgically insulted bladder muscle are painful. These can be successfully treated with B and O suppositories or other bladder relaxants.

The urine is observed for both quantity and quality. It may be pink-tinged, and small blood clots may be present in the early postoperative period and with early ambulation but should soon disappear. Daily urine tests include specific gravity, urinalysis, culture and sensitivity (midstream voiding), sugar, and acetone. Creatinine clearances may also be ordered along with 12- or 24-hour specimens. Nursing responsibility for obtaining specimens correctly and for patient teaching of the correct method cannot be overly stressed.

Fluid and Electrolyte Balance

Fluid balance depends upon the true urine output (T.U.O.), which is the total output minus the amount of bladder irrigation. Accurate fluid calculation and replacement are essential to prevent radical changes in volume balance.

The graft can function in two patterns:

1. Osmotic diuresis due to ischemic tubular lesions that prevent sodium and water reabsorption, hyperosmolar plasma with an increase in BUN and creatinine, or fluid overload from blood transfused during surgery. The nurse observes for electrolyte imbalances of hypokalemia and hyponatremia and plans for early treatment to prevent complications. Hypotensive episodes from dehydration or bleeding can cause a decrease in the oxygen and blood supply to the transplanted kidney, furthering the ischemic changes within the organ.

2. Oliguria due to acute tubular necrosis, technical complications, or a rejection crisis. Fluid overload can cause hypertension, congestive heart failure, and pulmonary edema. Two parameters examined in assessing the fluid status are daily weights (same time each day, same scales) and blood pressure (systolic, diastolic, and end-diastolic readings). The volume of urine output is assessed in relation to the degree of function of the patient's own kidneys if they are intact. Osmotic agents (such as Mannitol) and diuretics (such as furosemide or hydrochlorothiazide) may be given to increase urine output by increasing the glomerular filtration rate and by inhibiting sodium reabsorption in the tubules and in the loop of Henle. The transplanted kidney has a reversed circadian rhythm such that the volume is usually higher at night rather than in the daytime. The urine output from 10 P.M. to 6 A.M. indicate the status of renal function and may determine treatment for the remainder of the day. This cycle will change to normal (higher output during the day) within approximately one to two months. Rarely the patient will complain of sleep interruption to void. Recording must be strict and complete to insure adequate medical management of the patient's fluid balance. Intravenous fluids are discontinued as soon as oral fluids are begun in order to prevent the I.V. site from becoming a source of infection.

Gastrointestional System

The I.V. is usually discontinued as the patient begins to take oral fluids. Careful assessment of bowel sounds to detect an ileus is done routinely. A nasogastric tube may be inserted and connected to low Gomco suction if necessary. Appropriate fluid and electrolyte replacement is initiated to replace gastric losses. pH determinations and antacid therapy may be ordered to prevent the gastric irritation of high dosages of steroids.

Constipation is relieved by stool softeners or enemas. With the graft placed in the left iliac fossa, ileus and constipation may be a problem because of the reflexion and exposure of the sigmoid colon during surgery.

The patient usually progresses from NPO, to clear liquid, to renal diet and eventually to a transplant diet.

Pulmonary

With the use of general anesthesia and immunosuppressive drugs, the chance of pulmonary infections is increased. Turning, coughing, deep breathing, the use of blow bottles or Triflows, and early ambulation seek to decrease this problem. Care must be taken when turning the patient in order to protect the newly transplanted kidney. The patient should not be positioned on the side *opposite* the surgery because the force of gravity on the kidney can disrupt the vascular anastomosis. Long periods of sitting at a 90-degree angle can cause kinking of the ureter and should be avoided.

COMPLICATIONS OF RENAL TRANSPLANTS

The complications can be divided into two major categories: *1*) technical or surgical and *2*) clinical.

Technical Complications

Vascular Complications

Stenosis of the renal artery can be detected by hypertension, decreased renal function, and/or a bruit over the anastomosis site. This is hypothesized to be caused by the surgical technique of anastomosis or by the recipient's possible rejection of the artery. Revascularization includes resection and reanastomosis, anastomosis to another artery, or a "detour" graft around the stenotic area. The surgical procedure presents a challenge when the patient is on high-dose steroids or large doses of antihypertensive drugs.

Vascular leakage is usually caused by technical difficulty and/or poor tissue healing. Emergency transplant nephrectomy is done to save the patient's life.

Thrombosis caused by arterial emboli completely blocking the blood supply to the kidney results in renal infarction. The kidney usually cannot be saved, and an emergency nephrectomy is performed. Removal of the thrombus (endarterectomy) is dangerous and rarely successful. Renal vein thrombosis can also be a cause of graft failure. This condition is difficult to detect because it resembles an acute rejection episode. The kidney usually fails and is removed.

Graft Rupture

Rupture of the transplanted kidney is usually caused by swelling of the graft during a rejection crisis. Operative intervention is usually required, and repair of the renal capsule and graft may be attempted if the patient's condition warrants.

Wound Complications

Perinephric hematomas, urinomas, abscesses, and lymphoceles (an accumulation of lymph into the neorenal pocket) can cause deterioration of renal function by applying external pressure on the kidney and/or ureter. These can become a medium for infection. Wound infection is usually the most common complication of immunosuppresive drugs, and it can result in septicemia and death. With the use of preoperative skin washing with an antibacterial agent (Betadine), preoperative shaving, strict surgical technique, and prophylactic wound irrigation, the incidence of infection is on the decline. Each of these types of perinephric masses should be incised and drained, packed or irrigated with appropriate antibiotic or antibacterial agents, and closely monitored by repeated culture and sensitivity testing. Infection of the donor graft is usually prevented by strict organ procurement and preservation techniques. Negative cultures from all cadaveric donors seek to eliminate this problem.

Urological Complications

Ureteral obstruction, ureteral leakage, vesical fistula and ureteral fistula formation are caused by poor wound healing, poor vascularity, tissue necrosis, kinking, stricture of the anastomosis, blood clots, and stone formation. Reoperation and reconstruction are necessary to prevent infection in the kidney and to prevent leakage of urine around the kidney.

Other Complications

Other complications that may occur are lymphedema, bladder neck contracture, peripheral nerve injury, and scrotal problems. These are treated and corrected on an individual basis.

Clinical Complications

This section discusses changes in renal function, including rejection, and drug-induced complications. Refer to Chapter 1 for preexisting problems of the uremic patient. This section does not cover common postsurgical complications. Refer to a textbook of medical surgical nursing if information is needed.

Rejection

Nothing is more discouraging and distressing to the patient and the health team than to transplant a kidney that is rejected. The pathophysiology of the various types of rejection has already been discussed. This section discusses management of transplant rejection.

Early recognition and treatment of rejection can prevent the cellular death of the nephron and insure adequate renal function. Since rejection often mimics surgical complications or infection and its symptoms may be masked by steroids, diagnosis of rejection is very complicated. Careful monitoring of the patient's condition by the nurse will enhance early medical management and success of the graft.

Types of Rejection

Hyperacute. This type of rejection occurs immediately after surgical implantation of the kidney. Within minutes of the onset of arteriolar blood flow, circulating preformed cytotoxic antibodies attack, infiltrate, and infarct the foreign tissue. There is no treatment for this irreversible rejection. With advances in tissue typing and crossmatching of the donor and recipient, tissue rejection of this type is rare.

It is also thought that accelerated rejection (24 to 48 hours after transplant) is another form of hyperacute rejection.

The rejected kidney is removed early to prevent further complications.

Acute. This type of rejection crisis occurs within one week to two years of transplant. Almost every transplant candidate undergoes at least one to two acute rejection episodes. The majority of these crises can be halted and reversed if intervention occurs promptly. The ischemic changes of acute tubular necrosis can be reversed, and recovery occurs within a few days. In some instances, however, acute rejection cannot be reversed and renal function ultimately fails.

Treatment usually consists of large doses of intravenous Solumedrol (or prednisolone) and possible local graft irradiation to kill the invading lymphocytes. The speed of recovery (if it recovers) depends upon the length of time from onset of rejection and the initiation of treatment.

Chronic. This insidious form of rejection occurs over a period of months or years. The clinical picture is one of gradual increasing serum creatinine and blood urea nitrogen levels, electrolyte abnormalities, and fluid retention (weight gain, hypertension, and edema). This type of rejection is usually caused by antibody destruction of the graft. There is no treatment to reverse it. Adding or increasing immunosuppressive drugs at this time only compounds their debilitating side effects. Conservative management includes approprite medicine, diet, and fluid restrictions until renal function deteriorates and the patient resumes chronic dialysis.

The successful kidney graft can continue to function for years. The body covers the graft's foreign antigens with its own cells and accepts the kidney as its own.

If the rejection becomes irreversible, the patient is returned to dialysis. The graft may be left in place to allow a more liberal fluid allowance and to prevent an operation on the immunosuppressed patient.

A transplant nephrectomy must be done if the patient experiences any of the following:

1. Drug-induced complications. Adverse complications may occur due to prolonged, excessive use of steroids.
2. Infection. Nonviable tissue is an excellent medium for proliferation of pathogens. Sepsis may occur because steroids have decreased the body's resistance to infecting organisms.
3. Hypertension. Damaged kidneys often produce increased levels of renin.
4. Protein deficiency. Proteinuria occurs from the altered glomerular permeability in the damaged kidney. Low serum protein and albumin is usually controlled by diet.

The patient's immunosuppressive drugs should be discontinued as rapidly as possible before the transplant nephrectomy. Observations for acute adrenal insufficiency include signs and symptoms of fatigue, weakness, lethargy, hypoglycemia, and shock.

Complications following a transplant nephrectomy are wound infection, hematoma formation (use of heparin during dialysis), and hemorrhage from vascular injury or leakage.

The decision to sacrifice the graft to save the patient is based on the philosophy that the patient's life must be the primary consideration in renal transplantation. The immunosuppressive therapy is discontinued and/or the graft removed before the patient's life is in danger (usually after two to three nonreversible rejection crises).

The dialysis patient with a nonfunctioning graft in place or following a transplant nephrectomy may receive another transplant as soon as he desires and his health status is deemed suitable by the health team. The chance of success of a second transplant is decreased, and the patient can experience more drug-related complications.

Since the immune defense system is the primary cause of graft failure, clinical research is vital for the prevention and treatment of rejection.

Listed below are the major signs and symptoms of kidney rejection. The responses are variable and individual, depending upon the acute or chronic changes of the rejection.

1. Oliguria or possible anuria.
2. Temperature greater than 100°F (37.8°C) (may be masked by the high dosages of steroids).
3. Swollen, soft, tender kidney.
4. Fluid retention and hypertension.
5. Weight gain (two to three pounds in one day or five to seven pounds in one week).
6. Malaise.
7. Changes in blood chemistries.
8. Changes in urine components.
9. Renogram and other radiological test changes.

Immunosuppressive Drugs

The immunological responsiveness of the recipient is the most critical factor in determining whether or not he accepts the graft. The goal of immunosuppressive therapy is to alter the body's innate protective defense, a precarious balance of inducing specific immunological tolerance to foreign graft antigens, yet enabling the recipient to protect himself against environmental pathogens. The success of a transplanted kidney depends on the proper use of immunosuppressive therapy—drugs, lymphocyte depletion, and irradiation.

Imuran (azathioprine) alters the immune response by inhibiting DNA and RNA (nucleic acid) synthesis, thus decreasing or blocking antibody production or producing abnormal antibodies. Side effects are bone marrow depression (leukopenia, thrombocytopenia) and liver dysfunction. Imuran dosages are decreased or temporarily discontinued until the toxic effects are reversed.

Prednisone and Medrol are corticosteroids that act as an anti-inflammatory agent to stabilize the cell membrane (lysosome) and prevent infiltration of leukocytes into tissue during rejection. They also decrease antibody production and inhibit antigen-antibody complexing. Side effects are:

• Infection—viral, fungal, bacterial.
• Ulceration and G.I. bleeding.
• Diabetes mellitus.
• Acne.

- Delayed wound healing.
- Fat dystrophy.
- Aseptic necrosis of the femoral head.
- Cataracts.
- Pancreatitis.
- Arthropathy.
- Psychosis.

Cytoxan (cyclophosphamide) resembles Imuran in its action and can be used in conjunction with or in the place of Imuran. Cytoxan decreases antibody production and can destroy circulating lymphocytes. Side effects are those of bone marrow depression and of hair loss.

Antilymphocyte sera (ALS) (antihymocyte globulin) is another immunosuppressant drug. Synthesized from a sensitized horse, goat, sheep, or rabbit, this drug facilitates the production of immunological unresponsiveness by coating the antigens of the graft, making them unrecognizable, or by destroying circulating thymic-origin lymphocytes. ALS exerts little of no bone marrow depression. One side effect is anaphylactic shock from hypersensitivity to the injected foreign protein. With quality control and standardization of ALS, more transplant centers will use this drug routinely.

Appendix II is a compilation of the side effects of immunosuppressive drugs and the related nursing interventions.

Drug therapy is begun before transplantation, at the time of surgery, or at the first rejection crisis depending on the individual transplant center's drug protocol. The use of immunosuppressive drugs continues as long as the recipient has a functioning graft. The schedule and doses of all drugs are determined by each transplant center.

Other Methods of Immunosuppression
Many methods can be used in conjunction with drug therapy to prevent rejection of the kidney graft. Either before the actual transplant, during the transplant, or during a rejection crisis, irradiation, thoracic duct drainage, spleenectomy, or thymectomy can constitute an added "booster" to help a floundering kidney. These techniques along with drug therapy have increased the success of graft survival.

Irradiation. High doses of irradiation produce temporary depression of the immune response by destroying circulating peripheral lymphocytes and inhibiting formation of antibodies. The side effects are septicemia and bone marrow aplasia.

The various types of irradiation are:

1. Total body irradiation.
2. Radiation of blood via extracorporeal circulation.
3. Local radiation to the graft site. Lymphocytes within the graft are destroyed. This can cause radiation damage to the insulted kidney.
4. Irradiation to the thymus gland.

Spleenectomy. The aim of this surgical procedure is to decrease the lymphoid mass that would produce lymphocytes. It also increases the patient's tolerance to Imuran. Because this is a major operation and postoperative thrombolic complications may occur, transplant centers are reevaluating the benefits for graft survival of this procedure.

Thymectomy. The thymus produces immunoaggressive T-cells, which attack foreign protein. Removal of the thymus gland leads to some lymphoid cell ablation. This procedure is rarely performed today.

Thoracic Duct Drainage (TDD). This is the removal of lymph from the patient's right or left thoracic lymph duct via an indwelling catheter. This type of lymphocyte depletion carries the danger of septicemia. Though the benefit of an increased graft survival rate is present, most transplant centers do not perform this procedure, owing to the risks involved.

Other Methods. Other methods of specific immunodepression are being researched. Maybe one will prove to be successful in prolonging graft survival.

Specific Nursing Care of the Transplant Patient During a Rejection Crisis

Implementation of the ESRD management regimen may extend into the posttransplant period. The patient requires strong emotional and psychological support during this time. Yet, it can be beneficially used to teach the patient the signs, symptoms, and treatment of a rejection episode. The faster treatment is initiated to reverse a rejection, the less ischemic damage occurs within the graft.

The *immunosuppressive drug* dosages may be increased. Observe for exacerbated side effects and toxic changes in the patient.

Other means of immunosuppression may be implemented. Drugs (I.V. Solumedrol) or irradiation therapy should be carefully explained so the patient can understand their use and the procedure involved. Solumedrol given I.V. (500 mg) can cause acute personality changes, severe weakness, increased incidence of infection, a feeling of lightheadedness, or flushing. This infusion should be given slowly over a period of one to three minutes.

Medications. Amphojel may be used as an antacid as well as a phosphate binder. Administration with meals and between meals may be indicated. Close observations of serum phosphorus and calcium levels are necessary as renal function increases.

Diet. The renal diet consisting of limited protein and high carbohydrates and sugars can aggravate the steroid effects of muscle wasting and moon facies. The patient usually complains of not enough to eat, owing to the voracious appetite caused by steroids. Fluid restriction may present a problem if the patient had been unlimited before the rejection. A change to a transplant diet usually occurs as the BUN reaches 50 to 80 mg/100 ml.

Dialysis. Accurate monitoring of the patency of the patient's shunt is essential should dialysis be required during a crisis. The patient is usually dialyzed using a regional heparinization. Close observation for bleeding is required because of the recent surgery, low platelets due to the Imuran's bone marrow suppression, and the slower tendency of wound healing due to the effect of steroids. The nurse should closely observe for signs of hemorrhage following dialysis.

LONG-TERM CARE

The patient is usually discharged from the hospital in three to four weeks with an adequately functioning kidney. Patient teaching begins before surgery and is continued throughout the entire hospitalization. Large doses of intravenous Solumedrol may decrease the ability of some patients to concentrate. Careful observation of the patient's willingness and readiness to learn is essential for teaching.

The patient is given a record book, which he begins to fill out and update while in the hospital. He begins to take his own medications and records them in his book. (See Figure 9.9.) The patient, with careful observation by the nurse, learns the names, pill size and color, the dosage, time interval, action, and possible side effects of all his drugs. Should the patient require, the medications can be color-coded and then symbol-coded for easier identification. For example, Prednisone can be identified with a purple star. At Nashville the colors and symbols are standardized to prevent miscommunication between the patient and the

Medications	Week of _____						
	Sun	Mon	Tue	Wed	Th	Fri	Sat
6 a.m.							
8 a.m. (breakfast)							
12 noon (lunch)							
2 p.m.							
6 p.m. (supper)							
10 p.m. (bedtime)							

Figure 9.9. Medication schedule and record kept by the patient.

health team. Our blind patients with the help of a family member can dispense their own drugs from a prefilled container or use a Braille method with small pealike objects taped to their medication bottles.

The patient also begins to record other parameters of his health status in the book. (See Figure 9.10.) These include daily weight, temperature, blood pressure, urine for sugar and acetone, stools for occult blood, and the number of bowel movements per day. This clinical record is used as a teaching tool for recognizing a rejection episode. The book has the signs and symptoms of rejection listed on its front page along with the phone numbers of the physicians and transplant nurse.

A flow sheet with the laboratory blood and urine values recorded on it is kept in the patient's room. (See Figure 9.11.) This flow sheet serves as an invaluable tool for patient teaching. The patient may also take the responsibility of recording his own laboratory values.

Other health teaching includes the following:

Activity Level

The patient is encouraged to resume his pretransplant activity level and, with encouragement, increase his strength, endurance, and stamina.

Name _____

Date	Sun	Mon	Tue	Wed	Th	Fri	Sat
Weight—before breakfast							
Blood pressure — 8 a.m.							
Blood pressure — 8 p.m.							
Temperature — 8 a.m.							
Temperature — 8 p.m.							
Urine sugar/acetone—before breakfast							
Intake							
Output							
B.M.'s—number each day							
Stool guaiac tests—negative or positive							

Figure 9.10. Daily record kept by the patient.

Recipient Name _____ Race _____ Age _____

Transplant Date _____ Nephrectomy Date _____

	Date															
	Weight															
	Temp															
	B/P															
	Output															
	Platelet															
	Hct.															
	WBC															
	BUN															
	Serum Cr.															
	Na															
S	K															
E	Cl															
R	CO_2															
U	Glucose															
M	Uric acid															
	Ca															
	In. phos.															
	T.P.															
	Alb.															
	Chol.															
	T. bil.															
	Alk. phos.															
	SGOT															
	LDH															

Figure 9.11. Flow sheet used to record blood and urine laboratory values.

	Protein																		
U	Creatinine																		
R	Na																		
I	K																		
N	BUN																		
E	Cr. cl.																		
	U. culture																		
	Dialysis																		
M	Solumedrol																		
E	Imuran																		
D	Prednisone																		
S																			
	Radiation																		

Figure 9.11. (Continued)

The patient's energy increases as the uremic anemia disappears and the hemoglobin and hematocrit levels return to normal values. While the steroid doses are at a high level, any activity that produces stress on the joints of the hip is avoided. Long walks and jogging are discouraged. Swimming, bicycle riding, and the like are encouraged. Heavy lifting and all contact sports are also avoided.

Exercise Schedule

Each patient, providing no preexisting condition contraindicates, is given a series of exercises designed to maintain muscle strength of the quadriceps (thigh) muscle. (See Figure 9.12.) Prednisone's muscle-wasting effect is especially apparent in these muscles. Before discharge, the patient receives a schedule of total-body exercises for arms, legs, and stomach, which should also be done twice daily. As the patient's strength increases, he can add to this exercise schedule to reach his tolerance level.

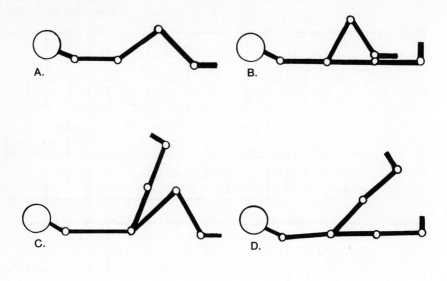

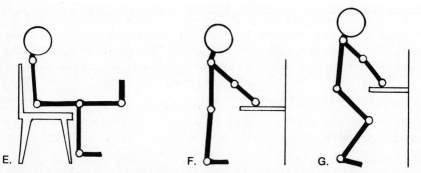

Figure 9.12. Exercise taught to transplant patients to maintain strength of the leg muscles, especially the quadriceps.

Sexual Activity

Usually fertility and libido return to men and women following transplantation. Women may ovulate before establishing a regular menstrual cycle (two to six months). Contraception, other than birth control pills, is encouraged. Men may father children at any time. Women are encouraged to prevent any pregnancies for up to two years posttransplant. There is some controversy concerning a vaginal delivery of the fetus versus Caesarean section. The woman with a transplanted kidney would be followed closely by her obstetrician, should she choose to have a baby. Depending upon the etiology of the individual's renal failure, genetic counseling may be required. Men and women may begin sexual relations as soon as they are discharged from the hospital (four to six weeks after surgery). There are no restrictions to the positions used or frequency of relations. Personal hygiene is encouraged before and after sexual intercourse to decrease the chance of infection. Men are instructed to merely bathe adequately. Women are instructed in douching with a mild vinegar solution or a solution of their own preference. Regular tub bathing is discouraged for about six months, owing to the increased chance of bladder infections from bacteria ascending into the short urethra of the female. The patient may shower as soon as the sutures are removed from his incision or when the skin has healed.

Female transplant patients, because of the increased risk of cancer, are instructed in the technique of self breast examination. This should be done once a month until menstruation begins, then after each menses. Women are encouraged to have a Pap smear twice a year.

Infection Control

The patient is instructed to avoid large groups of people for about three months postoperatively. He should wear a mask when returning for clinic visits. Should a family member become ill, the transplant patient should avoid that person until his health returns. Minor cuts should be treated promptly and should be observed closely for possible infection. The patient is instructed to contact the transplant center should he become exposed to a contagious disease, such as chicken pox or hepatitis.

Career

At the Nashville transplant center, we suggest that the patient not return to his career for about six months to a year. During this time, drug dosages and schedules are changed and renal function is evaluated closely. However, individual considerations are given to the financial need and type of employment for each patient. Children are encouraged to have a home tutor for approximately six months and then may return to school.

THE PSYCHOLOGICAL EXPERIENCE OF TRANSPLANTATION: FROM WONDER TO WISDOM

Within the span of a single lifetime technology has developed far beyond the dreams of the preceding generation. Science has unlocked secrets held for centuries by the oceans, the universe, as well as the single cell. Our understanding of nature has supplemented a sense of awe with a feeling of power—power to alter the course of nature in ways that benefit mankind and the quality of life.

Human organ transplantation has given man the power to change the natural course of disease and lengthen life. It is a procedure so taken for granted that we seldom reflect on its wonder. Beyond the mysteries of immunology and intricate surgical technique lies a whole area of transplantation where little is known or understood—an existential experience of those involved in the exchange of human organs so that life may go on. The donor and recipient as well as their families undergo an experience unique to most of us and one that is at present beyond our understanding.

Wonder is defined as a "feeling of mingled surprise and curiosity, astonishment. A strange thing; a miracle" (15). A sense of wonder prompts investigation so that the object of curiosity can be understood in a meaningful way. Only recently have we attempted to explore with transplant patients their experience of accepting an organ from another person. Hopefully, this pursuit will lead us to a greater understanding of the events that influence the success or failure of transplantation.

The following discussion attempts to conceptualize the transplant experience as a process involving three phases: *1*) anticipation, *2*) actualization, and *3*) reconciliation.

Anticipation Phase

At some point in the life of a chronically ill kidney patient the question of transplantation is entertained. Whether the decision to undergo the operation is conscious or deliberative, in the patient's own way the potential gains and losses are weighed. For most persons the transplant offers hope of recovery and freedom from illness, dialysis, and the restrictions of managing a chronic illness. Waiting for the surgery is a time fraught with many feelings; hope, fear, worry and conflict weigh heavy on the patient's mind and influence the quality of the decision in ways that are not always revealed to us. Most of the work of worry is done privately, as the patient does not readily share the burden of coming to terms with the quality of his own existence. Families may find the patient spending more time alone than before. There may be a preoccupation with one's own fantasies about what is to be: fantasies of recovery, the possible donor, the kidney; images of mutilation, loss of virility, strength, sexuality; and always the finality of death.

Recovery is not always viewed as a positive alternative to illness. Secondary gains one receives reinforce the comfort of dependency. Giving up the benefits of illness constitutes a crisis for the patient and his family (16,17,18). Marital problems that may have existed earlier are easily reactivated by problems created by the transplant, particularly when sexual fantasies predominate (19). Fantasies of sexual fears are not uncommon:

> Castration fears in both male and female patients are common and they reactivate latent conflicts concerning sexual identity; these difficulties are usually found to have pre-existed. Thus, transplantation is generally experienced as a "rephallicisation" or a refertilization. The female patient has fantasies of pregnancy, the male patient fantasizes the recovery of a phallus, sensed as lost because of the illness and dialysis, during which sexual impotence is a frequent finding (19).

Sexual fantasies become particularly troublesome postoperatively in the case of opposite-sex donors in situations where the recipient does not have a strong sexual identity (20). Exploration of fantasy content is extremely important preoperatively, especially when potential donors are discussed.

Donor-Recipient Relationship

The donor-recipient relationship is fraught with both real and imagined problems. Though actual emotional ties do not exist for the cadaver recipient, patients fantasize the origin of the donated kidney in a way that symbolizes intrapsychic conflict. Issues of femininity, masculinity, virility, power, and strength emerge as themes representing an idealized representation of the "new" self. It is important to help patients sort out realistic expectations from unrealistic wishes before transplant to help maintain psychological equilibrium in the reconciliation phase.

Assessment of the living-related donor-recipient relationship is often complex. The psychological experience of the donor has recently been given attention owing to the role of the family in selecting a donor, the motivations of the donor, the psychological rewards, and the post-transplant changes in the family relationships (18,20,21,22).

Kemph (21) has studied the emotional complications that develop as a result of ambivalent and conflictual relationships between donor and recipient. Conflict appears to exist between the conscious altruism of the donor and the unconscious hostility and resentment felt toward the recipient (21). The unconscious conflicts of the donor are expressed by Crombez and Lefebvre (19):

> The requirements of superego can be projected while the patient feels he is being used as an "object" or even a guinea pig; secondly, it seems that the donor gives his kidney and also everything that his kidney represented for him as links with aggressive and sexual trends—a loss of life, of strength, or virility or a gift of life or of death.

Just as in the case of the cadaver transplant patient, the conflict of the donor's inner life must be worked through, as fantasized distortions create complications in the actual real-life relationship with the recipient (19).

During the anticipation phase, donor and recipient appear to view the impending surgery very differently. While the recipient begins to feel hopeful and enthusiastic, the donor feels more doubtful, apprehensive, and exploited (21,22,23). Kemph (24) describes the donor's response:

> In contrast (to the recipient), the donor tended to withdraw emotionally and appear harassed as the operative date approached. The loss of a part of his body was rapidly becoming a reality. Previously he felt he compensated for the altruistic sacrifice he was making, but when surgery was imminent he realized more fully the significance of losing an organ through major surgery in terms of narcissistic threat, fear of damage to sexual organs, and the vital dangers of major surgery.

Concurrently, family members alternate their attention from donor to recipient. Preoperatively, the investment in the donor is considerable and supportive (23). After the surgery the attention turns to the recipient, leaving the donor isolated and bewildered. Fellner and Marshall (22) postulate that the crisis resolution of transplantation has the potential of ego growth when the following four positive factors are operative:

1. Belief in the good they felt they were doing.
2. Positive relationship with the physician.
3. Positive emotional reinforcement from recipient and family.
4. Attention derived from friends, acquaintances, and news media.

In order to promote the maximum benefit of crisis resolution it may be feasible for members of the treatment team to compensate for the postoperative diversion of attention from donor to recipient. Certainly more study is required to reveal ways to intervene in the loss experienced by the renal donor in this period. It may also be of benefit to explore those relationships where minimal difficulty exists, such as the maternal-child donor relationship. Ferris (25) points out that "the type of relationship and the presence or absence of ambivalence and its degree seems to be a far more important factor than the sex or age of the donor."

The Pretransplant Nephrectomy

Patients who undergo nephrectomy appear at times to be in turmoil beyond what may be expected at that point of the illness. Lefebvre (26) describes the nephrectomy as a highly cathected experience because it irrevocably commits the patient to transplantation and he must give up the solace of fantasies that by some magic the kidneys might recover. At transplantation the recovery fantasies may be experienced as a "rebirth"—a feeling fraught with a sense of purpose, mission, or responsibility in life. The theme of rebirth and redemption has been identified as a defense against overwhelming death anxieties (19). Crombez explains this behavior:

> ... confrontation with death is feared and avoided by all manner of pathological defense mechanisms—denial, strangulation of affects, a headlong flight into surgery, manic-like manifestations, or hypochondriacal symptoms. Anxieties about death tend to become focused and displaced onto the specific events of surgical interventions, and various cat-and-mouse type reactions are used to avoid these tensions.

Staff and family members respond to such behaviors by reducing contact with the patient. In a sense his anxieties serve only to isolate him further from those who could help most in dealing with the actual fears. As with other fantasies, the patient feels they are too bizarre or "crazy" to reveal.

A trusting relationship with members of the treatment team is invaluable to the recipient. The extent to which the patient and his family are helped to confront their fears and apprehensions influences their sense of well-being. Helping the potential recipient attain psychological equilibrium is an important treatment goal of this phase of the transplant experience.

Actualization Phase

The process of taking in and accepting the donated kidney represents a "psychological passage" or "emotional transplant" (27). Tasks confronting the recipient include dealing with rejection, the donor, an altered body image, and the incorporation of a new kidney. Muslin describes the patient's image of the kidney as:

> ... part of the psychological structures present in the psychic apparatus, finally becoming merged with the individual's self-representations. Through this psychological passage, we have seen the new kidney becoming invested with many meanings, becoming a symbol of important developmental conflicts and serving as an object for projection and displacement as well as an intermediary link between donor-transplant-recipient (27).

Three phases of integration are described by Muslin (27). The foreign-body stage is one of separateness marked by total body configuration changes. In the stage of partial incorporation the patient reports less interest in the transplant, until acceptance of the new organ comes in the stage of complete incorporation. The acceptance-rejection conflict has been widely discussed (25,28,29,30). Whether or not, and to what extent, psychological mechanisms operate in the physiological reaction of rejection is unclear. Viederman (30) writes, "Even in the absence of rejection, high anxiety levels as well as depression are related to fear of rejection and reflect the patient's unconscious view of the 'meaning' of the transplant."

On this level, the degree of psychic posttransplant distress is in direct relationship to unconscious conflict, but there is no evidence that this necessarily influences the likelihood of a physiological reaction.

One way to further understand the meaning of the transplant to the patient is to explore the concepts of incorporation, introjection, and internalization (18,26,29,30,31). To clarify, "Introjection refers to a process by which an inner presence is felt as separate from the self-representation, whereas incorporation describes a fantasy whereby an inner presence is experienced as somatically taken in and merged with the self-representation" (32). Internalization on the other hand, is a "generic describing the passage of an external object representation into that of an internal object" (19). One term or another may be most appropriate to describe the reaction, depending upon whether the patient experiences the kidney as separate from self (introjection) or as a fusion between self and the kidney (incorporation). Crombez and Lefebvre (19) suggest the more appropriate term "accorporation" to describe a "progressive internalization of the kidney on both the mental and somatic levels without implying that self-object differentiation exists at the beginning."

The perceptions of individual recipients are unique in the representations the kidney holds with respect to the self. Exploration of these perceptions indicate the degree to which the organ has been psychologically accepted. The manner in which the recipient views the kidney as a symbolic representative of another human being influences the post-operative course (33). Whether the representation is of a benevolent or hostile introject depends both on the actual and fantasized relationship with the donor. Viederman (33) postulated that "fear of loss will be most intense with the activation of a hostile introject. The activation of a benevolent introject will lead to a positive change in the self-concept, more specifically an enhancement of self-esteem coincident with the rapprochement between the self-concept and the ideal self."

As the recipient focuses on the new body part, in this event a kidney, a narcissistic cathexis occurs wherein tremendous psychic energy is directed toward integration and the development of a new body ego (34). Lefebvre (26) comments on the regressive nature of the narcissism and views the process as "reminiscent of a state of affairs in early childhood when body parts are not yet experienced as owned and merged with the self-representation."

Body Image

Recipients of transplanted internal organs undergo changes in body image, the process of which is not completely understood, as many variables are unique to the transplant experience. Body image is a term usually used to describe the body's inner representation and appears to be related to age, sex, time, and the level of ego integration (29). Ferris (25) comments that "transplant patients in their early or middle teens are usually more sensitive to body form since they are going through a time when they are undergoing many changes both in physical size and in secondary sexual characteristics."

The concept of the differences between inner and outer space and body boundaries also appears to play a role in the recipient's ability to achieve an integrated self-representation. A transplanted organ lies inaccessible within the body and is perceived in a much different way than an amputation or mastectomy. The mystery of internal organs gives rise in part to the active fantasies recipients create in an attempt to understand and accept the changes occurring within their body. Viederman (33) comments that in his experience patients rarely reported a sense of change inside the body except to speak of the form of the kidney, which is palpable from the outside. In his view, there is no internal body image, as our knowledge of the inside of our bodies is basically cognitive or intellectual.

Patients who undergo both nephrectomy and transplant experience conflicting perceptions of their inner body sense. Turokow (29) explains:

Life-saving operations (removing diseased or worn-out organs) appear to restrict the body image by removing a diseased part. What was ego must become nonego. The patient experiences a loss, typically manifested by depression and frequently by the phantom phenomena. Life-extending transplant operations necessitate enlarging the body image; a foreign part is added, and what previously was nonego now needs to be integrated into the ego.

During the actualization phase the recipient comes to an understanding within his mind of the changes that have occurred within his body. Some time passes before integration takes place at a social level and the patient begins to resume functioning as a well individual within the family and at work.

Reconciliation Phase

By the time the transplant patient is stabilized and begins to live again as a well person, he or she has undergone considerable stress. Confrontation with a prolonged illness, pain, innumerable losses, and possible death deplete the resources one needs for coping with a new life. Whatever fantasies, hopes, or dreams the patient may have had about life with a transplant are now gradually colored by reality. Most are hopeful of the future and truly sense a rebirth and renewal of energies and anticipation. Gradually, in ways that are not fully clear, the patient finds a peace within himself or herself. The turmoil is over for the moment, and the moment is precious. Most patients and their families, however, understand the tenuous nature of the transplant and learn to set short-term goals and realistic expectations of time.

Helping patients accept their fears and live around the fear without continually expressing it is an important function of the treatment team (35).

CONCLUSION

Prolonged life by transplanting healthy organs into diseased bodies is a wondrous event. For patients who have experienced transplantation, it is truly a miracle. For those of us who have witnessed the process, it is a phenomenon of great curiosity. How does a person accept an organ foreign to his or her own body? What does it mean to have your life extended by transplantation? What factors determine whether or not the organ will be accepted or rejected? And on a more personal level, how does a person find meaning in the transplantation experience?

Currently, these are unanswered questions. Yet, our wonder at the process leads us to further investigation. Organ transplantation offers a unique opportunity to study the mind-body relationship. As well it offers a way to understand psychic phenomena such as introjection and incorporation, body image, and fantasy and the part these events play in the process of rejection. Only with this knowledge can we appreciate the wisdom of the human body undergoing transplantation.

REFERENCES

1. J E Dunphy: The story of organ transplantation. *Hastings Law Journal* 21: 1, Nov 1969.

2. J Hamburger, J Crossier, J Dormont, et al.: *Renal Transplantation: Theory and Practice.* Baltimore, Williams & Wilkins Co, 1972, p 24.

3. B Sachs: *Renal Transplantation: A Nursing Perspective,* Flushing, N Y, Medical Examination Co, 1977.

4. F K Widmann: *Goodalis Clinical Interpretation of Laboratory Tests.* Philadelphia, F A Davis, 1973.

5. F Bach: Recent advances in immunogenetics and histocompatibility testing. *Dialysis and Transplantation* 7: 2, 1978.

6. K C Cochrun, A A Perkins, R D Payne, et al.: The correlation between MLC and graft survival. *Transplantation Proceedings* V: 1, March 1973.

7. J O Nepather, A E Katz, J L Lenth: The immune system: its development and function. *Am J Nursing* 76: 10, 1976.

8. K M H Butt, S L Kountz: Transplantation immunology. *A O R N Journal* 20: 4, 1974.

9. S K Dhar, E C Smith: Renal transplantation. *Heart and Lung* 4: 6, 1975.

10. R W Schwartz: *Immunosuppression.* Kalamazoo, Upjohn Co, 1972.

11. B Dupont, A Saejgaard: HLA and disease. *Transplantation Proceedings* IX: 1.

12. W Schumen, R Sperling: Shock and its effect on the cell. *JAMA* 205: July 22, 1968, pp. 215–219.

13. R A Sells: Physiological aspects of kidney transplants, in C Wells (ed): *Scientific Foundations of Surgery.* Philadelphia, Saunders, 1974, pp. 90–97.

14. J M Visel: Clinical aspects of renal biopsy. *Heart and Lung* 4: 6, 1975, pp 900–902.

15. Funk and Wagnall: *New Comprehensive International Dictionary.* New York, Publishers Guild, 1977.

16. D M Bernstein: After transplantation—the child's emotional reactions. *Am J Psychiatry* 127: 1189, 1971.

17. K M Hickey: Impact of kidney disease on patient, family, and society. *Social Casework* 53: 391, 1972.

18. R H Moos: The crisis of treatment: organ transplants, in R H Moos (ed): *Copying with Physical Illness.* New York, Plenum, 1977, p 329.

19. J C Crombez, P Lefebvre: The behavioural responses of renal transplant patients as seen through their fantasy life. *Can Psychiatr Assoc J* 17: 19, 1972.

20. W A Cramond: Renal transplantations—experiences with recipients and donors. *Seminars in Psychiatry* 3: 116, 1971.

21. J P Kemph: Renal failure, artificial kidney and kidney transplant. *Amer J Psychiatry* 122: 1270, 1966.

22. C H Fellner, J R Marshall: Twelve kidney donors. *JAMA* 206: 2703, 1968.

23. D R Freebury: The psychological implications of organ transplantation—a selected review. *Can Psychiatr Assoc J* 19: 593, 1974.

24. J P Kemph: Psychotherapy with patients receiving kidney transplant. *Am J Psychiatry* 124: 623, 1967.

25. G N Ferris: Psychiatric aspects of renal transplantation. *A Dialysis Symposium for Nurses.* U S Dept of H E W, 1969.

26. P Lefebvre, J C Crombez, J LeBeuf: Psychological dimension and psychopathological potential of acquiring a kidney. *Can Psychiatr Assoc J* 18: 495, 1973.

27. H L Muslin: On acquiring a kidney. *Amer J Psychiatr* 127: 105, 1971.

28. S Basch: The intrapsychic integration of a new organ: a clinical study of kidney transplantation. *Psychoanal Q* 42: 364, 1973.

29. L P Tourkow: Psychic consequences of loss and replacement of body parts. *J Am Psychoanal Assoc* 22: 170, 1974.

30. M Viederman: Psychogenic factors in kidney transplant rejection: A case study. *Am J Psychiatry* 132: 957, 1975.

31. P Castelnvovd-Tudesco: Organ transplant, body image, psychosis. *Psychoanal Q* 42: 349, 1973.

32. R Schafer: *Aspects of Internalization.* New York, International Universities Press, 1968.

33. M Viederman: The search for meaning in renal transplantation. *Psychiatry* 37: 283, 1974.

34. H L Muslin: The emotional response to the kidney transplant: the process of internalization. *Can Psychiatr Assoc J* 17: 3, 1972.

35. K S Felix: The team approach to transplantation. *Nurs Clinics N Amer* 4: 451, 1969.

BIBLIOGRAPHY

Bates B: *A Guide To Physical Examination.* Philadelphia, Lippincott, 1974.

_____ : Battered body: nursing grand rounds. *Nursing '78* 8(1): 36–41, 1978.

Belzer F O: Organ preservation. *Dialysis and Transplantation* 7(2): 128–137, 1978.

Brundage D J: *Nursing Management of Renal Problems*. St. Louis, Mosby, 1976.

Brunner L S, et al: *Medical Surgical Nursing*. Philadelphia, Lippincott, 1970.

Brunner L S: What to do (and what to teach your patient) about peptic ulcer. *Nursing '76* 6(11): 27–34, 1976.

Calne R V (ed): *Clinical Transplantation*. Oxford, Blackwell Scientific Pub, 1971.

Collins G M, Halasz N A: Current aspects of renal preservation. *Urology* 10(1 Supp): 22–32, 1977.

Ehrlich R M, Smith R B: Surgical complications of renal transplantation. *Urology* 10(1 Supp): 43–56, 1977.

Freedman P (ed): Renal disease—a symposium. *Heart and Lung* 4(6): 871–902, 1975.

Griffiths H J: *Radiology of Renal Failure*. Philadelphia, Saunders, 1976.

Guttman R D: Pretransplant evaluation and treatment of donors and recipients. *Dialysis and Transplantation* 7(2): 118–125, 1978.

Hamburger J: *Renal Transplantation: Theory and Practice*. Baltimore, Williams & Wilkins, 1972.

Hamdi ME: Nursing intervention for patients receiving corticosteroid therapy, in Kintzel K C: *Advanced Concepts of Clinical Nursing*. Philadelphia, Lippincott, 1971, pp. 236–245.

Juliani L, Reamer B: Kidney transplant: your role in after care. *Nursing '77* 7(10): 46–53, 1977.

Juliani L: Assessing renal function. *Nursing '78* 8(1): 34–35, 1978.

Karow A M, et al.: *Organ preservation*. Boston, Little, Brown, 1974.

Kobrzycki P: Renal transplant complications. *Am J Nurs* 77(4): 641–643, 1977.

_____: *Living With End Stage Renal Disease*. Washington D C, U S Dept H E W.

Long G D: G I bleeding. *Nursing '78* 8(3): 44–50, 1978.

MacBryde C M, Blacklow R S: *Signs and Symptoms*. Philadelphia, Lippincott, 1970.

Mannick J A: The current status of immunosuppressive therapy. *Surgery* 67(4): 711–719, 1970.

Martin D C: Nephrectomy. *Urology* 10(1 Supp): 11–15, 1977.

Meltzer L E, et al.: *Intensive Care For Nurse Specialists*. Philadelphia, Charles Press, 1969, pp. 437–442.

Napolitano L V, et al.: Immunology: clinical benefits coming. *Patient Care*, Jan 15, 1977, pp. 22–41.

Najarian J H, Simmons R L: *Transplantation*. Philadelphia, Lea & Febiger, 1972.

Newton D W, et al.: Cortiscosteroids. *Nursing '77* 7(6): 26–33, 1977.

Nysather J O, et al.: The immune system. *Am J Nurs* 76(10): 1614–1628, 1976.

Sachs B L: *Renal Transplantation: A Nursing Perspective*. Flushing, NY, Medical Examination Pub Co, 1977.

Schuman D: The renal donor. *Am J Nurs* 74(1): 105–110, 1974.

Shenasky J H: Renal transplantation in patients with urologic abnormalities. *J Urology* 115: 490–493, May 1976.

Starzl T E, Putnam C W: Renal Transplantation, in Wells C (ed): *Scientific Foundations of Surgery*. Philadelphia, Saunders, 1974, pp 82–90.

Strauss M B, Welt L G (eds): *Diseases of the Kidney*. Boston, Little, Brown and Co, 1971, pp. 1423–1456.

Thompson W L: The cell in shock. *Proceedings of a Symposium on Recent Research Developments and Current Clinical Practice in Shock*, April 25–27, 1974, pp 3–37.

Wolf Z R: What patients awaiting transplant want to know. *Am J Nurs* 76(1): 92–94, 1976.

10
Drug Dosages in Renal Disease and Dialysis

H. Earl Ginn, M.D.

Larry E. Lancaster, R.N., M.S.N.

One of the kidneys' major physiological functions is the elimination of many of the ordinary products of metabolism. It is also a major excretory route for a large number of frequently used drugs. As well, in some instances it is an important site for structurally altering compounds, either enhancing or diminishing their physiological or pharmacological activity. Because of the diverse medical problems to which patients with renal failure are predisposed, they are liable to be treated with several pharmacological agents. In order to reduce the frequency and severity of adverse drug reactions in patients with renal insufficiency it is imperative that those responsible for prescribing and administering drugs comprehend certain pharmacokinetic concepts as well as the potential complications of the agents used (1–6). Bergersen emphasizes the importance for the professional nurse of a sound scientific understanding of drug therapy:

> . . . The nurse's expanded role currently includes a variety of functions, all of which are predicated upon a sound understanding of drug action. . . . [H]er responsibility has shifted to assuring safe administration of drugs by a variety of specially educated health workers and to observing and interpreting the patient's response to drug therapy. The moral, ethical, and legal responsibility of drug administration remains the nurse's. . . . [T]he nurse has the responsibility of teaching patients about the drugs they are receiving. She has a data-gathering role in relation to the patient's previous drug therapy and present and past responses to drug therapy. . . . She is a decision-maker regarding p.r.n. medications. By virtue of her interpersonal skills, she may also function as a potentiator of drug effects. . . . [S]he is a communicator of her knowledge and observations to other health care professionals, notably the physician who prescribes drug therapy (7).

One of the important responsibilities of the nurse caring for the renal failure/dialysis patient is that of teaching the patient and family about the desired effect, side effects, and dosage interval for each drug the patient receives. In addition, the nurse. through observations, use of laboratory data, and patient interviews, is constantly alert to both desired and side effects of drug therapy. The nurse must be knowledgeable about dosage modifications in renal failure and dialysis and must periodically review each patient's drug list based on this knowledge. Also, the nephrology nurse is in a position to act as liaison between the patient and physician by relating her observations to the physician and interpreting the physician's orders to the patient. The success of drug therapy depends to a great extent on a well-informed patient and a knowledgeable nurse who work cooperatively with the physician.

To provide a basic knowledge for the nephrology nurse this chapter presents general concepts related to drug metabolism and elimination in patients with renal insufficiency, reviews some practical aspects to pharmacologic management of drugs commonly prescribed for patients with renal failure, and considers changes in therapy that may be required for patients on dialytic treatment.

DRUG METABOLISM

Although few studies have specifically concerned the gastrointestinal absorption of drugs in patients with renal failure, there is little evidence to suggest that this route is significantly affected in most instances. Notable exceptions include drugs that are best absorbed in an acid environment, such as iron and calcium compounds. Often uremic patients sustain an increase in gastric pH—that is, an alkaline environment—as a result of gastric urease activity upon the urea secreted by their salivary glands. As a consequence drugs, such as iron, that are best absorbed in an acid milieu may have impaired absorption in uremic patients. The absorption of calcium is influenced by the level of biologically active vitamin D, which is normally enhanced by hydroxylation of 1 (OH) vitamin D_3 to 1,25 $(OH)_2$ vitamin D_3 by the kidney. Consequently, unless the active form of vitamin D is administered to patients with renal failure, calcium absorption is reduced.

Once a drug is absorbed, it is usually bound to some extent to a fraction of plasma protein. The "free" unbound moiety can penetrate cell membranes, is pharmacologically active, and is usually the fraction that is metabolized and/or excreted. On the other hand, the protein-bound fraction is not readily filtered, metabolized, or dialyzed. Although most drugs have similar degrees of protein binding in uremic plasma compared to normal, some, including morphine, diphenylhydantoin, dicloxacillin, and penicillin, have reduced protein binding and increased levels of "free" active drug in uremia (4).

Within the body drugs are usually distributed in a volume greater than plasma volume. The apparent volume of distribution is defined as the theoretical volume, a mathematical expression, into which the drug is distributed in a concentration equal to that in the blood (8). The theoretical volume is usually calculated by dividing the amount of drug in the body by its plasma concentration. Drugs that have high lipid-to-water solubility ratios readily penetrate body tissues and have a large volume of distribution. As well, lipid-soluble drugs have larger volumes of distribution in fat people than in lean people of similar weight. For example, a larger quantity of heparin, a highly lipid-soluble drug, may be required to obtain a desired effect upon anticoagulation in an obese patient, yet in the same patient the biological half-life of heparin may be prolonged. On the other hand, drugs with a high degree of protein binding generally have a small volume of distribution. Additionally, uremia can affect the volume of distribution of certain drugs (4).

Water-soluble drugs, which are relatively few, do not readily diffuse intracellularly and, therefore, if kidney function is normal, are rapidly excreted in the urine. Most drugs, however, are not excreted unchanged by the kidney but require various pathways of metabolism, including oxidation, reduction, hydrolysis, acetylation, and synthesis (9). These routes tend to convert lipid-soluble drugs into water-soluble metabolites. If the required metabolic pathways are impaired by uremia, for example, for drugs that are metabolized by the processes of reduction, acetylation, or ester hydrolysis, then unmetabolized drug accumulation and potential toxicity may occur if standard doses of these agents are administered to patients with renal failure (4).

The means whereby the kidney handles the elimination of drugs and their metabolites include glomerular filtration, active reabsorption and/or secretion by the tubules, nonionic back diffusion, and metabolic alterations (4). Nevertheless, the problem of estimating the role of excretion by the kidneys can be simplified, because the elimination rates of most drugs by the kidney can be related to commonly used measurements of kidney function, such as creatinine clearance.

DRUG ELIMINATION IN RENAL DISEASE

Most drugs are eliminated at a rate proportional to the amount present in the body. Although there may be several routes of elimination for any nonvolatile drug (wherein the lungs are not involved in elimination), the overall elimination rate can be described as that due to excretion by the kidneys plus metabolic excretion (such as liver extraction and conversion to inactive metabolites) (5).

For many drugs there is a linear relationship between the endogenous creatinine clearance and the overall drug elimination rate constant (3,10,11). Depending upon the relationship of the renal elimination of the drug to creatinine clearance, the following three types of drugs may be distinguished (3,12):

Type A—when the drug is eliminated entirely by the kidney.

Type B—when the drug is eliminated entirely by extrarenal mechanisms.

Type C—when the drug is eliminated both by renal and extrarenal mechanisms.

The elimination half-life is the time required for the amount of drug in the body to decrease to one-half. Based on the linear relationship between the overall elimination rate constant and the endogenous creatinine clearance, the individual elimination rate constant of a drug in any patient with renal disease may be determined by simple linear inter-polation. If the elimination half-life for a specific drug has been estab-lished in anephric subjects as well as in people with normal renal func-tion, then the dose fraction for anephric patients and for any patient with renal disease can be determined. By the use of these principles, dosage regimen formulae and nomograns applicable to any drug in which serum half-life values are known for normal and anephric pa-tients have been constructed to permit simple calculation of the dose for any patient with impaired renal function, based on creatinine clearance (3,4,5,10,11,13).

The usual method of drug administration in patients without kidney impairment is to administer multiple doses at uniform dose intervals until a steady state of concentration is reached. To reach 90% of steady-state drug concentration requires 3.3 times the drug half-life. Since the half-life may be markedly prolonged in renal failure, particularly with Type A drugs, adjustments that involve the administration of a mainte-nance dose based on altered half-life may delay effective therapy. To rapidly achieve therapeutic drug concentrations a loading initial dose is often required. This is particularly applicable to digitalis and antibiotic therapy.

The two most commonly used maintenance dosage schedules in renal failure for drugs that have prolonged half-life (Type A and Type C drugs) are the constant dose-varying interval method and the reduced dose–constant interval method. The major disadvantage of the former is the profound peaks and troughs that occur in the serum drug concentration. The reduced dose–constant interval method, on the other hand, may necessitate impractical fractions of the usual dosage. In practice, both methods, either separately or in combination, will be useful when tempered with clinical judgment.

Before administering any drug to a patient with renal failure, Alfrey and Butkus (14) suggest that the nurse should review the following questions:

1. Does the drug depend on the kidney for secretion?
2. Does an excess blood level affect the kidney?
3. Does the drug add chemically to the pool of urea nitrogen?
4. Does the effect of the drug alter electrolyte imbalance?
5. Is the patient more susceptible to the drug because of kidney disease?

DRUGS AND DIALYSIS

Accurate quantification of drug removal during peritoneal dialysis or hemodialysis has not been done with most commonly used drugs. However, some qualitative studies have been done on drug removal involving drug overdoses. The data have shown whether or not a drug is substantially dialyzable but have not been useful for calculating precise changes in drug dosage following routine dialysis. Mostly, drugs of small molecular weight and low protein binding are readily removed by dialysis, provided that they are distributed in a small volume and are not metabolized rapidly. Studies are beginning to appear concerning the dialyzability of some drugs, particuarly antibiotics, based on changes in plasma half-time during dialysis as compared to a period when the patient is not on dialysis treatment. Although renal function is usually very low in dialysis patients, so long as any residual kidney function remains it is constantly present and is a significant aspect of drug removal. During dialysis the elimination of a drug depends not only upon residual renal function and nonrenal elimination but also upon removal by dialysis. Where accurate dialyzer clearance and plasma clearance in anephric patients are available for a compound, calculations can be accomplished to predict the amount of drug removal by dialysis (5).

In general, drugs whose predominant route of elimination from the body is via renal excretion (Type A drugs) will undergo significant decreases in concentration during clinical dialysis. Drugs that are normally filtered at the glomerulus usually are readily dialyzable across the membranes of artificial kidneys. On the other hand, Type B drugs, drugs with a high degree of protein binding or of large molecular size, will have insignificant loss during dialysis.

The following points may be used as guidelines in the drug treatment of renal-failure and dialysis patients (4):

1. Do not use drugs in renal-failure patients unless definite indications are present.
2. If the dosage regimen of a drug in renal failure has been determined by a well-controlled study, this regimen should be followed.
3. In a situation where the drug has not been carefully studied, but where information is available on the characteristics of its excretion in an unchanged form by the kidney, or on the elimination half-life in anephric patients and in subjects with normal kidney function, then the above-referenced formulae and nomograms may be used to make a rough estimate of the proper dose schedules in renal failure.
4. If an assay procedure for the drug is available, the periodical measurement of blood levels of the drug is advisable for any schedule.
5. Careful clinical monitoring for toxicity and pharmacological effect is mandatory in all cases.

Bennett, Singer, Golper, Feig, and Coggins recently published tables of data concerning the pharmacokinetic variables required to arrive at recommendations for drug therapy in patients with renal failure. In addition, the nephrotoxicity or adverse effects of drugs in patients with renal disease are noted, and adjustments are suggested for dialysis (15).

DRUGS USED FREQUENTLY IN PATIENTS WITH RENAL DISEASE
Antimicrobial Agents

Several recent reviews have published recommendations for antimicrobial therapy in renal failure (4,5,6,12,13,15). For Type A drugs that are excreted primarily by the kidneys, and particularly those with narrow toxic-therapeutic ratios such as the aminoglycoside antibiotics (gentamycin, tobramycin, kanamycin. amikacin), major modifications in dose interval are required. Sequential serum levels during the treatment period are most useful to insure efficacy. Tetacyclines should be avoided in renal failure because of their potent protein catabolic effect. Methenamine and nitrofurantoin should also be avoided in renal failure. Table 10.1 lists some commonly used antibiotics based on the need for dosage reduction in renal failure.

Table 10.1. Classification of Commonly Used Antibiotics Based on Need for Dosage Reduction

I. Major Modifications	II. Slight Modifications	III. No Modifications Required
Aminoglycosides	Amphotericin B	Chloramphenicol
Ampicillin	Isoniazid	Clindamycin
Carbenicillin	Lincomycin	Erythromycin
Cephalosporins	Nalidixic acid	Isoxazolyl penicillins
Colistimethate	Trimethoprim	(oxacillin, cloxacillin,
Cycloserine		dicloxacillin, nafcillin)
Ethambutol		Doxycycline
Chloroquine		Rifamycin
Methicillin		
Penicillin G		
Vancomycin		
Sulfonamides		
Quinine		
Paraminosalicylic acid		

Analgesic and Narcotic Drugs

Narcotics are predominantly metabolized in the liver to more polar metabolites. These metabolites potentially have pharmacologic activity and, more importantly, toxic manifestations if they accumulate in the presence of renal failure. Recently a metabolite of meperidine, normeperidine, has been shown to accumulate in patients with renal failure, producing seizures in some (16). The sensitivity of uremic patients to the respiratory depressant effects of morphine may be increased because of decreased plasma protein binding in uremic serum. Thus, morphine should be administered with caution in uremic patients. Codeine, pentazocine, and naloxone can be used without dose modifications in renal-failure patients. None of the narcotics undergo sufficient removal during dialysis to require dosage supplementation.

Salicylates should be used sparingly in patients with renal failure. In uremic patients receiving low-dose (250-mg) therapy the elimination half-life is relatively normal. Nevertheless, uremic platelet dysfunction may be enhanced. and gastrointestinal symptoms are common. Salicylate binding to plasma proteins is decreased in renal failure. With doses greater than 500 mg there is saturation of hepatic metabolic pathways, and renal elimination of unchanged drug becomes a more important pathway of salicylate removal.

Although acetaminophen metabolites accumulate in patients with kidney failure, they have no known pharmacologic activity or known toxic effects. There does not appear to be an increased incidence of toxicity to acetaminophen in uremia.

Cardiac Drugs

Two digitalis glycosides, digoxin and digitoxin, have been well studied in patients with renal failure. Excretion of digoxin is primarily by the kidney. In the anephric patient, the plasma half-life is lengthened to four to five days (normally 1.5 days), owing to a loss of only 15% of the body digoxin stores daily. A digitalizing dose of 10–20 μg per kilogram of body weight is usually associated with a low incidence of toxicity. Adjustments of the maintenance dosage for patients with varying degrees of renal failure have been previously reviewed (17). Digoxin is only slightly bound to plasma proteins and is dialyzable with a clearance of 10–20 ml per minute. This low rate of dialysance and the very large apparent volume of distribution mean that elimination during hemodialysis or peritoneal dialysis is insignificant. The usual maintenance dose for adult patients on dialysis is about 30% of the normal daily dose—that is, 0.1 to 0.15 mg per day.

Elimination of digitoxin depends much less on kidney excretion than on biotransformation by the liver to inactive metabolites. Only 12% of the body load of digitoxin is eliminated daily when renal and liver function are normal and 8% in anephric patients. The removal of digitoxin by dialysis is insignificant. Anephric patients on dialysis require a daily maintenance dose of digitoxin of about 70% of the normal maintenance dose.

In the cardiac patient on dialysis, a special consideration must be given to the body potassium stores and to changes in pH and in calcium concentration when either of these cardiac glycosides is required. Such changes increase the chance of digitalis intoxication.

Should antiarrhythmic agents be necessary for acute care, lidocaine, propranolol, and diphenylhydantoin are the drugs of choice, as their routes of elimination are substantially nonrenal and the dosage and precautions for their use are identical to those in patients with normal renal function. Quinidine or procainamide may be required for the treatment of ventricular irritability on a chronic basis. Quinidine half-life is the same in patients with renal failure as in normal subjects, and no adjustment of dosage is necessary. Procainamide is metabolized to n-acetylprocainamide, which has antiarrhythmic potency similar to that of the parent compound. Since n-acetylprocainamide has a long half-life and is eliminated almost entirely by the kidney, the interval between doses of procainamide should be increased to eight to 12 hours with advanced renal failure.

Diuretics and Antihypertensive Drugs

Diuretics form an essential part of most antihypertensive regimens for patients without renal failure. Most of the antihypertensive action of these drugs is thought to depend on achieving a natriuresis, thereby reducing the extracellular volume. In the presence of progressive renal failure they are less useful, as their effectiveness to produce natriuresis is blunted. Spironolactone and triamterene may cause fatal hyperkalemia when given to patients with advanced renal failure and should be avoided. Mercurials are ineffective and nephrotoxic in patients with renal failure and are therefore contraindicated. Thiazide diuretics are generally ineffective if glomerular filtration rate is below 25% of normal, and metholazone is ineffective with glomerular filtration rates less than 10% of normal. Furosemide and ethacrynic acid, which have sites of action in the loop of Henle, may, if large doses are used, produce a natriuresis in patients with glomerular filtration rates as low as 5% of mormal. The large doses required may produce ototoxicity. This potential side effect is particularly hazardous if ethacrynic acid is used in patients with severe renal failure. For patients with end stage renal disease desired reductions in extracellular volume are best achieved by salt restriction and dialysis or hemofiltration.

The use of antihypertensive agents in patients with renal failure should be based on titrating individual doses of the hypotensive drug against the patient's blood pressure. Several antihypertensive agents are in part eliminated by the kidneys. These include methyldopa, guanethidine, hydralazine, and diazoxide. Somewhat smaller doses of these agents may be required as renal function diminishes. Diazoxide also has decreased protein binding in uremia and therefore is often more potent in these patients. Methyldopa and diazoxide are significantly dialyzable. Other antihypertensive agents are not significantly excreted by the kidneys and are not dialyzable. These include reserpine, minoxidil, propranolol, clonidine, and prazosin. No dose adjustments for renal failure are required for these agents.

Drug treatment of hypertension for patients with renal failure requires careful attention to possible decrements in renal function, as well as to retention of salt and water as blood pressure is lowered. The additional unwanted side effects of the antihypertensive agents should be carefully monitored.

For urgent lowering of blood pressure in patients with renal insufficiency either diazoxide or nitroprusside is especially useful. The metabolism of nitroprusside to thiocyanate presents some risks to patients with renal failure unless blood levels of thiocyanate are monitored and maintained less than 5–10 mg/dl. Symptoms of thiocyanate toxicity include nausea, vomiting, myoclonic movements, and seizures. These can be rapidly alleviated by dialysis. Administration of nitroprusside infusions in patients with renal failure should be terminated within 48 hours.

Adequate dietary sodium restriction plus adequate ultrafiltration or hemofiltration for patients on maintenance hemodialysis will prevent or control hypertension in most patients. When such therapy is unsatisfactory, dosages of antihypertensive agents may be administered based on their blood pressure response. It is often wise to omit the dose of antihypertensive medication before dialysis in those patients who have problems with hypotension during the procedure, especially if fluid removal is required.

Psychotherapeutic Drugs

Insomnia and restlessness are frequent complaints of patients with renal failure. Although the habit of "reading oneself to sleep" is often effective and certainly the safest sedation, it may not suffice. Chloral hydrate, flurazepam, chlordiazepoxide, meprobamate, short-acting barbiturates, and diphenhydramine, an antihistamine, are eliminated principally by nonrenal routes and can be given in customary doses in renal failure. Because of significant renal elimination and potential drug accumulation, the use of long-acting barbiturates should be avoided in patients with renal failure.

In cases of psychosis or depression usual doses of phenothiazines and tricyclic compounds may be given. Although there are no unique side effects of these drugs in patients with renal failure, orthostatic hypotension can be a problem, especially when added to dialysis induced volume depletion. Tricyclic antidepressants may interfere with the antihypertensive action of guanethidine and may cause urinary retention by virtue of their anticholinergic effects. Imipramine is the drug of choice for a depressed patient who has psychomotor retardation, while amitriptyline may be more appropriate for more agitated individuals.

For seizure disorders standard doses of diphenylhydantoin may be used in patients with all degrees of renal impairment. Although uremia decreases diphenylhydantoin binding to plasma proteins, this effect appears to be counteracted by a shortened half-life of this drug in renal failure. For the other drugs frequently used in treatment of seizure disorders, such as long-acting barbiturates, trimethadione, and the succinimide derivatives, some dosage modifications are required. Empirical decreases in doses of these drugs with close monitoring of plasma levels and observation for toxic effects are required. The usual doses of parenteral diazepam may be administered for the treatment of status epilepticus.

Usual Drugs for Uncomplicated Dialysis Patients

Dialysis patients who have managed to cope with their life situation will require only a small number of medications. These usually include aluminum gel, water-soluble vitamins, calcium, iron, and stool softeners.

The dosage of aluminum gel required to maintain inorganic phosphorus at normal levels depends directly upon the quantity of phosphorus ingested in foods. Milk products are especially high in phosphorus. The major unwanted side effect of aluminum gels is constipation, hence the frequent requirement for stool softeners. This problem can be reduced by increasing bulk in the diet or by the ingestion of metamucil. Dioctyl calcium sulfosuccinate is an effective and safe stool softener. Laxatives containing dantron should be used sparingly, however, because this agent can cause hepatotoxicity in renal failure. Phosphate-containing enemas must be avoided, since they can precipitate abrupt severe elevations in serum phosphorus and decrements in serum calcium in patients with renal failure.

As already mentioned, iron is poorly absorbed by the gastrointestinal tract in uremic patients. Oral iron should not be taken at the same time as aluminum gels, as this further reduces its absorption. To obtain effective body stores of iron intravenous administration, as at the end of dialysis procedures, is often warranted.

Folic acid and pyridoxine are not present in some water-soluble vitamin preparations. Since these vitamins are removed by dialysis, they can be replaced by administration of 1–2 mg of folic acid and 25–50 mg of pyridoxine after each dialysis.

REFERENCES

1. J W Smith, L G Seide, L E Cluff: Studies on the epidemiology of adverse drug reactions. V. Clinical factors influencing susceptibility. *Ann Intern Med* 65: 629, 1966.

2. G Richet, J Fabre, J Freudevreich, R Podevin: La tolerance medicamenteuse des uremiques. *Presse Med* 74: 2339, 1966.

3. L Dettli: Individualization of drug dosage in patients with renal disease. *Med Clin-North Am* 58: 977, 1974.

4. R J Anderson, J G Gambertoglio, R W Schrier: Fate of drugs in renal failure, in B M Brenner and F C Rector Jr (eds): *The Kidney*. Philadelphia, Saunders, 1976.

5. R E Cutter, T G Christopher: Drug therapy during renal insufficiency and dialytic treatment, in S G Massry, A L Sellers (eds): *Clinical Aspects of Uremia and Dialysis*. Springfield, Ill, Charles C Thomas, 1976, pp 427–452.

6. W M Bennett, I Singer, C H Coggins: Guide to drug usage in adult patients with inpaired renal function. *JAMA* 223: 991–997, 1973.

7. B S Bergersen: *Pharmacology in Nursing*, ed 12, St Louis, Mosby, 1973, pp 75–87.

8. S Feldman: Drug distribution. *Med Clin-North Am* 58: 917, 1974.

9. M M Reidenberg: Kidney disease and drug metabolism. *Med Clin-North Am* 58: 1059, 1974.

10. L Dettli, P Spring, R Habersang: Drug dosage in patients with impaired renal function. *Postgrad Med J* Suppl 46: 32, 1970.

11. L Dettli, P Spring, S Ryter: Multiple dose kinetics and drug dosage in patients with kidney disease. *Acta Pharmacol* 29: Suppl 3, 211, 1971.

12. C M Kunin: A guide to use of antibiotics in patients with renal disease. *Ann Intern Med* 67: 151, 1967.

13. C S Bryan, W J Stone: Antimicrobial dosage in renal failure: a unifying nomogram. *Clinical Nephr* 7: 81, 1977.

14. A C Alfrey, D E Butkus: Renal failure: pathophysiology and management, in C M Hudak, T Lohr, B M Gallo: *Critical Care Nursing*, ed 2, Philadelphia, Lippincott, 1977, pp 326–327.

15. W M Bennett, I Singer, T Golper, P Feig, C J Coggins: Guidelines for drug therapy in renal failure. *Ann Intern Med* 86: 754, 1977.

16. C E Inturrisé: Disposition of narcotics in patients with renal disease. *Am J Med* 62: 528, 1977.

17. R W Jelliffe: An improved method of digoxin therapy. *Ann Intern Med* 69: 703, 1968.

APPENDICES

I.   Renal and Renal Transplant Diets

II. Complications of
    Immunosuppressive Therapy

APPENDIX I
Renal and Renal Transplant Diets*

RENAL DIETS

Purpose

The purpose of renal diets is to lower blood urea nitrogen, to control hypertension and electrolyte balance, and to prevent catabolism.

Description

Renal diets usually contain specified amounts of high- and low-biological-value protein. Sodium, potassium, phosphorus, and fluids are restricted as needed. To restrict the absorption of phosphorus, aluminum hydroxide gels are often prescribed. To be effective the diet must be adequate in calories.

Adequacy

The diet's adequacy is determined by the protein, sodium, and potassium allowances.

The 20-gm and 40-gm high-biological-value protein diets may not meet the Recommended Daily Dietary Allowances for calcium, iron, and vitamin B complex. Multivitamin, calcium, and iron supplements are often recommended.

Suggested Diet Prescriptions

Diet orders should include desired levels of protein, sodium, potassium, calories, and fluid. Some patients, however, do not require restriction of all of these elements.

*Nashville District Dietetic Association: *Diet Manual.* First edition, 1974. Reprinted with permission.

307

Initial Renal Failure: 20–40 gm high-biological-value protein (HBV).

15 gm or less low-biological-value
protein (LBV).

40–70 mEq potassium (average 60
mEq or 2346 mg).

500–2000 mg sodium.*

Calories to maintain desired body
weight (approximately 45–50
calories per kg of weight).

Fluid is not usually restricted if
sodium is controlled.

Hemodialysis: 60–80 gm high-biological-value protein (1 gm per kg ideal body
weight for adults, 1.5 gm per kg
for children).

15 gm or less low-biological-value
protein.

40–70 mEq potassium (average 60
mEq or 2346 mg).

500–2000 mg sodium.*

Calories to maintain desired body
weight (40–50 calories per kg for
adults, 80 calories per kg for
children).

Fluid (output plus 500 cc).

*It is critical that the patient consume all the sodium allowance.

RENAL MENU PLANNING FORM

High Biological Value Protein _____ Sodium _____
Low Biological Value Protein _____ Fluid _____
Potassium _____ Calories _____

MEAL PLAN

Breakfast
____Servings fruit or juice
____SC* cereal or substitute
____SC meat
____SC bread
____SC butter or margarine
____Milk or cream
____Sugar and jelly
____Coffee or tea

Dinner
____SC Meat
____SC potato or substitute
____SC vegetable
____SC bread
____Fruit or dessert
____SC butter or margarine
____Sugar and jelly
____Beverage: milk, juice, coffee
        or tea

Supper
____SC meat
____SC potato or substitute
____SC vegetable
____SC bread
____Fruit or dessert
____SC butter or margarine
____Sugar and jelly
____Beverage: milk, juice, coffee
        or tea

SAMPLE MENU

Breakfast
½ cup applesauce
½ cup SC grits
SC scrambled egg
SC bread
SC butter or margarine—any amount
**Milk or cream
Sugar and jelly—any amount
**Coffee or tea

Dinner
SC ground beef patty
SC mashed potato
½ cup SC carrots
SC bread
2 halves canned peaches
SC butter or margarine—any amount
Sugar and jelly—any amount
**Coffee or tea

Supper
SC wheatstarch fried chicken
½ cup SC rice
½ cup SC green beans
SC bread
2 halves canned pears
SC butter or margarine—any amount
Sugar and jelly—any amount
**Coffee or tea

*SC = sodium controlled
**Fluid according to output

RENAL DIETS

MEAT AND MILK CHOICES
High Biological Value Protein

High biological value (HBV) protein contains all of the essential amino acids and is from animal sources. The following foods are major sources of HBV protein in the diet and should be eaten in sufficient amounts to provide the number of grams of HBV protein prescribed per day. Meat portions must be weighed after cooking and after removing all fat, skin and bone. However, fats should be eaten because of the additional calories they provide. If skin is eaten count as part of total high biological value protein allowance.

FOOD	Amount	Weight Gm.	% Water	High Biological Value Protein Gm.	Sodium (Na) Mg.	Potassium (K) Mg.	Calories
Egg	1 large	54	74	7	60	65	75
Beef, lean	1 oz.	30	50	7	17	104	75
Lamb, lean	1 oz.	30	60	7	20	81	75
Pork, fresh, lean	1 oz.	30	37	7	18	109	75
Veal, lean	1 oz.	30	68	7	20	142	75
Chicken or Turkey	1 oz.	30	64	7	24	115	75
Fish	1 oz.	30	78	7	30	67	75
Shrimp	1 oz. (5 sm.)	28	70	7	56	69	68
Rabbit	1 oz.	28	60	7	12	110	65
Sausage, cooked	1 oz.	40	35	7	383	108	190
Tuna Fish, Low Sodium, canned	¼ cup	70	50	7	10	77	75
Salmon, Low Sodium, canned	¼ cup	70	50	7	15	90	75
Oysters, raw	5-7 med.	100	85	7	70	115	60
Milk, whole	1 cup	240	87	8	122	350	165
Milk, skim	1 cup	240	90	8	128	350	85
Cream, heavy whipping	1 cup	240	57	5.5	80	220	880
Cream, sour	1 cup	240	57	7	96	134	454
Ice Cream, Vanilla	1 cup	136	63	7	85	244	262
Cottage Cheese, Low Sodium	¼ cup	56	79	7	11	40	40
Yellow Cheese, Low Sodium	1 oz.	28	37	7	1	28	115

NOTE: 1 ounce ground beef, cooked, is 2 tablespoons.
      1 ounce chicken, cooked and cubed, is 3 tablespoons.
      1 ounce beef, cooked and cubed, is 3 tablespoons.
      1 ounce roast beef, all lean, is a slice 3'' x 2'' x ¼'' or 1½'' x 2'' x ½''.

BREAD CHOICES
Low Biological Value Protein

Low biological value (LBV) protein is low or lacking in one or more of the essential amino acids and comes from vegetable sources and gelatin. Low biological value protein is not well utilized by uremic patients and should be restricted.

As a substitute for flour, wheat starch may be used for making breads, desserts and pastas. Unlike foods made from regular flour, wheat starch products contain no LBV protein and may be eaten in unlimited quantities. They provide needed calories. Ingredients as eggs and milk which contain high biological value protein should be counted in the HBV protein allowance for the day. Fruits or other ingredients which contain low biological value protein should be included in the daily allowance.

The following foods are major sources of low biological value protein.

FOOD	Amount	Weight Gm.	% Water	Low Biological Value Protein Gm.	Sodium (Na) Mg.	Potassium (K) Mg.	Calories
Bread:							
Bread, S.C.	1 slice	23	36	2.0	9.0	24	62
Bread, regular	1 slice	23	36	2.0	117.0	24	62
Bread, wheat starch	1 slice	32	36	0.4	11.0	27	100
Doughnuts	Raised - 1	30	28	2.0	70.0	24	124
Cornbread, regular	Average Piece	45	54	3.0	270.0	68	89
Rolls (brown and serve)	1 Average	38	27	3.0	187.0	34	107
Cereal, cooked	½ cup	120	80	2.0	1.0	15-60	70
Cereal, dry:							
Puffed Rice	½ cup	65	4	0.5	0.2	5	25
Puffed Wheat	½ cup	6	3	1.0	0.5	18	22
Shredded Wheat	1 biscuit	22	7	2.0	0.5	80	84
Corn Flakes, regular	1 cup	13	4	2.0	165.0	40	95
Rice Krispies, regular	½ cup	14	3	1.0	140.0	15	50
SC Cornflakes	½ cup	75	3	1.0	10.0	40	50
Crackers:							
Saltines	5 each	16.	4	1.5	175.0	25	70
SC Crackers	5 each	36	4	1.5	1.9	18	65
Vanilla Wafers	5 each	16	3	1.0	42.0	12	75
Graham Crackers	4 each	20	6	1.6	134.0	77	77
Pasta:							
Macaroni, regular	⅓ cup cooked	50	64	2.0	0.5	30	70
Macaroni, wheat starch	1 cup cooked	150	64	tr.	tr.	tr.	207
Noodles, regular	½ cup cooked	53	70	2.0	1.0	29	66
Noodles, W.S.	1 cup	106	70	tr.	tr.	tr.	200
Spaghetti, regular	⅓ cup cooked	49	64	2.0	0.5	22	56

VEGETABLE CHOICES

Vegetables contain significant amounts of potassium and low biological value protein. Potassium in vegetables may be reduced by about half if they are soaked in a large amount of water for several hours (4-6), drained and then cooked in a large amount of water.

Tuberous vegetables as potatoes, beets, carrots, etc. should be peeled and sliced thinly before soaking. This does not reduce the amount of protein.

The vegetables in this list are low in protein. If sodium restriction is necessary use fresh, frozen or canned without salt. Vegetables are grouped according to potassium content.

FOOD	Amount	Weight Gm.	% Water	Low Biological Value Protein Gm.	Sodium (Na) Mg.	Potassium (K) Mg.	Calories
GROUP I 0-150 mg. K							
Asparagus	½ cup	75	93	2.0	2	125	15
Beans, Green, snap	½ cup	63	92	1.0	2.5	95	20
Beets	½ cup	83	91	1.0	36	139	30
Cabbage, raw	½ cup	50	92	0.7	10	116	12
Cauliflower	½ cup	60	93	1.3	6	124	13
Celery, raw	½ cup	50	94	0.4	63	170	8
Cucumber, raw	½ cup	50	95	0.5	3	80	8
Eggplant, cooked	½ cup	100	94	1.0	1	150	19
Endive, raw	½ cup	50	93	0.8	7	147	10
Lettuce	½ cup 3 leaves	30	96	0.6	5	53	5
Onions, mature, raw	1 Tbsp.	10	90	0.2	1	16	4
Onions, mature, ckd.	½ cup	100	91	1.2	7	110	30
Onions, spring	5	50	90	0.6	2	116	22
Peppers, Green, raw	½ cup	50	95	0.6	6.5	100	11
Squash, summer	½ cup	100	93	1.0	1	140	14

VEGETABLE CHOICES (continued)

FOOD	Amount	Weight Gm.	% Water	Low Biological Value Protein Gm.	Sodium (Na) Mg.	Potassium (K) Mg.	Calories
GROUP II 151-350 mg. K							
Broccoli	½ cup	75	91	3.0	7.5	200	20
Brussels Sprouts	½ cup	75	88	4.2	7.5	210	25
Carrots, cooked	½ cup	75	91	1.1	25	167	25
Carrots, raw	½ cup	55	88	1.1	25	188	35
Kale	½ cup	66	90	2.0	27	150	19
Mustard Greens, cooked	½ cup	100	92	2.2	18	220	23
Okra	½ cup 8 pods	85	91	2.0	2	164	25
Pumpkin	½ cup	100	90	1.0	2	240	33
Radishes	½ cup 10 sm.	100	94	0.5	18	320	15
Rutabagas	½ cup	100	90	1.0	4	167	35
Spinach, cooked	½ cup	90	92	2.7	45	292	24
Squash, winter	½ cup	100	89	1.2	1	260	35
Tomatoes, reg. cnd.	½ cup	100	94	1.0	130	217	20
Turnip Greens, cooked	½ cup	100	92	1.5	17	150	23
Turnips, white	⅔ cup	100	93	0.8	34	188	23
GROUP III Over 350 mg. K							
Cress	½ cup	100	92	1.9	8	353	23
Mushrooms	½ cup	100	93	2.7	15	414	20
Parsley	½ cup	100	85	3.6	45	727	44
Squash, Acorn, baked	½ cup	100	83	2.0	1	480	55
Tomatoes, raw	½ cup	150	93	1.6	5	366	33
Lima Beans (Fordhook, frozen)	½ cup	80	75	6.0	81	422	80
Canned	½ cup	80	74	5.4	190	222	77
*SC Corn Kernels	½ cup	83	75.9	2.0	1.7	81	70
SC Peas, Blackeyed	½ cup	80	70	5.1	8	229	76
SC Potatoes, Sweet, boiled	½ cup	100	64	2.0	10	164	130
SC Potatoes, white, boiled	½ cup	100	75	2.0	9	211	65
SC Potato Chips	15 chips	30	2	2.0	3	160	264
SC Green Peas	¼ cup	40	77	2.0	3	78	53
SC Mixed Vegetables, frozen	½ cup	80	82	2.5	42	152	52

FRUIT CHOICES

Fruits contain potassium and low biological value protein. Sodium content is minimal. They should be used as allowed on the diet. Canned fruits are higher in calories because of the sugar added and lower in potassium because of processing and are a better choice than fresh or frozen fruits. Fruits are grouped according to potassium content.

FOOD	Amount	Weight Gm.	% Water	Low Biological Value Protein Gm.	Sodium (Na) Mg.	Potassium (K) Mg.	Calories
GROUP I 40-150 mg. K							
Applesauce, sweet, canned	⅓ cup	100	75	0.5	2.0	65	90
Blackberries, heavy syrup	Scant ½ cup	100	76	1.0	1.0	110	90
Blueberries, fresh, frozen or canned	½ cup	120	73	0.5	1.0	75	120
Cherries, sweet or sour, heavy syrup	½ cup	100	78	1.0	1.0	125	90
Cranberries, raw	½ cup	50	88	0.5	1.0	40	20
Cranberry Sauce	Scant ¼ cup	50	62	0.1	0.5	15	60
Figs, canned	3 med.	100	77	0.5	2.0	150	85
Grapefruit, fresh	½ med.	100	89	0.5	1.0	135	40
Grapefruit, canned, syrup pack	½ cup	100	81	0.5	1.0	135	70
Grapes, Concord, Catawba, American	½ cup	75	82	1.0	2.5	120	55
Grapes, European, Muscat, Thompson Seedless, Emperor Flame, Tokay	½ cup	80	81	0.5	2.5	140	55
Peaches, heavy syrup, 2 halves	½ cup	100	79	0.5	2.0	130	80
Pears, heavy syrup, 2 halves	½ cup	120	80	0.5	1.5	100	90
Pineapple, heavy syrup	½ cup	100	80	0.5	1.0	100	75
Plums, Green Gage	½ cup	100	90	0.5	1.0	80	55
Plums, purple	½ cup	100	77	0.5	1.0	140	85
Raspberries, frozen sugar added	½ cup	123	74	1.0	1.0	125	120
Tangerine, fresh, 1 large	½ cup	100	87	1.0	2.0	125	45
Watermelon	½ cup	100	93	0.5	1.0	100	25

FRUIT CHOICES (continued)

FOOD	Amount	Weight Gm.	% Water	Low Biological Value Protein Gm.	Sodium (Na) Mg.	Potassium (K) Mg.	Calories
GROUP II 151-350 mg. K							
Apple, fresh, med.	½ cup	150	85	0.5	1.0	165	90
Apricots, heavy syrup, 3 halves	½ cup	100	77	0.5	1.0	235	85
Cantaloupe, ¼, 5'' diameter	½ cup	120	91	1.0	14.0	310	35
Fruit Cocktail, heavy syrup	½ cup	100	80	0.5	5.0	160	75
Honeydew Melon	½ cup	120	91	1.0	14.0	310	35
Nectarine, 1 med.	½ cup	50	82	0.5	0.5	150	30
Orange, 1 small	½ cup	100	86	1.0	1.0	200	50
Plums, raw, Damson, 2	½ cup	100	81	0.5	2.0	300	65
Prunes, cooked, 5 medium	½ cup	100	66	1.0	4.0	325	120
Pumpkin, canned	Scant ½ cup	100	90	1.0	2.0	240	35
Rhubard, cooked, sweetened	½ cup	100	63	0.5	2.0	200	140
Strawberries, raw	½ cup	75	90	0.5	1.0	125	30
Strawberries, frozen, sweetened	½ cup	128	71	0.5	1.0	145	140
GROUP III Over 350 mg. K							
Banana, 1 whole, small	½ cup	100	75	1.0	1.0	370	85
Dates, dried	½ cup	90	23	2.0	1.0	575	250
*Raisins	½ cup	80	18	2.0	20.0	610	230
*Raisins, Seedless	1 Tbsp.	10	18	0.5	3.0	75	30

*Use Sparingly for Seasoning.

FRUIT JUICE CHOICES

FOOD	Amount	Weight Gm.	% Water	Low Biological Value Protein Gm.	Sodium (Na) Mg.	Potassium (K) Mg.	Calories
Group I 0-150 mg. K							
Apple Juice	½ cup	120	87.8	1.0	2	120	60
*Awake (orange drink)	½ cup	124	—	tr	5	41	51
Cranberry Jc. Cocktail	½ cup	120	83.2	0.1	1	12	78
Grape Juice	½ cup	120	82.9	0.3	2	139	83
Grape Juice Drink	½ cup	120	86.0	0.1	2	42	65
Lemonade, fresh or frozen	½ cup	120	88.5	0.1	tr	19	55
Limeade, fresh or frozen	½ cup	120	88.9	tr	tr	16	49
Peach Nectar	½ cup	120	87.2	0.3	1	94	60
Pear Nectar	½ cup	120	86.2	0.3	1	47	65
*Pineapple and Orange Drink	½ cup	120	86.0	0.2	1	84	65
*Pineapple and Grapefruit Drink	½ cup	120	86.0	0.2	1	74	65
*Tang-Orange flavor	½ cup	120	—	tr	13	45	61
*Tang-Grape flavor	½ cup	120	—	tr	9	1	61
Group II 151-350 mg. K							
Apricot Nectar	½ cup	120	84.6	0.4	1	181	70
Grapefruit Juice, canned, sweetened	½ cup	120	86.2	0.6	1	196	65
Grapefruit and Orange Juice, canned, sweetened	½ cup	120	86.9	0.6	1	221	60
Lemon Juice	½ cup	120	91.0	0.6	1	169	30
Orange Juice, frozen (dilute 1 to 4)	½ cup	120	88.1	0.8	1	233	54
Pineapple Juice, canned	½ cup	120	85.6	0.5	1	179	66
Prune Juice	½ cup	120	80.0	0.5	3	282	92
Tomato Juice, regular	½ cup	120	93.6	1.0	240	272	23
Tomato Juice, SC	½ cup	120	94.2	1.0	84	272	24
Sherbet	½ cup	66	67.0	0.7	7	15	118
Tangarine Juice	½ cup	120	88.0	0.6	1	214	50

*Low in Potassium.

FREE FOODS

These foods may be used in unlimited quantities to furnish the desired amount of calories. These foods have negligible amounts of protein, sodium and potassium.

Each exchange contains 5 grams of fat and 45 calories:

Butter or margarine, unsalted	1 teaspoon
*Regular margarine	1 teaspoon
Oil or cooking fat, unsalted	1 teaspoon
French dressing, unsalted	1 tablespoon
Mayonnaise, unsalted	1 teaspoon

Each exchange has approximately 55 calories:

Sugar, white	1 Tablespoon
Jelly, jam, preserves	1 Tablespoon
Syrup, white	1 Tablespoon
Honey, strained	1 Tablespoon

Soft Drinks:

7-Up	6 ounces (180 cc.)
Gingerale	6 ounces (180 cc.)

Candies: (½ oz.)

Hard candies	4 pieces
Gum drops	3 medium, 14 small
Jelly beans	8
Stick candy (3"long)	3
**Marshmallows	3 large
Pillow Mints	10
Wheatstarch cookies	2 small
Wheatstarch crackers	2 small
Cornstarch pudding	⅓ cup

*Salted Margarine . . . . 1 teaspoon has 49 mg. sodium.
**Contains small amount of protein. Use only 2 exchanges per day.

317

RENAL TRANSPLANT DIET

Purpose

The renal transplant diet is used for the patient who has a functioning kidney transplant and is receiving high doses of glucocorticoid drugs to prevent rejection of the new kidney. When high doses of steroids are given, this diet may reduce side effects. When drug dosage is reduced to maintenance levels, this diet may no longer be necessary. Adverse effects of these drugs that may alter dietary needs are:

1. Accelerated protein catabolism resulting in negative nitrogen balance, protein wasting, muscle weakness, and ecchymoses.
2. Impaired carbohydrate metabolism resulting in decreased glucose tolerance and sometimes steroid diabetes.
3. Salt and water retention resulting in hypertension and/or edema.
4. Adverse effects on skeletal system: osteoporosis, impaired calcium absorption, suppression of growth in children due to impaired epiphyseal growth.

Description

Protein: 2 gm/kg ideal body weight
Sodium: 2–4 gm
Calcium: 800–1200 mg
Phosphorous;   800–1200 mg
Carbohydrate: 1.0–1.5 gm/kg ideal body weight

Restricting concentrated sources of carbohydrate and total carbohydrate (provided by bread and starch sources) has been found beneficial in controlling the hyperglycemia of patients who have developed steroid diabetes. This restriction may minimize the symptoms of a Cushingoid state caused by the steroid drugs. Adequate carbohydrate is essential to provide energy, to prevent ketosis, and to protect against excessive breakdown of body protein.

Adequacy

When a severely restricted carbohydrate diet is used, the following nutrients may be present in marginal amounts: calcium, vitamin D, thiamine, magnesium.

MEAL PLANNING FORM

This Meal Planning Form is designed to be used with the Post Transplant Diet.

Calories _____   Carbohydrate _____
High Biological Protein _____   Sodium _____

MEAL PLAN   **SAMPLE MENU**

Servings	Food Choices or Exchanges	Serving Size	Food	Sodium	Protein	Carbohydrate
Breakfast:						
_____	Milk Choice	_____	_____	_____	_____	_____
_____	Meat Choice	_____	_____	_____	_____	_____
_____	Fruit Choice	_____	_____	_____	_____	_____
_____	Bread Choice	_____	_____	_____	_____	_____
_____	Fat Choice	_____	_____	_____	_____	_____
	Coffee - Tea					
Lunch:						
_____	Milk Choice	_____	_____	_____	_____	_____
_____	Meat Choice	_____	_____	_____	_____	_____
_____	Vegetable A Choice	_____	_____	_____	_____	_____
_____	Vegetable B Choice	_____	_____	_____	_____	_____
_____	Fruit Choice	_____	_____	_____	_____	_____
_____	Bread Choice	_____	_____	_____	_____	_____
_____	Fat Choice	_____	_____	_____	_____	_____
	Coffee - Tea					
Dinner:						
_____	Milk Choice	_____	_____	_____	_____	_____
_____	Meat Choice	_____	_____	_____	_____	_____
_____	Vegetable A Choice	_____	_____	_____	_____	_____
_____	Vegetable B Choice	_____	_____	_____	_____	_____
_____	Fruit Choice	_____	_____	_____	_____	_____
_____	Bread Choice	_____	_____	_____	_____	_____
_____	Fat Choice	_____	_____	_____	_____	_____
	Coffee - Tea					

Snacks:

_____   _____ Choice
_____   _____ Choice

POST TRANSPLANT DIET
FOOD CHOICE OR EXCHANGE LISTS

MILK CHOICES

One milk choice contains 8 grams of high quality protein and 12 grams of carbohydrate. Four cups of milk each day are recommended for adequate calcium and phosphorus. _____ servings per day are needed.

	Amount	Sodium (mg.)
*Milk, whole or nonfat	1 cup	100
Evaporated	½ cup	150
1% fat	1 cup	150
2% fat	1 cup	150
*Yogurt, plain or unflavored, made from whole or nonfat milk	1 cup	150

*The following food should be used only if sodium is totaled daily.

*Buttermilk	1 cup	300

*High in calcium and phosphorus

MEAT CHOICES

One meat choice contains 7 grams of high quality protein, 75 calories, no carbohydrate and various amounts of sodium, depending on the particular food. All weights and measures apply to edible portions. _____ servings per day are needed.

	Amount	Sodium (mg.)
Cheese, cheddar and American	¾ oz.	150
Cheese, cottage, regular	¼ cup	125
Crab, tuna and salmon, canned, regular	¼ cup	250
Egg	1	50
Fresh fish, cod, herring, crab, oysters, clams, tuna and salmon canned without salt	1 oz. (¼ cup)	25
Liver	1 oz.	50
Lobster	2 oz.	50
Meat and Fowl		
beef, fresh pork, chicken and turkey, veal, lamb	1 oz.	25
Sausage, link or patty	1 oz.	200
Shrimp, fresh	1 oz.	50

The following foods should be used only if sodium is totaled daily.

Ham, sugar cured or regular canned	1 oz.	300
Ham, country	1 oz.	700

VEGETABLE A CHOICES

These vegetables contain little protein, carbohydrate, calories and sodium. If they are cooked and unsalted, up to one cup per meal may be eaten. Use fresh, frozen or canned without salt.

_____servings per day are needed.

Asparagus, fresh or frozen
  *Green or white, canned
Beans, green or wax, fresh or frozen
*Canned
Broccoli, fresh or frozen
Brussels sprouts, fresh or frozen
Cabbage, fresh
Cauliflower, fresh or frozen
Celery, fresh, limit to 2 small inner stalks
  Cooked, limit to ⅓ cup
Collards, fresh or frozen (limit to ½ cup)
Eggplant
Escarole
Kale, fresh or frozen
Lettuce, any variety
Mushrooms, fresh
Mustard greens, fresh or frozen
  *Canned
Okra, fresh or frozen
Parsley
Pepper, green
Radishes
Rhubarb
Squash, summer, fresh or frozen
Tomatoes, fresh
  *Canned
Turnip greens, fresh or frozen

The following foods should be used only if sodium is totaled daily.

		Sodium mg.
Sauerkraut, canned, well drained	½ cup	650

*A ½ cup serving of a regular canned vegetable, well drained, contains approximately 250 mg. sodium.

VEGETABLE B CHOICES

These vegetables contain a small amount of low quality protein, 7 grams of carbohydrate and 35 calories per ½ cup serving. Occasionally, one half of a bread exchange or one fruit exchange may be used to replace a serving of these vegetables.

_____SERVINGS PER DAY ARE NEEDED.

	Amount	Sodium (mg.)
Pumpkin, fresh or canned	½ cup	0
Onion	½ cup	0
Rutabagas	½ cup	0
Squash, winter	½ cup	0
Peas, small green, fresh	½ cup	0
Frozen	½ cup	75
*Canned		
Beets, fresh cooked	½ cup	50
*Canned		
Carrots, raw, fresh cooked	½ cup	50
*Canned, limit to ⅓ cup		
Turnips, raw, fresh cooked	½ cup	50

The following foods should be used only if sodium is totaled daily.

Catsup, regular	2 Tbsp.	400

*A ½ cup serving of a regular canned vegetable, well drained, contains approximately 250 mg. sodium.

FRUIT CHOICES

One fruit choice provides 10 grams of carbohydrate and 40 calories. Fruit juices should be unsweetened, and fruits, fresh, water-packed or juice-packed. Fresh fruits contain very little sodium.

_____servings per day are needed.

	Amount
Apple juice or cider	⅓ cup
Apple	1, 2-inch dia.
Applesauce	½ cup
Apricots, fresh or canned	2 medium
Apricots, dried (sun dried only)	4 halves
Banana	½ small
Blueberries, boysenberries	⅔ cup
Blackberries, raspberries, strawberries	1 cup
Cantaloupe	¼, 6-inch dia.
Cherries	10 large
Dates	2
Figs, Kadota	⅓ cup
Figs, fresh and canned	2 large
Figs, dried (sun dried only)	1 small
Fruit cocktail or mixed fruit cup	½ cup
Grapefruit	½ small
Grapefruit juice	½ cup
Grapes	12
Grape juice	¼ cup
Honeydew melon	⅛, 7-inch dia.
Mango	½ small
Nectarine	1 medium
Orange	1 small
Orange juice	½ cup
Papaya	⅓ medium
Peach	1 medium
Pear	1 small
Pineapple	½ cup
Pineapple juice	⅓ cup
Raisins	2 Tbsp.
Watermelon	1 cup

BREAD CHOICES

One carbohydrate choice provides approximately 2-4 grams of low quality protein, 15 grams of carbohydrate and 70 calories. Sodium values for different foods are listed below.

_____servings per day are needed.

	Amount	Sodium (mg.)
Biscuit, baking powder	1, 2'' diameter	200
From self-rising flour	1, 2'' diameter	250
Bread, white, whole wheat, cracked wheat, Roman Meal, Hollywood, French, rye	1 slice	150
Cereals, dry		
Cornflakes, Special K	¾ cup	150
Puffed rice, puffed wheat, shredded wheat	¾ cup	0
Cereals, regular, cooked without salt		
Cream of Wheat, farina, Maltex, Malt-o-Meal, *oatmeal, Pettijohn, Ralston	½ cup	0
Cornbread	1½'' cube	225
Hot water cornbread (from plain meal)	1½'' cube	0
Cornstarch	2½ Tbsp.	0
Crackers, sodium controlled	5	0
Flour, regular	2½ Tbsp.	0
Self-rising	2½ Tbsp.	200
Grits, rice, noodles, spaghetti, macaroni, cooked without salt	½ cup	0
Muffin	1 medium	200
Peanut butter, regular (limit peanut butter to one choice per day)	2 Tbsp.	150
Unsalted (limit peanut butter to one choice per day)	2 Tbsp.	0
Potato chips, sodium controlled	15 medium	0
Roll	1, 2'' diameter	200
Starchy Vegetables:		
*Beans, peas, dried, cooked and unsalted (lima, navy, split pea, cowpeas, etc.)	½ cup	0
**Canned	½ cup	250
Corn, fresh or frozen	⅓ cup	0
	½ cup	250
Parsnips	⅔ cup	0
Potato, instant, mashed	½ cup	100
Potato, sweet, fresh	¼ cup	0
**Canned	½ cup	250
Potato, white, baked or boiled	1, 2'' diameter	0

*High in phosphorus

**A ½ cup serving of a regular canned vegetable, well drained, contains approximately 250 mg. of sodium.

The following foods should be used only if sodium is totaled daily:

Cheerios, Kix, Rice Krispies	¾ cup	200
Wheaties, Wheat Chex	¾ cup	300
Bran Flakes	¾ cup	350

FAT CHOICES

Fat choices contain no protein or carbohydrate. A fat choice provides 45 calories.

_____servings per day are needed.

	Amount	Sodium (mg.)
Avocado	⅛, 4 inch dia.	0
Bacon	1 slice	75
Blue Cheese Dressing	1 Tbsp.	150
Butter or margarine, regular	1 tsp.	50
unsalted	1 tsp.	0
Cream cheese	1 Tbsp.	50
Cream, coffee or table	2 Tbsp.	10
Cream, heavy	1 Tbsp.	5
Mayonnaise, regular	1 tsp.	25
unsalted	1 tsp.	0
*Nuts, unsalted	6 small	0
Oil or cooking fat, unsalted	1 tsp.	0
Tartar sauce	1 Tbsp.	100
1000 Island Dressing	1 Tbsp.	100

The following foods should be used only if sodium is totaled daily:

French Dressing	1 Tbsp.	200
Olives, green	5 small	750

*High in phosphorus (¼ cup contains 250 mg. phosphorus).
¼ cup nuts contains 10 grams of carbohydrate.

BEVERAGE CHOICES

	Amount	Sodium (mg.)
Coffee, decaffeinated coffee, tea, artificially sweetened Kool Aid and lemonade may be used as desired		
Diet Big K	12 oz.	100
Diet Shasta, all flavors	12 oz.	100
Tab, Fresca, Sugar-free RC, Diet Pepsi, Diet Rite	10 oz.	25

325

CONDIMENTS

	Amount	Sodium (mg.)
Mustard, prepared	1 tsp.	50

The following foods should be used only if sodium is totaled daily.

Pickle, dill	1 large	2000
Pickle, sour or mixed	1 large	1500
Salt	¼ tsp.	500

FOODS TO AVOID

Do not eat the following foods except on the advice of the physician or dietitian.

Alcoholic beverages	Onion salt
Beer, wine	Pickles
Candy	Pie or cake
Celery salt	Potato chips
Chewing gum, regular	Preserves
Condensed milk	Pretzels
Cookies	Pudding or custard
Garlic salt	Relishes
Honey	Salted crackers
Horseradish	Salted popcorn
Ice cream	Soda or baking powder
Jam or jelly	Soft drinks, regular
Kosher meats	Sugar
Marmalade	Syrup
Molasses	

APPENDIX II
Complications of
Immunosuppressive
Therapy

The use of steroids (Prednisone and Medrol) and other drugs (such as Imuran and Cytoxan) to alter the body's immune defense system is necessary to the success of the kidney transplant. The effect is a nonspecific reduction in the defense lymphocytes ("blanket immunosuppression"). The side effects and toxic complications affect every system of the body.

PRINCIPLES OF IMMUNOSUPPRESSIVE THERAPY

1. Complications and side effects are more common with prolonged use of the drugs.
2. Complications and side effects are more common on high dosages of the drugs and many have a tendency to disappear as the dosages are lowered toward maintenance levels.
3. Toxic effects result from accumulation of drugs when the kidney transplant is functioning poorly. Drug dosages may need to be adjusted according to the kidney's ability to eliminate a drug or its active metabolites.
4. Prevention is the primary responsibility of the health team.

PRINCIPLES OF PREVENTION OF INFECTIONS
IN THE TRANSPLANT PATIENT

Preexisting uremic changes in the patient have already created an infection-prone individual. This clinical state, aggravated by immunosuppressive drugs, allows for possible reactivity of a latent infec-

327

tion and endogenous or exogenous spread of infection to the patient. Listed below are some infection control principles:

1. Eliminate the presence of endogenous sources of infection. The patient should be free of all sources of infection before the surgery (for example, decayed teeth should be extracted before the transplant).
2. Eliminate the presence of ectogenous sources of infection (for example, by using aseptic technique in venipunctures and a preoperative scrub with pHisohex).
3. Eliminate the presence of exogenous sources of infection. The patient is highly susceptible to environmental pathogens.
4. Prevent the spread of a pathogen by interrupting the infection cycle:
    a. Portal of entry.
    b. Susceptible host (unable to eliminate).
    c. Reservoir.
    d. Exit.
    e. Mode of transmission.

Some nursing responsibilities in infection control are the following:

1. Aseptic technique is used in the care of all entrance sites for infection (such as I.V., catheter). These should be eliminated as early as possible in the course of the treatment.
2. Signs and symptoms of local and systemic infection should be carefully observed and managed with early treatment. These may be masked by the use of immunosuppressive drugs. The use of antibiotics or antibacterial agents is advised, either specifically or prophylactically.
3. Meticulous handwashing is stressed.
4. The patient is taught to avoid large crowds and visitors or family members who show signs or symptoms of illness.
5. Housekeeping should be directed to prevent pathogens from being transmitted on dust particles.
6. The patient should not be cared for by a staff member who is ill or who is taking care of another patient on isolation.
7. Isolation techniques vary throughout the country:
    a. Gown, gloves, mask.
    b. Use of mask only.
    c. Use of common sense to avoid infections.

Immunosuppressive therapy can be initiated using any of the following regimens:

1. Drugs given with surgery and continued.

2. Drugs given with surgery and again during the first rejection episode and continued.

3. Drugs given before surgery and continued.

Prednisone and Medrol, once initiated, will be gradually decreased until a maintenance dose of about 10 mg per day is reached. The patient will continue to take this dosage for the life of the graft. Imuran and Cytoxan will be maintained at a higher level. Following a protocol established by the medical team, ALG may be administered for a short time. Each transplant center has its own protocol and treatment plans. It is not the purpose of this appendix to review all of them.

Achieving a balance—inducing specific immunologic tolerance to kidney grafts versus enabling the recipient to protect himself against environmental pathogens—is a challenge for the entire health team when immunosuppressive drugs are given. The patient cannot live in a sterile glass balloon. The following is a compiled list of the side effects of steroids, Imuran, and Cytoxan. Included are nursing or patient responsibilities in relation to each. Not all patients will get all side effects, yet the nurse must be aware of and assess each one individually.

ASSESSMENT FACTORS

NURSING INTERVENTIONS

I. *General Appearance*
   A. Centripetal weight gain—central obesity with thin extremities.

   A. 1. Exercise for muscle tone.
      2. Strict adherence to diet with decreased CHO and sugar.
      3. Use artificial sweetners and diet drinks.

   B. Fat deposits on abdomen, trunk, supraclavicular area, back (buffalo hump), and cheeks (chipmunk cheeks, moon facies).

   B. 1.Strict adherence to low CHO diet.
      2. Exercise program.

   C. Growth impairment in children due to a refractoriness of the tissues to the growth hormone.

   C. Growth hormone is of little value.

II. *Integumentary*
   A. Hirsutism of face (hypertrichosis), trunk, and ex-

   A. Hair can be bleached,

ASSESSMENT FACTORS

NURSING INTERVENTIONS

tremities. Hair can be slight
and downing or coarse.

B. Alopecia.

C. Striae due to the tearing of
the subcutaneous tissues.
   1. Recent ones are pur-
   plish-blue, because the
   vascularity of the subepi-
   dermis shows through the
   tear.
   2. Older ones appear as
   white scar tissue.

D. Ecchymoses, petechiae,
purpura due to capillary
fragility and low platelet
count.

E. Acne—papules and pus-
tules.

F. Thinning of skin (fragile
parchment).

shaved, or removed with
a depilatory agent.

B. 1. Support patient with
   the encouragement
   that it will grow back.
   2. Use a wig or toupee.

C. 1. Weight maintenance
   on low-calorie diet.
   2. Prevent rapid weight
   gain.

D. 1. Diet with high protein
   and vitamin C.
   2. Knox gelatin in diet.
   3. Avoid venipunctures,
   which can cause sub-
   cutaneous hemor-
   rhage.
   4. Observe for throm-
   bocytopenia.

E. 1. Personal hygiene using
   soap and water; al-
   cohol for drying.
   2. Use Basis soap or other
   acne soaps.
   3. Avoid oily lotion.
   4. Diet low in CHO,
   greasy foods, and
   chocolate.

F. 1. Avoid use of adhesive
   tape.
   2. Prevent decubiti formation by changing
   positions frequently.
   3. Caution against sun-
   burn.

ASSESSMENT FACTORS

NURSING INTERVENTIONS

G. Delayed wound healing due to:
  1. Granulocytopenia (interference with the fibroblast formation of granulation tissue).
  2. A decreased growth of blood vessels in the new tissue.

G. 1. Wound care:
    a. Strict aseptic technique.
    b. Observe dressing—keep dry and clean.
    c. Sutures remain in place longer.
  2. Avoid strain on incision (prevent valsalva maneuver).
  3. High-protein diet with vitamin supplements.
  4. Avoid   additional surgeries.
  5. Avoid injuries (such as razor cuts).

H. Wound and skin infections due to a decreased immunological resistance and attack by opportunistic pathogens—viral, fungal, bacterial.

H. 1. Observe for signs and symptoms of infection, which may be masked by drugs. Cultures may be the only clue.
  2. Appropriate antibiotic and antibacterial agent therapy.
  3. Discontinue portal-of-entry sites as soon as possible (such as I.V., Foley catheter).
  4. Prevent endogenous spread.
  5. Prevent   exogenous spread.

III. *Face, Eyes, Nose, Mouth, Gums*
  A. Infection (monilia, herpes)

A. 1. Antifungal agent (Amphotericin or Mycostatin mouthwash).
  2. Appropriate drug therapy.
  3. Good oral hygiene.

ASSESSMENT FACTORS	NURSING INTERVENTIONS
B. Ulceration.	B. Appropriate drug therapy.

C. Eye changes.
  1. Increased intraocular pressure
  2. Cataracts.
  3. Corneal lesions.
	C. 1. Ophthalmic examination.
	  2. Long-term cataract surgery.
	  3. Prevent injury and infections.

D. Bleeding due to low platelet count.	D. 1. Soft toothbrush.
	  2. Oral hygiene.
	  3. Observe for epistaxis.

IV. *Respiratory System*

A. Tuberculosis exacerbation due to bacilli breakdown and active manifestation of the disease.	A. 1. Prophylactic use of Isoniazid (INH). 2. Pyridoxine therapy along with INH.

B. Opportunistic infections.
  1. Nocardia virus.
  2. Cytomegalic virus.
  3. Pneumocystis.
  4. Pneumonia.
  5. Lysteria.
  6. Others.
	B. 1. Observe for signs of infection.
	  2. Strict pulmonary toilet.
	  3. No smoking.
	  4. Mask isolation.
	  5. Staff members with respiratory problems should not care for the patient.
	  6. Medical asepsis in housecleaning.

V. *Cardiovascular System*

A. Hypertension due to:
  1. Sodium and water retention.
  2. Renin produced from ischemic transplanted graft.
  3. Renin produced from patient's own kidney.
  4. Renal artery stenosis.
	A. 1. Low-sodium diet.
	  2. Fluid restriction—I.V. and P.O.
	  3. Renin studies.
	  4. Bruit heard over graft's renal artery.
	  5. Antihypertensive and diuretic drug therapy.

B. Fluid retention.	B. 1. Observe for signs of edema in the feet, sac-

ASSESSMENT FACTORS	NURSING INTERVENTIONS
	rum, scrotum, fingers, and eyelids.
2. Observe for signs of congestive heart failure and pulmonary edema.
3. I.V. and P.O. fluid restriction.
4. Daily weights at same time each morning.
5. Accurate blood pressure measurements.
6. Low-sodium diet.
7. Diuretic drug therapy.
C. Accelerated atherosclerotic vascular disease due to metabolic changes. ASCVD may cause an increased incidence of cerebral vascular accidents and myocardial infarctions.	C. Appropriate diet restrictions.
D. Thromboembolic formation.	D. 1. Observe for signs of thromboembolism (such as pain in calf).
2. Blood stasis preventive measures:
a. Support stockings correctly applied.
b. Elevate legs.
c. No crossing of legs at knees.
d. Frequent ambulation.
3. Heparin therapy.
E. Capillary fragility.	E. 1. Diet of high protein and Knox gelatin.
2. Avoid injury.
F. Increased atrioventricular node conduction rate.	F. 1. Observe for arrhythmias.
2. Observe for EKG changes.

ASSESSMENT FACTORS	*NURSING INTERVENTIONS*

VI. *Gastrointestinal System*

A. Excessive weight gain due to a voracious appetite.

A. Calorie-controlled diet.

B. Irritation, ulceration, and perforation due to:
1. Increased hydrochloric acid production.
2. Altered resistance of gastroduodenal mucosa.
3. Inhibited secretion of mucus barrier.

B. 1. Observe for bleeding:
   a. Check all stools for gross and occult blood.
   b. Check vomitus for gross or occult blood.
   c. Daily hemoglobin and hematocrit.
2. Observe for epigastric pain.
3. Prophylactic use of antacids with steroids and when stomach is empty (Riopan, Titralac, Amphojel, milk).
4. Drug therapy—Cimetadine (Tagamet)—inhibits hydrochloric acid production.
5. Frequent and regular meals.
6. Control anxiety and stressful environment.
7. Prevent constipation.
8. Upper gastrointestinal series test and barium enema.
9. Nasogastric tube inserted.
10. Gastrectomy and vagotomy.

C. Pancreatitis.

C. 1. Observe for signs and symptoms.
2. Observe stools.
3. Blood amylase levels.
4. Surgery.

D. Viral hepatitis.

D. 1. Daily liver enzyme

ASSESSMENT FACTORS   *NURSING INTERVENTIONS*

studies (SGOT, SGPT, alkaline phosphatase, bilirubin).

2. Hepatitis Associated Antigen (HAA) drawn every week.
3. Clotting times.
4. Precautionary measures for staff.
5. Rapid decrease of drug dosages.

VII. *Genitourinary System and Reproductive System*
  A. Infection:
    1. Bladder.
    2. Vagina.
    3. Perineum.

  A. 1. Discontinue Foley catheter.
    2. Frequent voiding.
    3. Strict personal hygiene.
    4. Appropriate drug therapy.

  B. Oligomenorrhea or amenorrhea in the female.

  B. Menses should become regular as drug dosages are decreased.

  C. Impotence in the male.

  C. Males should become potent as drug dosages are decreased.

  D. Fertility may not be affected.

  D. Birth control counseling.

VIII. *Musculoskeletal System*
  A. Muscle atrophy—wasting and weakness due to protein breakdown, especially the quadriceps muscles of the thigh.

  A. 1. Diet with high protein and adequate potassium.
    2. Prevent immobility.
    3. Exercise:
      a. Physical therapy.
      b. Active and passive range of motion.
      c. Ad lib ambulation.
      d. Exercise program.

ASSESSMENT FACTORS	NURSING INTERVENTIONS
B. Arthralgia.	B. Appropriate analgesia therapy.
C. Myopathy.	C. Appropriate analgesia therapy.
D. Osteoporosis, compression fractures of the spine and spontaneous fractures of the ribs and extremities (hips).	D. 1. Adequate calcium in diet. 2. Safety. 3. Exercise.
E. Aseptic necrosis of the femoral and humeral heads.	E. 1. Observe for pain and limping. 2. Avoid stress on hip (as in jogging). 3. Long-term surgical hip replacement.
F. Arrest of linear growth in children.	

IX. *Central Nervous System*

A. Infections (meningitis).	A. 1. Observe for neurological changes.
B. Muscular rigidity: convulsions due to a lowering of ectopic threshold of seizures.	B. 1. Patient safety. 2. Anticonvulsant drug therapy. 3. Avoid overexciting stimulation. 4. Quiet environment.
C. Possible increased intracranial pressure (ICP).	C. 1. Observe for signs and symptoms of ICP. 2. Observe for papilledema.

X. *Metabolic and Electrolyte*

A. Glucogenesis and gluconeogenesis. Insulin antagonized, producing an impaired CHO tolerance.	A. 1. Observe for
	   a. Hyperglycemia.
	   b. Glucosuria.
	2. Observe for signs and symptoms of diabetes—polydipsia, polypolyphagia, polyuria.

ASSESSMENT FACTORS   *NURSING INTERVENTIONS*

                                          3. Obtain history of family diabetes.

                                          4. Glucose tolerance test.

                                          5. Diabetic urines every four hours.

                                          6. Insulin or oral hypoglycemic therapy.

                                          7. Diabetic diet.

B. Protein breakdown, causing a negative nitrogen balance.

B. 1. High-protein diet.
     2. Observe for muscle wasting.

C. Fatty acid breakdown.

C. 1. Observe for hyperlipidemia.
     2. Diabetic urines for ketosuria.
     3. Control fat in diet.

D. Hypokalemia due to increased excretion in urine.

D. 1. Observe for signs and symptoms.
     2. Adequate potassium in diet.
     3. Potassium supplement.
     4. Observe effects of digitalis drug therapy and dose alterations.

E. Hypochloremic alkalosis due to the loss of potassium and hydrogen ions.

E. Appropriate medical therapy.

F. Hypercalcemia due to:
   1. Low serum phosphate.
   2. Hyperparathyroidism.
   3. Antivitamin D effect promoting calcium excretion.

F. 1. Manage calcium and phosphorus in diet or by drug therapy.
     2. Vitamin therapy.
     3. Subtotal parathyroidectomy.

G. Bone marrow depression, producing:
   1. Leukopenia.
   2. Thrombocytopenia.
   3. Anemia.

G. 1. Observe for infection.
     2. Protective isolation technique if the WBC is less than 1000 per cubic millimeter.
     3. Observe for bleeding.
     4. Iron supplements.

H. Increased incidence or recurrence of malignancies of

H. 1. Observe major signs of cancer:

ASSESSMENT FACTORS	NURSING INTERVENTIONS
the epithelial tissues and deep tumors due to the inhibition of the immune surveillance mechanism (lips, skin, bowel, breast, cervix).	*a.* Wound not healing. *b.* Change in wart or mole. *c.* Lump or thickening of skin. *d.* Persistent hoarseness. *e.* Persistent indigestion. *f.* Change in bowel habit. 2. Monthly self breast examination for females. 3. Biannual gynecological examination.

XI. *Mental Status*

A. Emotional lability and mood swings: 1. Euphoria. 2. Restlessness. 3. Irritation. 4. Excitability. 5. Apathy. 6. Depression. 7. Crying. 8. Personality changes.	A. 1. Emotional support. 2. Drug therapy.
B. Insomnia.	B. 1. Quiet environment. 2. Drug therapy.
C. Psychosis, mania, paranoia, delusions, and suicidal behavior.	C. 1. Patient safety. 2. Suicide precautions. 3. Report any unusual behavior. 4. Psychological consultation. 5. Possible removal of graft.

Index